Textbook of Pediatrics

Textbook of Pediatrics

Edited by **Alice Kunek**

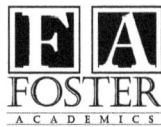

FOSTER ACADEMICS

New Jersey

Published by Foster Academics,
61 Van Reypen Street,
Jersey City, NJ 07306, USA
www.fosteracademics.com

Textbook of Pediatrics
Edited by Alice Kunek

International Standard Book Number: 978-1-63242-453-2 (Hardback)

Printed in the United States of America.

Contents

Preface

This book is a valuable compilation of topics, ranging from the basic to the most complex advancements in the field of pediatrics. This area of medicine generally focuses on providing complete care for infants, children, adolescents and young adults. Reducing infant mortality rate, controlling infections, treating genetic defects and malignancies, promoting a healthy lifestyle are the different areas covered under this discipline. From theories to research to practical applications, case studies related to all contemporary topics of relevance to this field have been included in this book. The extensive content of this book provides the professionals, pediatricians and students with a thorough understanding of the subject.

This book is the end result of constructive efforts and intensive research done by experts in this field. The aim of this book is to enlighten the readers with recent information in this area of research. The information provided in this profound book would serve as a valuable reference to students and researchers in this field.

At the end, I would like to thank all the authors for devoting their precious time and providing their valuable contributions to this book. I would also like to express my gratitude to my fellow colleagues who encouraged me throughout the process.

Editor

Paraneoplastic Recurrent Hypoglycaemic Seizures: An Initial Presentation of Hepatoblastoma in an Adolescent Male—A Rare Entity

Irappa Madabhavi,[1] Apurva Patel,[1] Mukesh Choudhary,[1] Suhas Aagre,[1] Swaroop Revannasiddaiah,[2] Gaurang Modi,[1] Asha Anand,[1] Harsha Panchal,[1] Sonia Parikh,[1] and Shreeniwas Raut[1]

[1] Department of Medical and Paediatric Oncology, GCRI, Ahmedabad, Gujarat 380016, India
[2] Department of Radiotherapy, Government Medical College, Haldwani, India

Correspondence should be addressed to Irappa Madabhavi; irappamadabhavi@gmail.com

Academic Editor: Pietro Strisciuglio

Hepatoblastoma (HB) is a rare malignant tumour of the liver and usually occurs in the first three years of life. Hepatoblastoma in adolescents and young adults is extremely rare; nevertheless the prognosis is much worse than in childhood, because these kinds of tumours are usually diagnosed late. Characteristic imaging and histopathological and AFP levels help in the diagnosis of hepatoblastoma. Paraneoplastic features of hepatoblastoma are not uncommon at presentation and include erythrocytosis, thrombocytosis, hypocalcaemia, isosexual precocious puberty, and rarely hypoglycaemia. Even though hypoglycaemia is commonly seen in hepatocellular carcinoma, its association with hepatoblastoma is very rare. We present a case of 15-year-old male patient presenting with complaints of recurrent hypoglycaemic seizures ultimately leading to diagnosis of hepatoblastoma. Managed successfully with neoadjuvant chemotherapy, surgery and adjuvant chemotherapy with adriamycin and cisplatin based regimens. An extensive review of literature in the PubMed and MEDLINE did not reveal much data on paraneoplastic recurrent hypoglycaemic seizures as an initial presentation of hepatoblastomas in adolescents and young adults.

1. Introduction

Hepatic tumours represent approximately 0.5–2% of all the tumours in children and are responsible for 1–4% of all the solid tumours. Approximately 90% of the cases occur in patients under 5 years of age and two- thirds of the cases occur in the first 2 years of life. In adolescents and adults, hepatoblastomas are extremely rare, and the initial symptoms are nonspecific and the usual presentation is failure to thrive, loss of weight, and a rapidly enlarging abdominal mass.

Paraneoplastic features of hepatoblastoma are not uncommon at presentation and include erythrocytosis, thrombocytosis, hypocalcaemia, isosexual precocious puberty, and rarely hypoglycaemia. About 10–30% of hepatic cancer may lead to hypoglycaemia. Plasma insulin, C-peptide, and proinsulin levels are low and free IGF-II levels will be elevated during hypoglycaemia.

The initial diagnosis of HB is mainly based on imaging, histopathology, and AFP levels. The complete surgical resection is the cornerstone of treatment; however, the tumour is often unresectable at the time of diagnosis. Chemotherapy has been proven effective in both an adjuvant and neoadjuvant treatment and can shrink tumours. AFP level is a valuable tumour marker to see response of presurgical chemotherapy, in the evaluation of the excision result and for the precocious diagnosis of the hepatoblastoma relapse.

2. Case Report

Our patient was an otherwise healthy 15-year-old adolescent male who was referred to us from a local physician. The patient initially presented with giddiness and syncope for three weeks followed by recurrent multiple episodes of

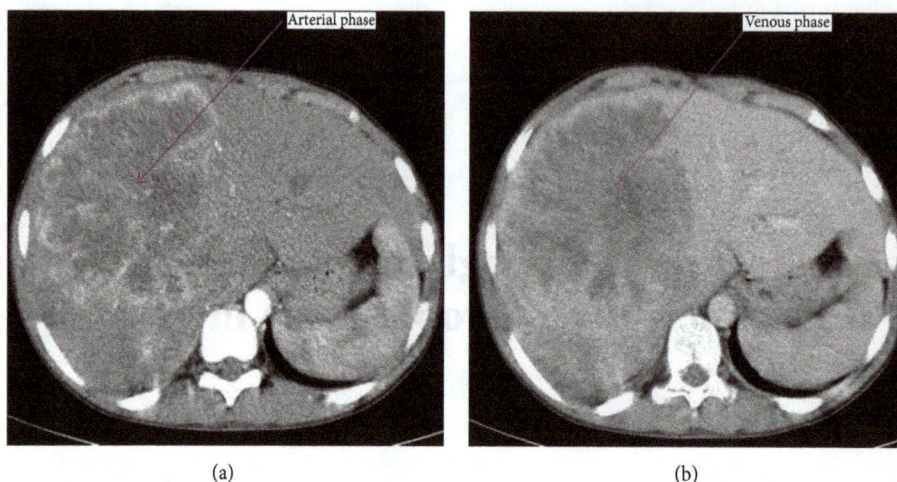

(a)   (b)

FIGURE 1: Ill-defined soft tissue density lesion of size 12×10 cm in right lobe of liver which shows marked heterogeneous enhancement on arterial phase (a) and shows washout of the contrast in the venous phase (b).

abnormal body movements, associated with frothing from the mouth, and postictal confusion. These symptoms used to subside with glucose tablets and local made glucose solutions. In view of the classical history of seizures and drastic improvement in the symptoms with glucose solutions, patients serum was sent for glucose level estimation and it was found to be 17 mg/dL. Patient was investigated for severe hypoglycaemia with serum insulin levels, C-peptide levels, fasting blood sugar, and postprandial blood sugar levels which were within the normal range. Ultrasonography of the abdomen was showing hepatomegaly for which he has been referred to us for further management. There was no history suggestive of diabetes or oral hypoglycaemic drug intake.

On clinical examination his height, weight, body mass index, blood pressure, pulse rate, and respiratory rate were within the normal range for his age and sex. There was no icterus, pallor, lymphadenopathy, or any other signs of liver disease. On per abdominal examination he was found to have moderate hepatomegaly, not associated with any bruit or venous hum.

His blood investigations revealed normal complete blood counts, renal function tests, and liver function tests. His serum sample was negative for hepatitis B surface antigen, antihepatitis B antibody, and antihepatitis C antibody. Alpha-fetoprotein (AFP) level was 155920 ng/Ml. In view of symptomatic hypoglycaemic episodes with normal insulin, C-peptide levels, patient's serum was sent for free insulin-like growth factor-II (IGF-II) levels which showed very high levels.

Computed tomography (CT) of abdomen shows an ill-defined soft tissue density lesion of size 12×10 cm in right lobe of liver which shows marked heterogeneous enhancement on arterial phase (Figure 1(a)) and washout of the contrast in the venous phase (Figure 1(b)). USG-guided biopsy sample was obtained with an 18 G tru-cut needle. Histopathology examination of the biopsy specimen shows atypical cells arranged in 1-2 layers of trabeculae separated

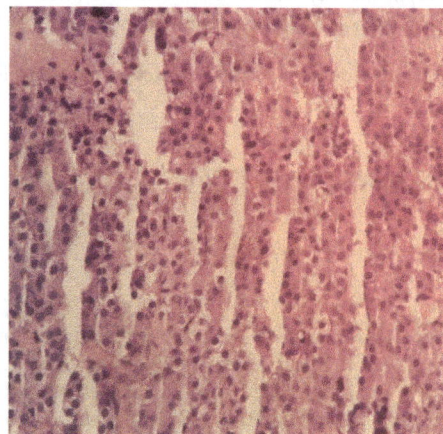

FIGURE 2: Atypical cells arranged in 1-2 layers of trabeculae separated by sinusoids. Individual cells are having round nucleoli with moderate granular cytoplasm.

by sinusoids. Individual cells are having round nucleoli with moderate granular cytoplasm and some cells showing clear cytoplasm. Overall findings were suggestive of foetal type of hepatoblastoma (Figure 2).

After the results of biopsy, four cycles of neoadjuvant chemotherapy with adriamycin 25 mg/m^2/day for 3 days and cisplatin 20 mg/m^2/day for 5 days were given. After two cycles of chemotherapy there was significant improvement in hypoglycaemic episodes. Neoadjuvant postchemotherapy abdominal CT image shows a heterogeneously enhancing soft tissue density lesion of size 45×65 mm, with internal foci of calcification involving right lobe of liver, suggesting a partial response as compared to prechemotherapy image according to RECIST criteria (Figure 3). There was a 2-log reduction in AFP levels. A right partial hepatectomy was performed without any postprocedural complications. Postoperative adjuvant systemic chemotherapy with adriamycin and cisplatin was continued for another 4 cycles.

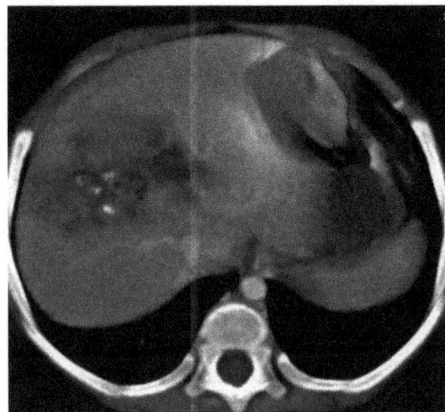

FIGURE 3: Postchemotherapy CT image shows a heterogeneously enhancing soft tissue density lesion of size 45 × 65 mm, with internal foci of calcification involving right lobe of liver.

Posttreatment imaging study did not show any residual lesion and AFP levels were within normal limits. Patient is under regular followup with 3 monthly ultrasound abdomen and AFP levels in our centre since one year without any abnormal findings.

3. Discussion

Hepatic tumours represent approximate 0.5–2% of all the tumours in child and are responsible for 1–4% of all the solid tumours. Hepatoblastoma represents the most common malignant hepatic tumour in childhood. Most cases of hepatoblastoma are sporadic; however, it might be associated with Beckwith-Weidman syndrome, familial adenomatous polyposis (FAP) coli, low birth weight, and genetic syndromes.

Hepatoblastoma (HB) is a rare malignant tumour of the liver and usually occurs in the first three years of life [1]. Approximately 90% of the cases occur in patients under 5 years of age and two-thirds of the cases occur in the first 2 years of life [2]. Most of these tumours arise in the embryo; hence it seems to be unusual that hepatoblastoma occurs in adolescents. HB in adolescents and young adults is extremely rare; nevertheless the prognosis is much worse than in childhood, because these kinds of tumours are usually diagnosed late. Since Bartok in 1958 described the first hepatoblastoma case in an adult patient, about 45 cases have been reported in the literature [3, 4].

The aetiology of HB has been elusive. Present investigations of the cytogenetic and molecular genetic abnormalities in HB revealed involvement of chromosomal loci on 1q, 2 (or 2q), 4q, 8 (or 8q), and 20. Loss of heterozygosis imprinting at locus 11p 15.5 also suggests a common genetic basis for HB [5]. The detection of nuclear β-catenin accumulation implies an oncogene alteration of the wnt/β-catenin pathway. Furthermore, nuclear p53 accumulation indicates that p53 mutation is also involved in the molecular pathogenesis of the malignancy [6].

Histologically, hepatoblastomas may present in two variants: (a) the epithelial type, which consists of foetal and embryonic cells presenting alone or in combination; (b) the epitheliomesenchymal mixed type, in which mesenchymal elements are present along with the epithelial component. It has been thought that hepatoblastoma develops during intrauterine life, but the same histological pattern has been seen in hepatic tumours in adults.

Hepatoblastoma usually develops in the right hepatic lobe. The left hepatic lobe receives oxygenated blood from the umbilical vein, while the right lobe receives oxygenated blood from the portal vein, with lower oxygen saturation. The lower oxygen saturation could favour the embryonic differentiation of the hepatoblastoma in certain conditions, this explaining the more frequent localization in the right hepatic lobe.

In adolescents and adults, the morbidity of HB is extremely rare, and the initial symptoms are nonspecific and the usual presentation is failure to thrive, loss of weight, and a rapidly enlarging abdominal mass. Systemic symptoms are rare and very rarely symptoms of hypoglycaemia may be present, such as in our case. The serum AFP level is almost invariably high [7].

Paraneoplastic features of hepatoblastoma are not uncommon at presentation and include erythrocytosis, thrombocytosis, hypocalcaemia, isosexual precocious puberty, and rarely hypoglycaemia [8]. Our patient had history of recurrent hypoglycaemic seizures as the only sole manifestation of the symptom complex leading to diagnosis of hepatoblastoma in an adolescent male.

Nonislet cell tumour induced hypoglycaemia has been reported with tumours of mesenchymal, epithelial, or haemopoietic origin. Hepatic tumour and gastric and lung cancer are common epithelial cancers that can cause hypoglycaemia. Hypoglycaemia disappears with definitive treatment of nonislet cell neoplasm.

The definition of the hypoglycaemia is defined as blood glucose levels less than 54 mg/dL. The metabolism in brain almost completely depends upon oxygen and glucose; when brain is deprived of the glucose, patients would show a series of neurological and psychological disorders. The mild symptoms are lack of concentration, behaviour changes, dizziness, vertigo, blurred vision, hallucination, and tics. When these symptoms get worse, patients develop convulsion and may fall into a coma or even die.

About 10–30% of hepatic cancer may lead to hypoglycaemia [9, 10]. Two types of hypoglycaemia (Types A and B) have been described in hepatic tumour. Type A occurs in terminal stages, especially in large tumours, when the energetic metabolism of the cancer cells would consume large amount of glucose and the glycogen storage would be seriously deficient, so it is hard to maintain glucose stability. And abnormalities in liver function cause the metabolism of insulin in liver to slow down and the function time of insulin prolongation, which results in the fact that liver could not convert nonglucose substances into glycogen and the ability of glycogenesis is reduced.

Type B occurs in 5% of the cases and is early in the course of the disease due to increased production of IGF-II by the tumour suggesting a paraneoplastic manifestation. Overproduction of insulin-like growth factor II (IGF-II) specifically as incompletely processed does not complex normally with circulating binding proteins and thus more readily bind to target tissue, is the cause of hypoglycaemia in most patients. Plasma insulin, C-peptide, and proinsulin levels are low and free IGF-II levels will be elevated during hypoglycaemia. Growth hormone and IGF-I concentration will be reduced due to negative feedback mechanism mediated by IGF-II [11].

Other reports found that in hepatic tumour patient with paraneoplastic syndromes, both the AFP and tumour size are higher than those without paraneoplastic syndromes. The possible hypothesis to explain it is that hepatic tumour patients with paraneoplastic syndromes have higher level of serum AFP and this is mainly because of the overexpression of AFP gene in hepatic cells which leads to the increase of serum AFP value. Meanwhile, tumour cells stimulate the biosynthesis of hormone like substances, such as IGF-II, parathyroid hormone-related protein (PTHrP), and erythropoietin, which leads to the expression of paraneoplastic syndromes such as hypoglycaemia, hypocalcaemia, and erythrocytosis [12].

The initial diagnosis of HB is mainly based on imaging. Proper diagnosis, staging, and treatment of HB require accurate imaging studies like ultrasound (US), computed tomography (CT), and magnetic resonance imaging (MRI). Other standard investigation includes serum AFP. However, the final diagnosis relies on tumour biopsy.

The complete surgical resection is the cornerstone of treatment for patients with HB and is the only chance of an optimal clinical result; however, the tumour is often unresectable at the time of diagnosis. Chemotherapy has been proven effective in both an adjuvant and neoadjuvant treatment and can shrink tumours. It makes them less prone to bleed and delineates the tumour from the surrounding normal parenchyma and vascular structures so as to facilitate the resections. HB is sensitive to such chemotherapy drugs as doxorubicin, cisplatin, vincristine, 5-FU, and cyclophosphamide [13].

There are two different strategies regarding the treatment of HB. The SIOPEL Group recommends the preoperative chemotherapy followed by the tumoral excision and then postoperative chemotherapy [14]. The American study group consider the surgical intervention when diagnosed (applicable to 50% of the patients) followed by postsurgical chemotherapy [15].

The SIOPEL established the PRETEXT (pretreatment tumour extension) staging system, reflecting the number of liver sections with or without tumour, that is,

> PRETEXT I: three adjoining liver sections free, one section involved;
>
> PRETEXT II: two adjoining sections free, two sections involved;
>
> PRETEXT III: two nonadjoining sections free or just one section free, in the latter case three sections involved;
>
> PRETEXT IV: no free section, all four sections involved.

The aim of the PRETEXT classification is to assess the operability prior to any treatment. This approach has shown reliable interobserver reproducibility and an excellent prognostic value. Its main limitation is the difficulty in accessing between actual invasion of a liver segment and displacement of an anatomical border [16].

PRETEXT I–III tumours are treated with partial hepatectomy and PRETEXT IV or unifocal, centrally located tumours with total hepatectomy, that is, liver transplantation [17]. Hepatoblastoma is considered to be unresectable, when the tumour is extremely large, involving the risk of severe haemorrhage; when both hepatic lobes are altered; when the hepatic vein or the inferior vena cava is affected. Gold standard chemotherapy—popularized by SIOPEL with acronym PLADO (cisplatin and doxorubicin).

Lung metastases are not an absolute contraindication to liver resection or even liver transplantation. Pulmonary metastases should be removed first either by surgery or by chemotherapy and then subsequently primarily tumour-resected—either by partial hepatectomy or by liver transplantation. The hepatic transplant is indicated either initially for the unresectable hepatoblastoma or after the relapse.

AFP level is a valuable tumour marker to see response of presurgical chemotherapy, in the evaluation of the excision result and for the precocious diagnosis of the hepatoblastoma relapse [18]. The complete excision of the hepatoblastoma determines the decrease of the AFP serum level, which will be normalized after 4–6 weeks. The persistency or secondary increase of the AFP values represents a residual tumour, metastases, or a relapse. The prognosis of patients with HB varies with the histology and stage. The favourable outcome associated with pure foetal histology and the poor prognosis of anaplastic (small-cell undifferentiated) hepatoblastomas.

Because of the lack of experience of hepatoblastomas in adolescent and adult patients, tumours can be treated with surgical resection (if it is possible) and chemotherapy as in children. However, mean survival time in adult patients is 3.5 months. Liver transplantation has recently been associated with significant success in the treatment of children with unresectable hepatic tumors.

4. Conclusion

Hepatoblastoma in adolescent and adult patients has an aggressive presentation and a poor prognosis compared to childhood patients. The symptoms of hepatic tumours patients with complicated hypoglycaemia tend to be erroneously diagnosed as central nervous system diseases, intracranial metastases of tumours, or hepatic encephalopathy. So when giving clinical treatments to hepatic cancer patients, it is necessary to pay attention to the change of their blood glucose levels, especially for those patients who have fallen into a coma.

5. Learning Points

(1) Hepatoblastoma (HB) is a rare malignant tumour of the liver and usually occurs in the first three years of life.

(2) Characteristic imaging and histopathological and AFP levels help in the diagnosis of hepatoblastoma.

(3) Paraneoplastic features of hepatoblastoma are not uncommon at presentation and include erythrocytosis, thrombocytosis, hypocalcaemia, isosexual precocious puberty, and rarely hypoglycaemia.

(4) Chemotherapy has been proven effective in both an adjuvant and neoadjuvant treatment and can shrink tumours.

(5) HB is sensitive to such chemotherapy drugs as doxorubicin, cisplatin, vincristine, 5-FU, and cyclophosphamide.

(6) The complete surgical resection is the cornerstone of treatment for patients with HB and is the only chance of an optimal clinical result; however, the tumour is often unresectable at the time of diagnosis.

Conflict of Interests

The authors declare no conflict of interests.

References

[1] L. Bortolasi, L. Marchiori, I. Dal Dosso, R. Colombari, and N. Nicoli, "Hepatoblastoma in adult age: a report of two cases," *Hepato-Gastroenterology*, vol. 43, no. 10, pp. 1073–1078, 1996.

[2] J. M. Schnater, S. E. Köhler, W. H. Lamers, D. von Schweinitz, and D. C. Aronson, "Where do we stand with hepatoblastoma? A review," *Cancer*, vol. 98, no. 4, pp. 668–678, 2003.

[3] H. J. Ahn, K. W. Kwon, Y. J. Choi et al., "Mixed hepatobiastoma in an adult—a case report and literature review," *Journal of Korean Medical Science*, vol. 12, no. 4, pp. 369–373, 1997.

[4] J. M. Remes-Troche, A. Montaño-Loza, J. Meza-Junco, J. García-Leiva, and A. Torre-Delgadillo, "Hepatoblastoma in adult age. A case report and literature review," *Annals of Hepatology*, vol. 5, no. 3, pp. 179–181, 2006.

[5] T. Nagata, M. Nakamura, H. Shichino et al., "Cytogenetic abnormalities in hepatoblastoma: report of two new cases and review of the literature suggesting imbalance of chromosomal regions on chromosomes 1, 4, and 12," *Cancer Genetics and Cytogenetics*, vol. 156, no. 1, pp. 8–13, 2005.

[6] W. Prange, K. Breuhahn, F. Fischer et al., "Beta-catenin accumulation in the progression of human hepatocarcinogenesis correlates with loss of E-cadherin and accumulation of p53, but not with expression of conventional WNT-1 target genes," *Journal of Pathology*, vol. 201, no. 2, pp. 250–259, 2003.

[7] H. Y. Ke, J. H. Chen, Y. M. Jen et al., "Ruptured hepatoblastoma with massive internal bleeding in an adult," *World Journal of Gastroenterology*, vol. 11, no. 39, pp. 6235–6237, 2005.

[8] K. Ha, T. Ikeda, S. Okada et al., "Hypoglycemia in a child with hepatoblastoma," *Medical and Pediatric Oncology*, vol. 8, no. 4, pp. 335–341, 1980.

[9] I. Ambulkar, P. Jagannath, and S. Advani, "Hepatocellular carcinoma presenting with troublesome hypoglycemia," *Indian Journal of Medical and Paediatric Oncology*, vol. 27, pp. 32–35, 2006.

[10] H. P. Lee, W. S. Hung, Z. Chen et al., "Study on the disturbance of glucose metabolism in hepatocellular carcinoma," *Journal of Practical Oncoloy*, vol. 18, pp. 217–219, 2003.

[11] P. R. Larsen, "Hypoglycemic disorders," in *William Text Book of Endocrinology*, WB Saunders, 10th edition, 2003.

[12] J. C. Luo, S. J. Hwang, J. C. Wu et al., "Paraneoplastic syndromes in patients with hepatocellular carcinoma in Taiwan," *Cancer*, vol. 86, no. 5, pp. 799–804, 1999.

[13] M. Reynolds, "Pediatric liver tumors," *Seminars in Surgical Oncology*, vol. 16, no. 2, pp. 159–172, 1999.

[14] G. Perilongo, E. Shafford, R. Maibach et al., "Risk-adapted treatment for childhood hepatoblastoma: final report of the second study of the International Society of Paediatric Oncology—SIOPEL 2," *European Journal of Cancer*, vol. 40, no. 3, pp. 411–421, 2004.

[15] J. A. Ortega, E. C. Douglass, J. H. Feusner et al., "Randomized comparison of cisplatin/vincristine/fluorouracil and cisplatin/continuous infusion doxorubicin for treatment of pediatric hepatoblastoma: a report from the children's cancer group and the pediatric oncology group," *Journal of Clinical Oncology*, vol. 18, no. 14, pp. 2665–2675, 2000.

[16] D. C. Aronson, J. M. Schnater, C. R. Staalman et al., "Predictive value of the pretreatment extent of disease system in hepatoblastoma: results from the International Society of Pediatric Oncology Liver Tumor Study Group SIOPEL-1 study," *Journal of Clinical Oncology*, vol. 23, no. 6, pp. 1245–1252, 2005.

[17] P. Czauderna, J.-B. Otte, D. J. Roebuck, D. von Schweinitz, and J. Plaschkes, "Surgical treatment of hepatoblastoma in children," *Pediatric Radiology*, vol. 36, no. 3, pp. 187–191, 2006.

[18] M. Kubota, M. Yagi, S. Kanada et al., "Effect of postoperative chemotherapy on the serum alpha-fetoprotein level in hepatoblastoma," *Journal of Pediatric Surgery*, vol. 39, no. 12, pp. 1775–1778, 2004.

2

A Challenge for Diagnosing Acute Liver Injury with Concomitant/Sequential Exposure to Multiple Drugs: Can Causality Assessment Scales Be Utilized to Identify the Offending Drug?

Roxanne Lim, Hassan Choudry, Kim Conner, and Wikrom Karnsakul

Division of Pediatric Gastroenterology and Nutrition, Johns Hopkins University School of Medicine, Baltimore, MD 21287, USA

Correspondence should be addressed to Wikrom Karnsakul; wkarnsa1@jhmi.edu

Academic Editor: Nan-Chang Chiu

Drug-induced hepatotoxicity most commonly manifests as an acute hepatitis syndrome and remains the leading cause of drug-induced death/mortality and the primary reason for withdrawal of drugs from the pharmaceutical market. We report a case of acute liver injury in a 12-year-old Hispanic boy, who received a series of five antibiotics (amoxicillin, ceftriaxone, vancomycin, ampicillin/sulbactam, and clindamycin) for cervical lymphadenitis/retropharyngeal cellulitis. Histopathology of the liver biopsy specimen revealed acute cholestatic hepatitis. All known causes of acute liver injury were appropriately excluded and (only) drug-induced liver injury was left as a cause of his cholestasis. Liver-specific causality assessment scales such as Council for the International Organization of Medical Sciences/Roussel Uclaf Causality Assessment Method scoring system (CIOMS/RUCAM), Maria and Victorino scale, and Digestive Disease Week-Japan were applied to seek the most likely offending drug. Although clindamycin is the most likely cause by clinical diagnosis, none of causality assessment scales aid in the diagnosis.

1. Introduction

Acute drug-induced liver injuries (DILI) predominate (about 90% of cases) [1] and are classified into 3 categories [2], acute hepatocellular injury, acute cholestatic liver injury, and mixed pattern acute liver injury. When a single drug is involved, the diagnosis is relatively simple. The administration of multiple concomitant drugs however can pose a difficult implication for which a specific agent would be the cause of DILI. The administration of multiple concomitant drugs can, however, pose a conundrum as to which specific agent is the cause of DILI. Several algorithms/clinical scales have been developed to improve the accuracy, consistency, and objectiveness in identifying the offending drug for the causality assessment of adverse drug reactions. Examples include the Maria and Victorino scale [3] and Council for the International Organization of Medical Sciences/Roussel Uclaf Causality Assessment Method scoring system (CIOMS/RUCAM) scale [3–5], which are used primarily to quantify the strength of association between a liver injury and a particular drug being

implicated. However, it must be emphasized that these diagnostic scales should not be substituted for clinical judgment.

We report a 12-year-old boy who received multiple antibiotics for the treatment of cervical lymphadenitis, retropharyngeal cellulitis, and developed signs and symptoms of cholestatic hepatitis. Causality assessment scales of adverse drug reactions including Council for the International Organization of Medical Sciences/Roussel Uclaf Causality Assessment Method scoring system (CIOMS/RUCAM), Maria and Victorino scale, and Digestive Disease Week-Japan (DDW-J) were utilized to identify the most probable offending drug.

2. Case Report

A previously healthy 12-year-old Hispanic boy presented with a history of sore throat and swelling in the right submandibular region without history of sick contact, travel, tick bites, or uncooked or raw food consumption. Amoxicillin was started to treat a probable streptococcal infection. Three days later he developed anorexia, dysphagia with liquids, and neck swelling with fever. He was brought to the Emergency Department of a nearby hospital and subsequently admitted. A computed tomography scan of the neck and chest showed a retropharyngeal fluid collection without features of an abscess or foreign body and lymphadenopathy throughout the neck and upper mediastinum. Ceftriaxone and vancomycin were started to treat diffuse facial and neck cellulitis for 3 days. While the neck swelling progressed, he was intubated. Ceftriaxone and vancomycin were discontinued, and ampicillin/sulbactam and steroid were started. The following day he was extubated due to improved neck swelling. Results from laboratory tests were all within normal limits except for mild anemia (hemoglobin 9.9 g/dL); however, liver function tests (LFT) were not performed at the time. Ampicillin/sulbactam and steroid were given for 2 days and discontinued. He was discharged home with a planned 10-day course of oral clindamycin 300 mg three times a day.

Over 5 days after the hospital discharge, he had developed fever, fatigue, headache, and dark urine. At the Emergency Department he had severe dehydration, fever (maximum temperature of 101°F), physical findings of mild hepatosplenomegaly, and right upper quadrant tenderness. LFT results included alanine aminotransferase (ALT), 406 IU/L (normal range 0–40); aspartate aminotransferase (AST), 98 IU/L (normal range 0–37); alkaline phosphatase (ALP), 404 IU/L (normal range 100–390); total bilirubin, 3.0 mg/dL (normal range 0.1–1.2); direct bilirubin, 2.7 mg/dL (normal range 0.0–0.4); prothrombin time (PT), 15.3 seconds; international normalized ratio (INR), 1.12; activated partial thromboplastin time (aPTT), 35.2 seconds. At this point, clindamycin was suspected as a cause of hepatic injury and ampicillin/sulbactam was started for 2 weeks because of the lower risk of hepatotoxicity. Infectious workups were all negative for hepatitis A, B, C, and E, Herpes, Epstein-Barr virus and cytomegalovirus viruses, Leptospira, *Bartonella henselae*, and blood culture. Three days after his admission in the Emergency Department, repeat LFTs were ALT, 232 IU/L; AST, 94 IU/L; ALP, 465 IU/L; total bilirubin (TB), 4.0 mg/dL; direct bilirubin (DB), 2.8 mg/dL. The patient was discharged home with clinical improvement.

Two days later at a follow-up with his pediatrician due to abdominal pain, enlarged liver was noted on examination and LFTs worsened: ALT, 152 IU/L; AST, 120 IU/L; ALP, 737 IU/L; TB, 8.8 mg/dL with peripheral eosinophilia with an absolute count of 900/μL. Referral was made to pediatric liver specialist 5 days later when TB was at 9.9 mg/dL.

At the Pediatric Liver Center at Johns Hopkins Hospital the patient complained of chest pain, fatigue, pruritus, and a recent onset of acholic stools. Physical examination was unremarkable except icteric sclera and mild hepatomegaly. Further investigation was promptly started; ALT, 185 IU/L with upper limit normal of normal ULN at 34; AST, 208 IU/L; ALP, 812 IU/L; TB, 11.8 mg/dL; PT, 11 seconds; INR, 1.1; aPTT, 28.6 seconds; amylase, 26 U/L; lipase, 33 U/L; normal ammonia level, glucose, and thyroid function tests. Since serum ALT elevated > 3X ULN and serum bilirubin > 2X ULN and DILI is one of the possible liver injury causes, by Hy's Law he had the potential for development of acute liver failure. However

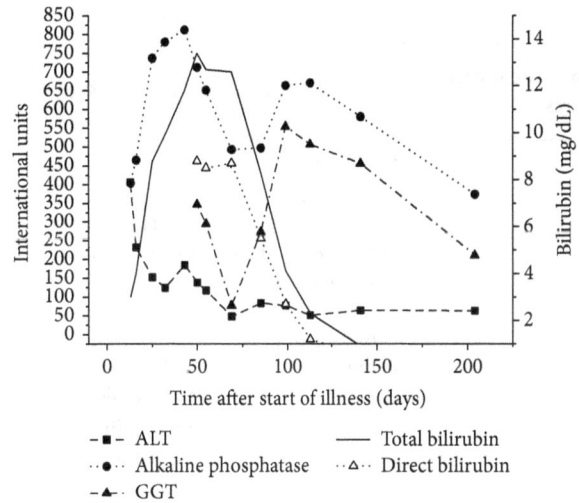

ALT, alanine aminotransferase; GGT, gamma glutamyl transferase; all values except direct and total bilirubin are given in international units.

FIGURE 1: Evolution of laboratory values of liver function tests of patients with time.

his other liver synthetic function was normal and clinically he did not have hepatic encephalopathy. All-out efforts were made to look for every possible contributing cause of his acute liver injury. Specific liver investigations revealed normal ceruloplasmin, serum ferritin level, normal alpha-1 antitrypsin level, negative alpha-1 antitrypsin mutation analysis, and negative liver autoantibodies (antimitochondrial, antinuclear, antismooth-muscle, and antiliver-kidney microsomal antibodies).

Magnetic resonance cholangiopancreatography excluded abnormal gallbladder, intra- and extrahepatic bile duct system, and intrahepatic lesions as possible causes of cholestasis. Vanishing bile duct syndrome was suspected. At approximately day 48 after illness a percutaneous liver biopsy was performed. Histopathologic findings demonstrated moderate lobular cholestasis, mild patchy lobular chronic inflammation, and mild portal fibrosis without features of viral cytopathic effects, autoimmune hepatitis, bile duct injury or loss, and iron storage. Ursodeoxycholic acid was used to treat cholestasis (20 mg/kg/day). Fat soluble vitamins were supplemented. At six-month and 4-year follow-up after the onset of illness his liver chemistry profiles did not indicate ongoing cholestatic jaundice or hepatocellular injury.

Over the following 5 months, jaundice and pruritus gradually improved with a more than 50% improvement in transaminases and bilirubin values. Clindamycin-induced hepatic injury is highly suspected with evidence of previous reports in the literature, and using clinical judgement as displayed in Table 1, Figure 1 summarizes correlation between clinical/biochemical manifestations and drug administration, trends of transaminases and bilirubin values, and timeline of events. The question of drugs other than clindamycin possibly causing DILI in this case was raised for the appropriate information for future drug use in the future. Since multiple antibiotics were administered in the same

TABLE 1: Correlation between clinical and biochemical manifestations and drug administration.

Time from onset of illness	Signs/symptoms	Drug exposure	Laboratory values				
			ALT	ALP	Total bilirubin	Direct bilirubin	Misc.
−5	Sore throat	Amoxicillin started					
0	Fever, anorexia, dysphagia, neck swelling, and cervical lymphadenopathy	Ceftriaxone and vancomycin started					
3–5	Worsening of neck swelling	Ceftriaxone and vancomycin discontinued, and ampicillin/sulbactam and steroid started					
5–10	Diarrhea	Ampicillin/sulbactam and steroid discontinued, and clindamycin and probiotics started					
10	Fever, headache, dizziness, chest pain on coughing, and dark urine. Hepatosplenomegaly, RUQ tenderness	Clindamycin switched to ampicillin/sulbactam	406	404	3.0	2.7	
16–23	Generalized maculopapular rash and pruritus	Ampicillin/sulbactam	152	737	8.8		
25–30	Abdominal pain, vomiting. Hepatomegaly	Ampicillin/sulbactam	124	780	9.9		AST 130
48	Chest pain, fatigue, pruritus, acholic stools, and jaundice		138	713	13.4	8.8	Cholesterol 1044, GGT 347,
53	Increasing pruritus, anorexia		117	651	12.7	8.5	GGT 294
67	Anorexia, pruritus		48	493	12.6	8.7	GGT 77
83	Anorexia		83	497	8.3	5.5	GGT 273
111	No anorexia		51	670	2.3	1.2	GGT 507

Time is in days. ALP = alkaline phosphatase, units used for ALT, ALP, and GGT used are IU. Bilirubin and cholesterol are displayed in mg/dL. Misc. = miscellaneous lab values.

temporal sequence, the probability of the hepatotoxicity being secondary to an adverse drug reaction from the other antibiotics administered prior to clindamycin was assessed using 3 scales (Table 2). Liver-specific causality assessment scales including CIOMS/RUCAM scoring system, Maria and Victorino scale, and DDW-J scale were applied to seek an offending drug but rated all the antibiotics as being equally "possible" and "probable" in causing the liver damage except amoxicillin showing lower score in Maria and Victorino clinical diagnostic scale.

3. Discussion

A period of 5–10 days after administration of multiple antibiotics, our patient had an acute presentation of cholestasis described by dark urine, icteric sclerae, and abnormal liver chemistry. Based on his history and physical examination,

all known causes for cholestasis in the pediatric population were excluded by extensive investigations. Therefore, drug-induced liver injury (DILI) was proposed as a probable etiology. This was further supported as follows: (1) the development of cholestasis after the introduction of the antibiotics, (2) clinical and biochemical improvement after withdrawal of the drugs, (3) hepatotoxicity as a known adverse side effect of each of the antibiotics, and (4) histopathologic findings excluding other causes of cholestatic hepatitis.

DILI is a well-recognized problem that accounts for up to 10 percent of all adverse drug reactions. Two main mechanisms of DILI have been proposed: predictable injury (intrinsic hepatotoxins) and unpredictable injury (idiosyncratic reactions). In our case, an idiosyncratic reaction is likely to be the case. Many experts would suggest that the liver injury could have been primarily caused by clindamycin and that subsequent medications played no role in the presentation. Although fever, abdominal pain, and hepatomegaly followed

TABLE 2: Comparison of three liver-specific causality assessment scales on multiple sequential drug exposure.

Causality assessment scales and criteria	CIOMS/RUCAM	Maria and Victorino clinical diagnostic scale	(DDW-J) scale
Chronological criteria			
From drug intake until onset	Score range: +1 to +2 (i) 5–90 days: +2 (ii) <5 or >90 days: +1	Score range: +1 to +3 (i) 4 d–8 wks: +3 (ii) <4 d or >8 wks: +1	Score range: +1 to +2 (i) 5–90 d/1–90 days: +2 (ii) <5 or >90 d/>15 days: +1
Withdrawal until onset	Score range: 0 to +1 (i) ≤30 d: +1 (ii) 0–29 d: 0	Score range: −3 to +3 (i) 0–7 d: +3 (ii) 8–15 d: 0 (iii) >15 d: −3	Score range: 0 to +1 (i) ≤30 d: +1 (ii) >30 d: 0
Course of the reaction	Score range: −2 to +3 Improvement in 180 days: (i) >50%: +2 (ii) <50%: +1 (iii) Lack of info or no improvement: +0	Score range: 0 to +3 (i) <6 mths (cholestatic/mixed) or <2 mths (hepatocellular): +3 (ii) >6 or 2 mths: +0	Score range: −2 to +3 After cessation of drug Difference in ALP peak and ULN (i) not applicable: +3 (ii) decrease in liver enzymes ≥50% in 180 d: +2 decrease <50% in 180 d: +1 (iii) no information/persistence/increase: +0 (iv) N/A: −2
Extrahepatic manifestations	N/A	Score range: 0 to +3 (rash, fever, arthralgia, eosinophilia >6%, and cytopenia) (i) ≥4: +3 (ii) 2 or 3: +2 (iii) 1: +1 (iv) None: 0	Score range: 0 to+1 Eosinophilia (≥6%) (i) present: +1 (ii) absent: +0
Risk factors	Score range: 0 to +2 (i) Age ≥55: +1 (ii) Alcohol or pregnancy: +1	N/A	Score range: 0 to +1 (i) alcohol/pregnancy: +1
Concomitant therapy	Score range: −3 to 0 Time to onset: (i) incompatible: +0 (ii) compatible but with unknown reaction: −1 (iii) compatible but known reaction: −2 (iv) role proved in this case: −3 (v) none or information not available: +0	N/A	N/A
Exclusion of other causes	Score range: −3 to +2 (i) ruled out: +2 (ii) "possible" to "not investigated": −2 to +1 (iii) probable: −3	Score range: −3 to +3 (i) complete: +3 (ii) partial: +0 (iii) possible alt cause: −1 (iv) probable alt cause: −3	Score range: −3 to +2 (i) ruled out: +2 (ii) 6 causes of Group I ruled out: +1 (iii) 5/4 causes of Group I ruled out: +0 (iv) <4 causes of Group I ruled out: −2 (v) nondrug cause highly probable: −3
Previous information or known reaction	Score range: 0 to +2 Reaction: (i) unknown: +0 (ii) published but unlabelled: +1 (iii) labeled in the product's characteristics: +2	Score range: −3 to +2 (i) yes: +2 (ii) no (drug marketed for ≤5 yrs): +0 (iii) no (drug marketed for <5 yrs): −3	Score range: 0 to +1 (i) reaction labelled in product characteristics or published: +1 (ii) reaction unknown: +0

TABLE 2: Continued.

Causality assessment scales and criteria	CIOMS/RUCAM	Maria and Victorino clinical diagnostic scale	(DDW-J) scale
Rechallenge	Score range: −2 to +3 (i) positive: +3 (ii) compatible: +1 (iii) negative: −2 (iv) Not available/interpretable: +0 (v) plasma conc. of drug toxic: +3	Score range: 0 to +3 (i) positive: +3 (ii) negative/absent: +0	Score range: 0 to +3 (i) ALP/TB ≥ 2x with drug alone: +3 (ii) ALP/TB ≥ 2x with drug already given at time of 1st reaction: +1 (iii) ALP/TB increases but $< N - 2$: −2 (iv) Other situations: +0
DLST	N/A	N/A	Score range: 0 to +2 DLST (i) positive: +2 (ii) semipositive: +1 (iii) negative/unavailable: +0
Scores interpretation	(i) >8 points: definite (ii) 6–8 points: probable (iii) 3–5 points: possible (iv) 1-2 points: unlikely (v) <0 points: excluded	(i) >17 points: definite (ii) 14–17 points: probable (iii) 10–13 points: possible (iv) 6–9 points: unlikely (v) <6 points: excluded	(i) >4 points: definite (ii) 3-4 points: probable (iii) <3 points: unlikely
Our case scores			
Amoxicillin	7 probable	10 possible	7 high possibility
Ceftriaxone	7 probable	13 possible	7 high possible
Vancomycin	7 probable	13 possible	7 high possibility
Ampicillin/sulbactam	7 probable	13 possible	7 high possibility
Clindamycin	7 probable	13 possible	7 high possibility

CIOMS, Council for the International Organization of Medical Sciences; DDW-J, Digestive Disease Week-Japan; DLST, Drug lymphocyte stimulation test; N/A, not available; d, days.

5–10 days after administration of several antibiotics, clindamycin is the immediate agent that started right before the presentation. The causality assessment scales for DILI were used as tools, for this reason, to give more clues as to which antibiotic would more likely be the offending agent.

In order to facilitate causality assessments for DILI, several methods have been developed, including expert judgement, probabilistic approaches, and algorithms/scales [6–8]. The latter can be divided into general and liver-specific scales. As strength in general any of standardized causality assessment scales enhance objectivity in case assessments, grade the strength of probability in broad categories, and can provide warning signs for drug regulatory measurements. However these scales are often complex and time consuming to operate. They do not provide a certain diagnosis of DILI. Each of these has its own strengths and weaknesses. For example, although the CIOMS/RUCAM scale is cumbersome and lacks intra- and interrater reliability, it is however the preferred method as a result of simple and practical use [9–11]. Absolute agreement between the scales could be low [3]. All scales are not designed to evaluate DILI when concomitant drugs are used to solve this particular problem. Therefore the scales do not replace clinical judgement. Exposure to multiple drugs during the same period is a challenging factor in identifying a single agent as a probable offending drug and poses a dilemma for future recommendation for drug use.

At the time of consultation on this case, we recommended holding off the use of clindamycin unless there was no available option for the prospective infection patient might have. Unfortunately, even for IgE mediated drug allergy, testing is very limited, and for this kind of situation there is not any commercial testing that would be helpful given most likely idiosyncratic mechanism in nature. When we look at cases like this, all that can be done is to consider which drugs are more likely to have this type of side effect and then proceed cautiously. However for an idiosyncratic reaction, it is unpredictable as the same drug(s) may not do the same thing in the future. DDW-J was the recently proposed scale in Japan which was modified from CIOMS adding in vitro drug lymphocyte stimulation test (DLST) [12]. The test demonstrates an immunological mechanism for the DILI by demonstrating the existence of a subset of T lymphocytes which recognize and are activated by the drug [13]. Recent findings on HLA allele associations with DILI via adaptive immune response suggested the benefit of DLST utilization [13]. DLST was not performed in their patient as it is not currently commercially available in the United States. The pros of DLST are that we will have a clue which drugs would be the prime candidate causing the reaction and the information could be used as a guide for an avoidance of the suspected drug. In theory DLST is the ideal and objective way to understand the immunologic response to the offending drug; however, many reactions are idiosyncratic, so the same drug(s) may not cause the same reaction in the future. As demonstrated in Table 2, each of the antibiotics administered has an almost equal probability of causing DILI. When we assessed the causality by different scales for ceftriaxone, vancomycin, clindamycin, and ampicillin/sulbactam (Table 2), scores for each were in similar category as a "possible" or "probable" cause of liver injury.

A search of the literature revealed that all five antibiotics have been known to be implicated in DILI. Most of isolated adult cases, however, may not reflect on the clinical aspect in children [14]. Although the reports in pediatric cases were limited, there was a recent pediatric report comparing several antibiotic uses with a focus on hepatic injury [14].

Maraqa et al. reported a 13-year-old child with clindamycin related DILI. The time to onset was 17 days and time to resolution was 10 days [15]. As for LiverTox database it only speaks of case reports in adults for hepatic toxicity from clindamycin. The rest of journal articles only relate hepatotoxicity to clindamycin in adult patients. A 42-year-old woman developed fatigue, nausea, vomiting, anorexia, pruritus, and jaundice 6 days after administration of the last clindamycin dose for a dental infection [16]. Transaminases were markedly elevated and liver biopsy revealed centrilobular and portal cholestatic hepatitis without fibrosis or necrosis. There is also another case of a 67-year-old man who received a 10-day course of oral clindamycin for a skin abscess. One week after the last clindamycin dose, he developed icterus accompanied by pale stools, dark urine, and pruritus [17]. Liver biopsy revealed marked cholestasis, portal inflammation, bile duct injury, and ductopenia. A second biopsy five months after the first one showed resolved cholestasis but persistent ductopenia.

Molleston et al. reported two cases of DILI secondary to amoxicillin use among pediatric patients in the DILIN prospective study [18]. Kim et al. presented a case of a 39-year-old woman who developed cholestatic hepatitis with bile duct damage and hepatocellular injury eight weeks after initiation of amoxicillin treatment for abdominal actinomycosis [19] and became asymptomatic fourteen weeks after drug discontinuation.

Several articles have been published in the literature documenting the association between ceftriaxone and DILI. Peker et al. reported a 12-year-old boy who complained of weakness 3 days and had elevated transaminases 6 days after ceftriaxone was given for tonsillitis [20]. Transaminases eventually returned to baseline within 10 weeks after discontinuing the drug. Bickford and Spencer described a case of a 53-year-old man who had elevated total and direct bilirubin levels after a week therapy of ceftriaxone [21]. Discontinuing ceftriaxone led to normalization of the LFTs within 2 weeks.

Chen et al. conducted a meta-analysis of 20 published randomized controlled trials involving 7419 patients [22]. An increased incidence of hepatic events, specifically elevated serum aminotransferase levels, was observed in patients receiving vancomycin (6.8%) compared to those who were not (3.9%). The majority of events were mild to moderate in nature and progressive or severe DILI has not been associated with vancomycin use.

Ampicillin/sulbactam, in a rare incident, was reported in a 74-year-old man with Hodgkin's disease in remission, who developed a 3-month period of cholestasis after a week treatment with ampicillin/sulbactam 750 mg twice daily for sore throat [23]. Abnormal liver enzymes prompted liver biopsy showing diffuse canalicular and mild hepatocellular cholestasis, mild and mixed inflammation in the portal area, and diffuse necroinflammatory areas in the liver parenchyma. Liver function tests eventually normalized 7 months after discontinuing the drug.

In DILI cases with concomitant or sequential drug exposure the CIOMS/RUCAM scale may not be able to differentiate between offending drugs and would require individual assessments for each of the drugs. These causality assessment scales disregard differences in metabolic pathways utilized by concomitant drugs and potential pharmacokinetic drug-drug or drug-disease interactions [3]. DLST in DDW-J scale on any drugs could predict the hepatotoxic potential of such a drug making it the prime candidate causing DILI. CIOMS has many shortcomings which render it inaccurate in assessing causality in a multipharmacy situation. A consensus on criteria for excluding nondrug-related cases will establish a standardized evidence based database of drugs causing DILI. This knowledge would allow physicians to apply a uniform scoring system in the sections of "concomitance therapy" and previous information on hepatotoxicity [24]. A "multihit" process could explain idiosyncratic drug reaction in this patient as a result from a succession of events or exposure to multiple drugs [25]. It is unlikely that genetic variants in isoenzymes or cytochrome 450 pathway alone would predispose to severe hepatotoxicity from toxic byproducts given that severe liver toxicity is a rare event. In addition there could be suppressor or attenuator pathways which could play a role in idiosyncratic hepatotoxicity.

In summary, we report on a case of probable DILI with concomitant use of several antibiotics. None of the known causality assessment scoring systems was developed for identifying an offending drug for DILI cases with concomitant drug use in the same temporal sequence. Close monitoring of liver functions could eliminate certain drugs as offending agents if an abnormal LFT is present before and after certain drugs. Obviously this still continues to pose us a challenge in determining which of the drugs is/are allowed to be utilized in this child in the future. Whenever suspected, the offending drug should be discontinued immediately as complete recovery is still possible with prompt drug discontinuation. A different model using knowledge of drug metabolism and interaction via genetic variant isoenzymes, cytochrome P450 pathway, and application of in vitro DLST could be considered to aid in identifying offended drug causing DILI.

Ethical Approval

All procedures followed were in accordance with the ethical standards of the responsible committee on human experimentation (institutional and national) and with the Helsinki Declaration of 1975, as revised in 2008 (5).

Consent

Informed consent was obtained from all patients for being included in the study.

Conflict of Interests

The authors declare that there is no conflict of interests regarding the publication of this paper.

References

[1] H. J. Zimmerman, *Hepatotoxicity: The Adverse Effects of Drugs and Other Chemicals on the Liver*, Lippincott Williams & Wilkins, 1999.

[2] C. Benichou, J. P. Benhamou, and G. Danan, "Criteria of drug-induced liver disorders," *Journal of Hepatology*, vol. 11, no. 2, pp. 272–276, 1990.

[3] M. Garcia-Cortes, C. Stephens, M. I. Lucena, A. Fernandez-Castañer, and R. J. Andrade, "Causality assessment methods in drug induced liver injury: strengths and weaknesses," *Journal of Hepatology*, vol. 55, no. 3, pp. 683–691, 2011.

[4] G. Danan and C. Benichou, "Causality assessment of adverse reactions to drugs—I: a novel method based on the conclusions of international consensus meetings: application to drug-induced liver injuries," *Journal of Clinical Epidemiology*, vol. 46, no. 11, pp. 1323–1330, 1993.

[5] C. Benichou, G. Danan, and A. Flahault, "Causality assessment of adverse reactions to drugs—II: an original model for validation of drug causality assessment methods: case reports with positive rechallenge," *Journal of Clinical Epidemiology*, vol. 46, no. 11, pp. 1331–1336, 1993.

[6] D. Larrey, "Drug-induced liver diseases," *Journal of Hepatology*, vol. 32, supplement 1, pp. 77–88, 2000.

[7] B. K. Gunawan and N. Kaplowitz, "Mechanisms of drug-induced liver disease," *Clinics in Liver Disease*, vol. 11, no. 3, pp. 459–475, 2007.

[8] P. Zapater, J. Such, M. Pérez-Mateo, and J. F. Horga, "A new poisson and Bayesian-based method to assign risk and causality in patients with suspected hepatic adverse drug reactions: a report of two new cases of ticlopidine-induced hepatotoxicity," *Drug Safety*, vol. 25, no. 10, pp. 735–750, 2002.

[9] P. H. Hayashi, "Causality assessment in drug-induced liver injury," *Seminars in Liver Disease*, vol. 29, no. 4, pp. 348–356, 2009.

[10] M. A. Shapiro and J. H. Lewis, "Causality assessment of drug-induced hepatotoxicity: promises and pitfalls," *Clinics in Liver Disease*, vol. 11, no. 3, pp. 477–505, 2007.

[11] M. García-Cortés, M. I. Lucena, K. Pachkoria, Y. Borraz, R. Hidalgo, and R. J. Andrade, "Evaluation of naranjo adverse drug reactions probability scale in causality assessment of drug-induced liver injury," *Alimentary Pharmacology and Therapeutics*, vol. 27, no. 9, pp. 780–789, 2008.

[12] H. Takikawa, Y. Takamori, T. Kumagi et al., "Assessment of 287 Japanese cases of drug induced liver injury by the diagnostic scale of the International Consensus Meeting," *Hepatology Research*, vol. 27, no. 3, pp. 192–195, 2003.

[13] P. B. Watkins, "Biomarkers for the diagnosis and management of drug-induced liver injury," *Seminars in Liver Disease*, vol. 29, no. 4, pp. 393–399, 2009.

[14] D. Serranti, C. Montagnani, G. Indolfi, E. Chiappini, L. Galli, and M. de Martino, "Antibiotic induced liver injury: what about children?" *Journal of Chemotherapy*, vol. 25, no. 5, pp. 255–272, 2013.

[15] N. F. Maraqa, M. M. Gomez, M. H. Rathore, and A. M. Alvarez, "Higher occurrence of hepatotoxicity and rash in patients treated with oxacillin, compared with those treated with nafcillin and other commonly used antimicrobials," *Clinical Infectious Diseases*, vol. 34, no. 1, pp. 50–54, 2002.

[16] C. Aygün, O. Kocaman, Y. Gürbüz, Ö. Şentürk, and S. Hülagü, "Clindamycin-induced acute cholestatic hepatitis," *World Journal of Gastroenterology*, vol. 13, no. 40, pp. 5408–5410, 2007.

[17] I. Altraif, L. Lilly, I. R. Wanless, and J. Heathcote, "Cholestatic liver disease with ductopenia (vanishing bile duct syndrome) after administration of clindamycin and trimethoprim-sulfamethoxazole," *The American Journal of Gastroenterology*, vol. 89, no. 8, pp. 1230–1234, 1994.

[18] J. P. Molleston, R. J. Fontana, M. J. Lopez, D. E. Kleiner, J. Gu, and N. Chalasani, "Characteristics of idiosyncratic drug-induced liver injury in children: results from the DILIN prospective study," *Journal of Pediatric Gastroenterology and Nutrition*, vol. 53, no. 2, pp. 182–189, 2011.

[19] J. S. Kim, Y. R. Jang, J. W. Lee et al., "A case of amoxicillin-induced hepatocellular liver injury with bile-duct damage," *The Korean Journal of Hepatology*, vol. 17, no. 3, pp. 229–232, 2011.

[20] E. Peker, E. Cagan, and M. Dogan, "Ceftriaxone-induced toxic hepatitis," *World Journal of Gastroenterology*, vol. 15, no. 21, pp. 2669–2671, 2009.

[21] C. L. Bickford and A. P. Spencer, "Biliary sludge and hyperbilirubinemia associated with ceftriaxone in an adult: case report and review of the literature," *Pharmacotherapy*, vol. 25, no. 10 I, pp. 1389–1395, 2005.

[22] Y. Chen, X. Y. Yang, M. Zeckel et al., "Risk of hepatic events in patients treated with vancomycin in clinical studies: a systematic review and meta-analysis," *Drug Safety*, vol. 34, no. 1, pp. 73–82, 2011.

[23] S. Köklü, A. Ş. Köksal, M. Asil, H. Kiyici, Ş. Çoban, and M. Arhan, "Probable sulbactam/ampicillin-associated prolonged cholestasis," *Annals of Pharmacotherapy*, vol. 38, no. 12, pp. 2055–2058, 2004.

[24] R. J. Fontana, L. B. Seeff, R. J. Andrade et al., "Standardization of nomenclature and causality assessment in drug-induced liver injury: summary of a clinical research workshop," *Hepatology*, vol. 52, no. 2, pp. 730–742, 2010.

[25] W. M. Lee, "Drug-induced hepatotoxicity," *The New England Journal of Medicine*, vol. 349, no. 5, pp. 474–485, 2003.

3

Atypical Presentation of Cat-Scratch Disease in an Immunocompetent Child with Serological and Pathological Evidence

Serkan Atıcı,[1] **Eda Kepenekli Kadayıfcı,**[1] **Ayşe Karaaslan,**[1] **Muhammed Hasan Toper,**[2] **Cigdem Ataizi Celikel,**[2] **Ahmet Soysal,**[1,3] **and Mustafa Bakır**[1]

[1]Department of Pediatrics and Division of Pediatric Infectious Diseases, Marmara University Medical Faculty, Pendik Training and Research Hospital, Fevzi Cakmak Mah. Mimar Sinan Cad., Ust Kaynarca, Pendik, 34899 Istanbul, Turkey
[2]Department of Pathology, Marmara University Medical Faculty, Pendik Training and Research Hospital, Fevzi Cakmak Mah. Mimar Sinan Cad., Ust Kaynarca, Pendik, 34899 Istanbul, Turkey
[3]Marmara University Medical Faculty, Pendik Training and Research Hospital, Fevzi Cakmak Mah. Mimar Sinan Cad., Ust Kaynarca, Pendik, 34899 Istanbul, Turkey

Correspondence should be addressed to Ahmet Soysal; ahsoysal@yahoo.com

Academic Editor: Bibhuti Das

Typical cat-scratch disease (CSD) is characterized by local lymphadenopathy following the scratch or bite from a cat or kitten. An atypical presentation which includes liver and/or spleen lesions is rarely reported in an immunocompetent child. Systemic CSD may mimic more serious disorders like malignancy or tuberculosis. Although a diagnosis is difficult to establish in systemic CSD, an early diagnosis and an appropriate treatment are important to prevent complications. Bartonella henselae is difficult to culture, and culture is not routinely recommended. Clinical, serological, radiological, and pathological findings are used for the diagnosis of CSD. Herein we present a case of systemic CSD presenting with hepatic mass in an immunocompetent child. The differential diagnosis is made by serological and pathological evidence. He was successfully treated with gentamicin (7.5 mg/kg) and rifampin (15 mg/kg) for six weeks.

1. Introduction

Cat-scratch disease (CSD) is an infectious disease caused by the *Bartonella henselae*. It is a small, curved, aerobic, slow-growing, fastidious, gram-negative, intracellular *Bacillus* that causes granulomatous inflammation of the tissue and it can be painted with silver stain [1].

CSD is usually associated with a previous history of exposure to cats or kittens. Although a history of scratch, bite, or licking from a cat or kitten is important, it is not necessary for the diagnosis. Typical CSD is characterized by local lymphadenopathy with or without skin rash and is usually self-limited. Systemic CSD may present in a more disseminated form which usually occurs in immunocompromised children. Atypical presentations which include hepatic and/or splenic lesions, osteomyelitis, discitis, granulomatous conjunctivitis, endocarditis, myocarditis, neuroretinitis, and encephalomeningitis may mimic more serious disorders such as malignancy and could be an important differential diagnostic problem [1, 2]. Isolated hepatic lesions of CSD are a rare clinical condition especially in an immunocompetent child.

We report the case of an immunocompetent child diagnosed as systemic CSD with serological and pathological evidence. He had multiple hepatic lesions. He was successfully treated with intravenous gentamicin and oral rifampin. The aim of this study was to report the management of hepatic CSD in an immunocompetent child.

2. Case Report

A 12-year-old boy was admitted to another hospital with 7-day history of fever, abdominal pain, headache, and weight loss. Empirical antibiotics therapy including ceftriaxone and

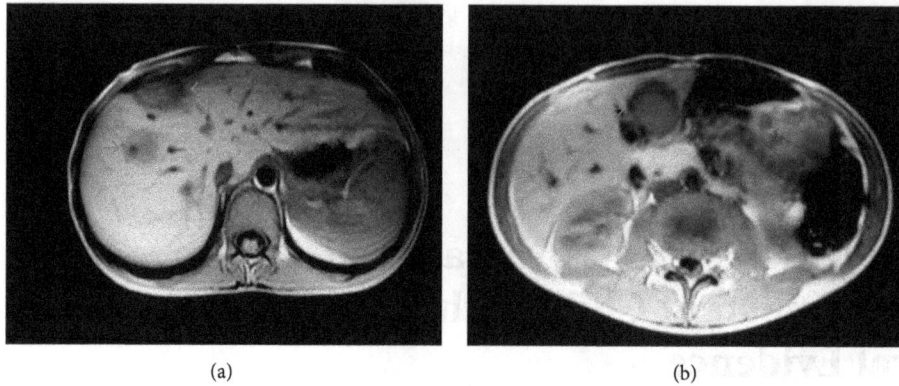

(a)   (b)

FIGURE 1: T1 (a) and T2 (b) weighted magnetic resonance imaging shows multiple lesions in the liver.

clindamycin had been administered. After the abdominal ultrasound demonstrated multiple hypoechoic liver lesions, he was transferred to our department on the eleventh day of hospitalization. Fever and abdominal pain continued and he had lost 8 kilograms. He had a history of playing with a kitten. Physical examination revealed bilateral inguinal lymphadenopathy. There was not any scratch or papule on his skin. His past medical history was not consistent with any primary or secondary immunodeficiency or any other underlying disease. Laboratory findings included the following: white blood cell count, 10 400/mm^3; hemoglobin, 11.9 g/dL; platelets, 385 000/mm^3; C-reactive protein (CRP), 10.1 mg/dL; erythrocyte sedimentation rate (ESR), 57 mm in 1 h; aspartate aminotransferase (AST), 168 U/L; alanine aminotransferase (ALT), 67 U/L. Blood and urine cultures were negative. Serology of human immunodeficiency virus was also negative. Abdominal magnetic resonance imaging (MRI) showed multiple hepatic lesions (Figure 1). Cranial and thoracal imaging revealed no distinct abnormality. Serological analyses by indirect fluorescent antibody (IFA) method detected the presence of immunoglobulin (Ig) G and IgM antibodies to Bartonella henselae positive with a titer of 1 : 320 and 1 : 100, respectively. He was assessed to the pediatric immunology department with suspected immunodeficiency. Lymphocyte subset analysis, dihydrorhodamine 123 flow cytometry, and the serum immunoglobulins levels were normal. Ultrasound guided liver biopsy was performed. Histopathological analyses of the lesions showed granulomas surrounded with palisade histiocytes and non calcified necrosis with hematoxylin and eosin (H&E) staining (Figure 2(a)). Acid-fast Bacilli were not detected with Ehrlich-Ziehl-Neelsen (EZN) staining (Figure 2(b)). Warthin-Starry silver stain was positive which was compatible with CSD (Figure 2(c)).

He was treated with intravenous gentamicin (7.5 mg/kg) and oral rifampin (15 mg/kg) for six weeks. His symptoms were resolved and abnormal laboratory findings including elevated CRP, ESR, and liver transaminases were normalized after antibiotic therapy. Contrast enhanced abdominal MRI was repeated on 30th day of antibiotic therapy and showed that hepatic lesions had regressed.

3. Discussion

Bartonella henselae is the etiologic agent of cat-scratch disease and cats are the major reservoir for the bacteria. A study in our country determined Bartonella henselae IgG antibody seroprevalence was 18.8% in cats. Seropositivity was observed as 27.5% for stray cats. The seropositivity was 14.3% and 11.4% in outdoor and indoor domestic cats in Turkey, respectively [3]. History of scratch or bite from a cat or kitten is helpful for the diagnosis. Our patient had a history of playing with a kitten.

Although most patients with CSD typically presented with fever and lymphadenopathy, atypical clinical manifestations may be seen. Atypical clinical presentations of CSD include a broad spectrum of clinical syndromes ranging from prolonged fever of unknown origin to hepatosplenic, ocular, and neurological manifestations [4, 5]. Hepatosplenic disease is an unusual clinic presentation occurring in only 0.3% to 0.7% of patients, mostly in children [6]. Hepatic involvement is an uncommon clinical presentation in immunocompetent children. Patients with hepatic lesions present episodic abdominal pain with prolonged fever. Although liver enzymes are usually normal, erythrocyte sedimentation rate is often increased.

Abdominal imaging is an important diagnostic step in patients with suspected hepatosplenic CSD [4]. Ultrasonography (US), computed tomography (CT), or MRI may show multiple and variable size and shape lesions in the liver or spleen. Lesions are usually hypoechoic on US and hypoattenuated on CT. Multiple hepatic lesions may be due to lymphoma, histoplasmosis, granulomatous processes, and metastatic disease [7, 8].

Bartonella henselae is difficult to culture, and culture is not routinely recommended. Clinical, serological, radiological, and pathological findings are used for the diagnosis of CSD. In history, the exposure to animals, especially cats, is important medical information to suspect from CSD [9]. Serological testing for Bartonella henselae antibodies is the most cost-effective diagnostic modality with IFA to be most frequently used [4, 10]. Granulomatous inflammation is not specific to CSD, so other granulomatous diseases such as tuberculosis should be considered. Although tuberculosis

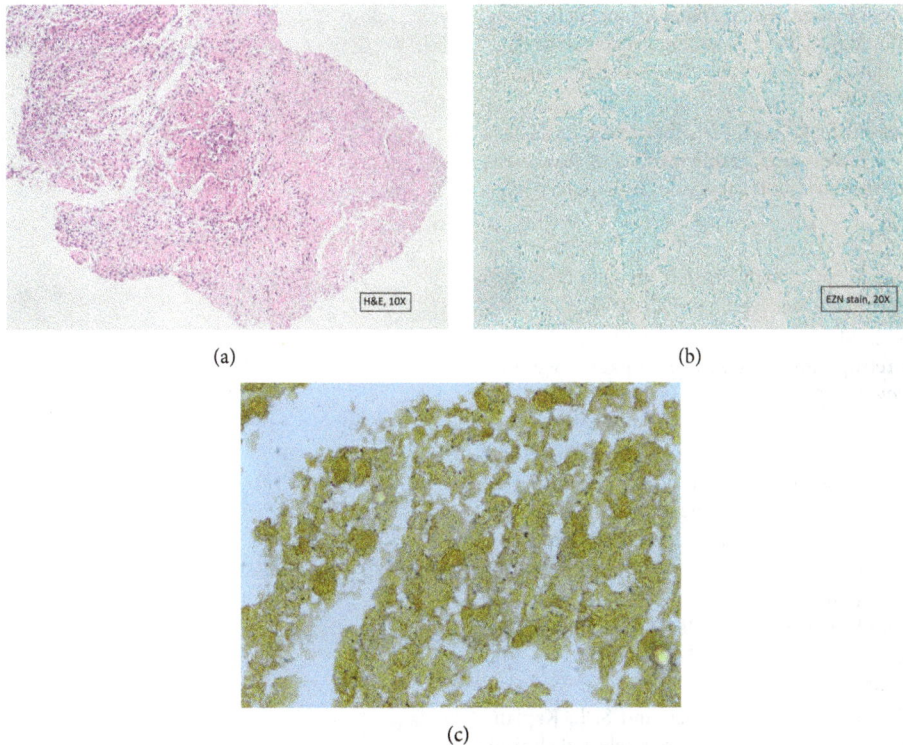

FIGURE 2: (a) The liver lesion is characterized by multiple granulomas hematoxylin and eosin ×10, (b) acid-fast Bacilli was not detected with EZN staining ×10, and (c) *Bartonella henselae* was demonstrated by Warthin-Starry silver stain ×10.

is still common in Turkey, isolated hepatic lesions are unusual. We have investigated for tuberculosis and ruled out histopathological findings and laboratory tests including IFN-gamma releasing assay (QuantiFERON-TB), EZN staining, and mycobacterial culture of gastric lavage fluids. Acid-fast *Bacillus* was not detected on liver biopsy with Ehrlich-Ziehl-Neelsen staining but *Bartonella henselae* has been demonstrated as short rods by using Warthin-Starry silver stain (Figure 2(c)). Previous history of contact with kitten, the positive serology for *Bartonella henselae*, and radiological and pathological findings were used for the diagnosis of our patient.

Systemic CSD has a high morbidity rate in immunocompromised children. There is no consensus about the type of antimicrobial drug and the duration of the therapy for the diagnosis of systemic CSD in an immunocompetent child [11]. Rifampin, trimethoprim-sulfamethoxazole, gentamicin, macrolides, extended spectrum cephalosporins, and ciprofloxacin all have *in vitro* activity against *Bartonella henselae* [11, 12]. Arısoy et al. published a large series including 19 children with hepatosplenic cat-scratch disease and all patients were treated with one or more antibiotics including gentamicin (7.5 mg/kg), rifampin (15–20 mg/kg), and trimethoprim-sulfamethoxazole (10–12 mg/kg) for 10 to 21 days. Thirteen patients were treated with rifampin alone and 3 patients were treated with rifampin plus gentamicin or trimethoprim-sulfamethoxazole. Rifampin was proposed in the antimicrobial treatment of hepatosplenic CSD in that study [12]. We used a rifampin plus gentamicin combination

therapy in our case for 6 weeks. His symptoms were resolved and the hepatic lesions regressed. A relapse was not determined during the follow-up.

Conflict of Interests

The authors declare that they have no conflict of interests.

References

[1] S. A. Klotz, V. Ianas, and S. P. Elliott, "Cat-scratch disease," *American Family Physician*, vol. 83, no. 2, pp. 152–155, 2011.

[2] M. Kojić, D. Mikić, D. Nožić, and L. Zolotarevski, "Atypical form of cat scratch disease in immunocompetent patient," *Vojnosanitetski Pregled*, vol. 70, no. 1, pp. 72–76, 2013.

[3] B. Celebi, S. Kilic, N. Aydin, G. Tarhan, A. Carhan, and C. Babur, "Investigation of *Bartonella henselae* in cats in Ankara, Turkey," *Zoonoses and Public Health*, vol. 56, no. 4, pp. 169–175, 2009.

[4] T. A. Florin, T. E. Zaoutis, and L. B. Zaoutis, "Beyond cat scratch disease: widening spectrum of *Bartonella henselae* infection," *Pediatrics*, vol. 121, no. 5, pp. e1413–e1425, 2008.

[5] E. Eskow, R.-V. S. Rao, and E. Mordechai, "Concurrent infection of the central nervous system by *Borrelia burgdorferi* and *Bartonella henselae*: evidence for a novel tick-borne disease complex," *Archives of Neurology*, vol. 58, no. 9, pp. 1357–1363, 2001.

[6] G. M. Marsilia, A. la Mura, R. Galdiero, E. Galdiero, G. Aloj, and A. Ragozzino, "Isolated hepatic involvement of cat scratch

disease in immunocompetent adults: enhanced magnetic resonance imaging, pathological findings, and molecular analysis—two cases," *International Journal of Surgical Pathology*, vol. 14, no. 4, pp. 349–354, 2006.

[7] A. Rohr, M. R. Saettele, S. A. Patel, C. A. Lawrence, and L. H. Lowe, "Spectrum of radiological manifestations of paediatric cat-scratch disease," *Pediatric Radiology*, vol. 42, no. 11, pp. 1380–1384, 2012.

[8] O. Danon, M. Duval-Arnould, Z. Osman et al., "Hepatic and splenic involvement in cat-scratch disease: imaging features," *Abdominal Imaging*, vol. 25, no. 2, pp. 182–183, 2000.

[9] T. Koga, J. Taguchi, M. Suzuki et al., "Cat scratch disease presenting with a retroperitoneal abscess in a patient without animal contacts," *Journal of Infection and Chemotherapy*, vol. 15, no. 6, pp. 414–416, 2009.

[10] D. Anyfantakis, M. Kastanakis, A. Papadomichelakis, G. Petrakis, and E. Bobolakis, "Cat-scratch disease presenting as a solitary splenic abscess in an immunocompetent adult: case report and literature review," *Infezioni in Medicina*, vol. 21, no. 2, pp. 130–133, 2013.

[11] C. Scolfaro, G. G. K. Leunga, S. Bezzio et al., "Prolonged follow up of seven patients affected by hepatosplenic granulomata due to cat-scratch disease," *European Journal of Pediatrics*, vol. 167, no. 4, pp. 471–473, 2008.

[12] E. S. Arisoy, A. G. Correa, M. L. Wagner, and S. L. Kaplan, "Hepatosplenic cat-scratch disease in children: selected clinical features and treatment," *Clinical Infectious Diseases*, vol. 28, no. 4, pp. 778–784, 1999.

Sanjad-Sakati Syndrome and Its Association with Superior Mesenteric Artery Syndrome

Osamah Abdullah AlAyed

King Faisal Specialist Hospital Research Centre, P.O. Box 280581, Riyadh 11392, Saudi Arabia

Correspondence should be addressed to Osamah Abdullah AlAyed; usamah222@hotmail.com

Academic Editor: Doris Fischer

Sanjad-Sakati syndrome (SSS) is an autosomal recessive disorder found exclusively in people of Arabian origin. It was first reported in the Kingdom of Saudi Arabia in 1988 and confirmed by a definitive report in 1991. The syndrome comprises of congenital hypoparathyroidism, seizures, severe growth and developmental retardation, low IQ, and atypical facial features. Supportive treatment in the form of vitamin D and growth hormone supplementation is often offered to patients suffering from SSS. This case study focuses on the steps taken to help a patient who was found to have very unusual symptoms and was later found to have superior mesenteric artery syndrome.

1. Introduction

Sanjad-Sakati syndrome (SSS) is a newly described syndrome found mainly in the Middle East and Arabian Gulf countries. The condition was first reported by Sanjad et al. in 1988 [1]. Three years later, its inheritance and configuration were confirmed by the same team from King Faisal Specialist Hospital and Research Centre, Saudi Arabia [2]. Later on, the syndrome was also described by Richardson and Kirk in 1990 [3] and in 1992 by Kalam and Hafeez [4]. SSS is listed in OMIM (241410) as HRD, that is, hypoparathyroidism-retardation-dysmorphism Syndrome. Parvari et al. reported a gene location on chromosome number 1 at 1q42-43, this syndrome can be caused by mutations in the gene encoding tubulin-specific chaperone E (*TBCE*) [5]. Children affected with this condition develop poorly in the mother's womb (IUGR) and therefore, after birth, suffer from various conditions such as hypocalcemic tetany or seizures due to hypoparathyroidism at an early stage in their lives [2]. They have atypical physical features, namely, long narrow faces, deep set small eyes, beaked noses, and large ears that have tendency to droop and undersized jaws (micrognathia). Along with the physical abnormalities, children suffering from SSS also exhibit mild to moderate mental retardation, leading to poor life prospects.

Less superficial symptoms have also been documented, namely, skeletal defects (medullary stenosis), hypocalcaemia, hyperphosphatemia, and low concentration of immunoreactive parathyroid hormone. In some rare cases, there may even be complete respiratory failure eventually [6, 7].

2. Case Report

An 8-year-old girl was diagnosed with Sanjad-Sakati syndrome (SSS) and was prescribed calcium and vitamin D supplements (one-alpha drops). She was in her usual state of health until January 2013 when she suddenly began to suffer from frequent vomiting with no apparent reason. She immediately went to her local hospital where she was diagnosed with gastroenteritis and treated accordingly. However, the problem persisted for a time and then worsened, adding severe constipation (only passing stool every three days) to the list of symptoms. She was once again admitted to the hospital and, once again, treated for the same condition. As her problem did not improve, she went to her local clinic and demanded the opinion of an expert. A gastroenterology team was consulted and, following their advice, she undertook a barium follow through. The results showed all the symptoms of severe superior mesenteric artery syndrome, a condition that causes almost complete intestinal obstruction at the level of the third part of the duodenum. With this new information, she was readmitted to the hospital on January 11 and underwent an upper esophagogastroduodenoscopy and NJ tube insertion. A biopsy was also taken because of the severe difficulties in performing the endoscopy. Despite all this, her condition worsened and, on January 15, she suffered an episode of vomiting, choking, and aspiration pneumonia, which required an ICU admission of 10 days for a course of antibiotics. After this, she was allowed to start gradual NJ feeding with a small amount administered initially (2 cc) and an incremental increase until the full dose (45 cc) was reached. She tolerated this well and it was deemed safe to prescribe her Movicol for the constipation. The medication worked and her bowel obstruction began to clear in the form of diarrhea 3 times a day, which required various readjustments of the NJ tube and even the insertion of an NG tube for drainage.

3. Discussion

Sanjad-Sakati syndrome tends to have severe growth retardation which is usually the predisposing factor in developing superior mesenteric artery (SMA) syndrome.

SMA syndrome is an uncommon but well-recognized clinical entity characterized by compression of the third, or transverse, portion of the duodenum between the aorta and the superior mesenteric artery. This results in chronic, intermittent, acute, complete or partial duodenal obstruction [8]. Superior mesenteric artery syndrome was first described in 1861 by Von Rokitansky, who proposed that its cause was obstruction of the third part of the duodenum as a result of arteriomesenteric compression. Some studies report the incidence of superior mesenteric artery syndrome to be 0.1–0.3% [9].

But the diagnosis of SMA syndrome is difficult. Confirmation usually requires radiographic studies, such as an upper GI series, hypotonic duodenography, and CT scanning. Therefore, there are very few studies that report the incidence of superior mesenteric artery syndrome (0.1–0.3%) and approximately 0.013–0.78% of barium upper GI studies evaluating the condition support the diagnosis [10, 11].

What can be confirmed from this study is that the insertion of an NJ to bypass the obstruction proved very helpful, allowing the patient to tolerate food, to gain weight, and to increase the angle between the superior mesenteric artery and the third part of the duodenum, thus relieving the symptoms. Reversing or removing the precipitating factor is usually successful in a patient with acute superior mesenteric artery (SMA) syndrome.

Conservative initial treatment is recommended in all patients with superior mesenteric artery syndrome; this includes adequate nutrition, nasogastric decompression, and proper positioning of the patient after eating (i.e., left lateral decubitus, prone, knee-to-chest position, or Goldthwaite maneuver). Enteral feeding using a double lumen nasojejunal tube passed distal to the obstruction under fluoroscopic assistance is an effective adjunct in treatment of patients with rapid severe weight loss and also eliminates the need

for intravenous fluids and the risks associated with total parenteral nutrition.

In some instances, both enteral and parenteral nutritional support may be needed to provide optimal calories. The patient's weight should be monitored daily. Subsequently, the patient can be started on oral liquids followed by slow and gradual introduction of small and frequent soft meals as tolerated. Finally, regular solid foods are introduced.

Metoclopramide treatment may be beneficial.

Surgical intervention is indicated when conservative measures are ineffective, particularly in patients with a long history of progressive weight loss, pronounced duodenal dilatation with stasis, and complicating peptic ulcer disease. A trial of conservative treatment should be instituted for at least 4–6 weeks prior to surgical intervention.

Options for surgery include a duodenojejunostomy or gastrojejunostomy to bypass the obstruction or a duodenal derotation procedure (otherwise known as the Strong procedure) to alter the aortomesenteric angle and place the third and fourth portions of the duodenum to the right of the superior mesenteric artery.

4. Conclusion

To the best of our knowledge and as far back as we go through previous case reports, this is the first case that showed that there could be a relation between SSS and SMA syndrome. It was therefore the aim of this case report to emphasize the importance of considering superior mesenteric artery syndrome when dealing with Sanjad-Sakati syndrome sufferers who present symptoms of intestinal obstruction. We hope that, by doing so, we may enable medical practitioners to better assess and treat future situations of this nature.

Conflict of Interests

The author declares that there is no conflict of interests regarding the publication of this paper.

References

[1] S. Sanjad, N. Sakati, and Y. Abu-Osba, "Congenital hypoparathyroidism with dysmorphic features: a new syndrome," *Pediatric Research*, vol. 23, abstract 271A, 1988.

[2] S. A. Sanjad, N. A. Sakati, Y. K. Abu-Osba, R. Kaddoura, and R. D. G. Milner, "A new syndrome of congenital hypoparathyroidism, severe growth failure, and dysmorphic features," *Archives of Disease in Childhood*, vol. 66, no. 2, pp. 193–196, 1991.

[3] R. J. Richardson and J. M. W. Kirk, "Short stature, mental retardation, and hypoparathyroidism: a new syndrome," *Archives of Disease in Childhood*, vol. 65, no. 10, pp. 1113–1117, 1990.

[4] M. A. Kalam and W. Hafeez, "Congenital hypoparathyroidism, seizure, extreme growth failure with developmental delay and dysmorphic features—another case of this new syndrome," *Clinical Genetics*, vol. 42, no. 3, pp. 110–113, 1992.

[5] R. Parvari, E. Hershkovitz, A. Kanis et al., "Homozygosity and linkage-disequilibrium mapping of the syndrome of congenital hypoparathyroidism, growth and mental retardation, and dysmorphism to a 1-cM interval on chromosome 1q42-43," *The*

American Journal of Human Genetics, vol. 63, no. 1, pp. 163–169, 1998.

[6] R. Parvari, E. Hershkovitz, N. Grossman et al., "Mutation of TBCE causes hypoparathyroidism-retardation-dysmorphism and autosomal recessive Kenny-Caffey Syndrome," *Nature Genetics*, vol. 32, no. 3, pp. 448–452, 2002.

[7] R. Parvari, E. Hershkovitz, N. Grossman et al., "Mutation of TBCE causes hypoparathyroidism-retardation-dysmorphism and autosomal recessive Kenny-Caffey Syndrome," *Nature Genetics*, vol. 32, no. 3, pp. 448–452, 2002.

[8] T. Gerasimidis and F. George, "Superior mesenteric artery syndrome," *Digestive Surgery*, vol. 26, no. 3, pp. 213–214, 2009.

[9] J.-R. Shiu, H.-C. Chao, C.-C. Luo et al., "Clinical and nutritional outcomes in children with idiopathic superior mesenteric artery syndrome," *Journal of Pediatric Gastroenterology and Nutrition*, vol. 51, no. 2, pp. 177–182, 2010.

[10] U. Baltazar, J. Dunn, C. Floresguerra, L. Schmidt, and W. Browder, "Superior mesenteric artery syndrome: an uncommon cause of intestinal obstruction," *Southern Medical Journal*, vol. 93, no. 6, pp. 606–608, 2000.

[11] B. Ünal, A. Aktaş, G. Kemal et al., "Superior mesenteric artery syndrome: CT and ultrasonography findings," *Diagnostic and Interventional Radiology*, vol. 11, no. 2, pp. 90–95, 2005.

Necrotizing Fasciitis of the Chest in a Neonate in Southern Nigeria

Oluwafemi Olasupo Awe,[1,2] **Emeka B. Kesieme,**[3] **Babatunde Kayode-Adedeji,**[4] **and Quinzy O. Aigbonoga**[1]

[1]*Plastic Surgery Unit, Department of Surgery, Irrua Specialist Teaching Hospital, Irrua, Edo State, Nigeria*
[2]*Plastic Surgery Unit, Department of Surgery, Ambrose Alli University, PMB 08, Ekpoma, Edo State, Nigeria*
[3]*Cardiothoracic Surgery Unit, Department of Surgery, Irrua Specialist Teaching Hospital, Irrua, Edo State, Nigeria*
[4]*Special Care Baby Unit, Department of Paediatrics, Irrua Specialist Teaching Hospital, Irrua, Edo State, Nigeria*

Correspondence should be addressed to Oluwafemi Olasupo Awe; olasupoawe06@yahoo.com

Academic Editor: Carmelo Romeo

We discuss the successful saving of a male neonate with necrotizing fasciitis of the chest following a hot fomentation of the umbilicus with exposure of the ribs and the pleural space on the right side. He recovered 5 weeks after admission. We stressed the need to recognize necrotizing fasciitis extending from the upper anterior abdominal wall to the chest following hot fomentation of the umbilicus. The need for multidisciplinary cooperation for excellent outcome is very important, that is, neonatologist, medical microbiologist, and plastic and chest surgeons.

1. Introduction

Necrotizing fasciitis (NF) is a life-threatening infection and necrosis of the skin, subcutaneous tissue, deep fascia, and sometimes underlying muscles, with a fulminant course and a high mortality rate. NF can be a complication of minor soft tissue infection, or it can occur after a trauma or surgical procedure. It is commoner in the lower extremities, perineum, and lower anterior abdominal wall but rare in retroperitoneal space, the chest, neck, and the scalp. Much more rare is necrotizing fasciitis in a neonate. We report a case of a male neonate with necrotizing fasciitis of the chest and the upper anterior abdominal wall. The importance of early aggressive serial surgical debridement, repeated sterile dressing, and antibiotics in the control of the disease is highlighted.

2. Case Report

A week-old male neonate was admitted via the paediatric emergency unit with complaint of swelling and discoloura-tion of the chest and upper abdomen, excessive crying, and fever of 2-day history. The swelling was first noticed at the umbilicus but spread to the chest within few hours, and the swelling was associated with reddish discolouration of the overlying skin. The child was crying excessively particularly when the abdomen or the chest was touched.

There was 2-day antecedent history of hot water massage of the umbilicus by the grandmother before the onset of the symptoms. No other risk factor for sepsis was identified.

On examination, he was a male neonate, was febrile, and was anicteric. Pitting edema was over the chest and anterior abdominal wall extending from the clavicles superiorly, midaxillary lines laterally, and umbilicus inferiorly. There are one (1) necrotic area over the midsternum (2 cm × 4 cm) and two (2) on the right chest (about 2 cm × 2 cm each). The swelling was hyperaemic and tender. He was tachypneic (88 cpm) and dyspneic. Also he had tachycardia (186 bpm). Diagnosis of necrotizing fasciitis (NF) of the chest and upper anterior abdominal wall was made.

He was admitted to the Special Baby Care Unit and comanaged with both plastic and cardiothoracic surgeons. Blood culture and wound biopsy report yielded coagulase negative *Staphylococcus aureus* sensitive to azithromycin,

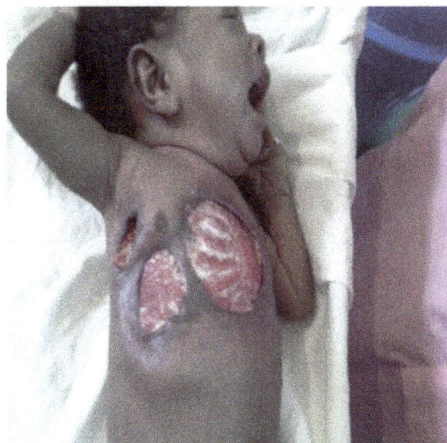

FIGURE 1: Immediate post-op.

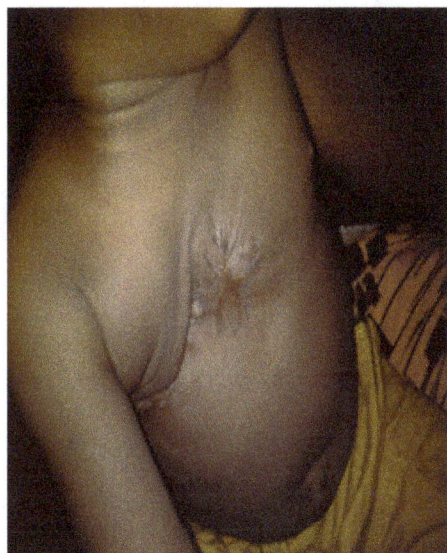

FIGURE 2: 10 months after discharge.

erythromycin, and gentamicin. He had 4 spikes of fever and hypothermia in the first week of admission. The complete blood count on admission was packed cell volume 47%, white blood cell count of 7200/cmm, with relative neutropenia (30%). Electrolyte and urea results were normal.

Following resuscitation, packed cell volume was 27% and maternal retroviral screen was negative. C-reactive protein was not done because it is not available in the hospital. Empirical antibiotics were I.V. imipenem, metronidazole, Gentamycin, and I.M. ibuprofen. He had two (2) aliquots of blood transfused and serial wound debridement resulting in three (3) wounds interspersed by 3 cm wide skin tags. The wounds were 6 cm × 6 cm and two of 3 cm × 4 cm each over the sternum and right chest, respectively, with raised edge, granulating base exposing 3rd to 7th ribs, and pleural cavity (Figure 1). He had regular dressing with 1% povidone iodine and diluted honey. He was discharged home to continue dressing at the outpatient clinic on the 42nd day of admission when the wound was almost completely healed.

He attended clinic twice over the next 3 months and 10 months thereafter for scar treatment (Figure 2).

3. Discussion

Necrotizing fasciitis is a severe soft tissue infection associated with rapidly progressive necrosis of the subcutaneous tissue and superficial fascia [1]. The disease is also characterized by early development of systemic toxicity [2]. NF is infrequent and is usually fatal in infants and children. There are reports of childhood NF resulting from appendicitis, intra-abdominal abscess, omphalitis, balanitis, and mammitis. Also predisposing factors vary with age, diabetes, and immune-suppressed status [3–6]. The NF of the chest wall has been secondary to some form of trauma, tumor resection, irradiation, or surgical procedure especially in the adults. There have been reported cases related to chest catheter drainage [7].

The early diagnosis of NF is very important in the management. The clinical symptoms and signs, such as erythematous rashes and other signs of sepsis, are important for differential diagnosis. In many cases, it is very difficult to distinguish early NF from cellulitis since fever, skin rashes, and other clinical findings are common symptoms of infection and sepsis.

The recent clinical classification of NF is distinguished into four types: NF type I (polymicrobial/synergistic, 70–80%), NF type II (20% of cases, usually monomicrobial), NF type III (Gram-negative monomicrobial, including marine-related organisms), and NF type IV (fungal) [8].

Our patient is a neonate who presented with most likely omphalitis being the leading point, though the eventual ulcers were closely related to the right nipple. It seems to be a monomicrobial NF with *Staphylococcus aureus*. The monomicrobial NF is common in patients with immuno-suppression. The neonate is considered to be immune-suppressed because his immune system is not yet well developed [3, 4].

Aggressive surgery and debridement are usually required in combination with antibiotic therapy to limit the spread of the disease and increase the chance of survival. Our patient had early serial debridement done, and which may have been the keys to success in avoiding wide spread of the infection. The extent of the skin debridement at the early stage is very difficult because the skin may often appear normal, though when investigated microscopically, the normal-appearing soft tissue showed extensive vascular microthromboses as well as vasculitis. This finding indicated that this tissue which has a normal external appearance has a high risk of full thickness necrosis [9, 10].

There was no need for any reconstruction of the chest wall of the patient unlike most of the reported cases of chest wall necrotizing fasciitis where reconstruction has been either by flaps or by skin grafts. Our patient is a neonate and most wounds at this age are forgiven with less scaring, which most likely prevented limitation in respiratory excursion.

The early multidisciplinary management of this patient may also have contributed to good outcome, that is, neonatologist, medical microbiologist, and plastic and chest surgeons.

The use of hyperbaric oxygen therapy was not applied in this case because we have no experience in using hyperbaric oxygen in a critically ill young patient, although its application is supported in the management of NF in some reports [7, 8].

In conclusion, NF is a life-threatening infection especially in the neonate in which early diagnosis with high index of suspicion, prompt resuscitation, aggressive surgical debridement, appropriate antibiotics therapy, and nutritional support with multidisciplinary approach will give a better outcome.

Conflict of Interests

None of the authors have any conflict of interests to declare in relation to this work.

References

[1] R. J. Green, D. C. Dafoe, and T. A. Raffin, "Necrotizing fasciitis," *Chest*, vol. 110, no. 1, pp. 219–229, 1996.

[2] W. M. Tang, P. L. Ho, W. P. Yau, J. W. Wong, and D. K. Yip, "Report of 2 fatal cases of adult necrotizing fasciitis and toxic shock syndrome caused by *Streptococcus agalactiae*," *Clinical Infectious Diseases*, vol. 31, no. 4, pp. e15–e17, 2000.

[3] A. Lodha, P. W. Wales, A. James, C. R. Smith, and J. C. Langer, "Acute appendicitis with fulminant necrotizing fasciitis in a neonate," *Journal of Pediatric Surgery*, vol. 38, no. 11, pp. E5–E6, 2003.

[4] E. A. Ameh and P. T. Nmadu, "Major complications of omphalitis in neonates and infants," *Pediatric Surgery International*, vol. 18, no. 5-6, pp. 413–416, 2002.

[5] C. Bodemer, A. Panhans, B. Chretien-Marquet, M. Cloup, D. Pellerin, and Y. De Prost, "Staphylococcal necrotizing fasciitis in the mammary region in childhood: a report of five cases," *Journal of Pediatrics*, vol. 131, no. 3, pp. 466–469, 1997.

[6] W. S. Hsieh, P. H. Yang, H. C. Chao, and J. Y. Lai, "Neonatal necrotizing fasciitis: a report of three cases and review of the literature," *Pediatrics*, vol. 103, no. 4, article e53, 1999.

[7] M.-S. Lu, C.-M. Chen, Y.-K. Huang, Y.-H. Liu, and C.-L. Kao, "Devastating chest wall necrotizing fasciitis following pigtail catheter drainage," *Respiratory Medicine CME*, vol. 1, no. 2, pp. 90–92, 2008.

[8] M. S. Morgan, "Diagnosis and management of necrotising fasciitis: a multiparametric approach," *Journal of Hospital Infection*, vol. 75, no. 4, pp. 249–257, 2010.

[9] Z. Roje, Ž. Roje, D. Matić, D. Librenjak, S. Dokuzović, and J. Varvodić, "Necrotizing fasciitis: literature review of contemporary strategies for diagnosing and management with three case reports: torso, abdominal wall, upper and lower limbs," *World Journal of Emergency Surgery*, vol. 6, article 46, 2011.

[10] T. J. Andreasen, S. D. Green, and B. J. Childers, "Massive infectious soft-tissue injury: diagnosis and management of necrotizing fasciitis and purpura fulminans," *Plastic and Reconstructive Surgery*, vol. 107, no. 4, pp. 1025–1035, 2001.

Perilobar Nephroblastomatosis: Natural History and Management

S. Stabouli,[1] N. Printza,[1] J. Dotis,[1] A. Matis,[1] D. Koliouskas,[2] N. Gombakis,[1] and F. Papachristou[1]

[1] 1st Department of Pediatrics, Aristotle University of Thessaloniki, Hippokration Hospital of Thessaloniki, 49 Kostantinoupoleos Street, 54642 Thessaloniki, Greece

[2] Pediatric Oncology Clinic, Hippokration Hospital of Thessaloniki, 49 Kostantinoupoleos Street, 54642 Thessaloniki, Greece

Correspondence should be addressed to S. Stabouli; sstaboul@auth.gr

Academic Editor: Denis A. Cozzi

Nephroblastomatosis (NB) has been considered as a precursor of Wilms tumor (WT). The natural history of NB seems to present significant variation as some lesions may regress spontaneously, while others may grow and expand or relapse and develop into WT later in childhood. Although, most investigators suggest adjutant chemotherapy, the effect and duration of treatment are not well established. Children with diffuse perilobar NB, Beckwith-Wiedemann syndrome, and hemihypertrophy seem to particularly benefit from treatment. We discuss our experience on two cases of NB and we review the literature for the management of this rare condition.

1. Introduction

Nephroblastomatosis (NB) defines the presence of diffuse or multiple nephrogenic rests (NRs). NRs are clusters of embryonic metanephric cells, which normally disappear after 36 weeks of gestational age. These lesions have been considered as precursors of Wilms tumor (WT). They can be present in about 1% of unselected infant kidneys at postmortem biopsies, while they are found in about 40% of kidneys with unilateral WTs and in nearly 100% of kidneys with bilateral WTs [1]. NB has also significant implications for the prognosis of pediatric patients with WTs, as its presence in the nontumoral part of the kidney may favor subsequent relapse of WTs [2].

NB can occur in any age, but it is most frequent in infants. NB in about of 40% of cases is bilateral, while unilateral presentation may be implicated with the presence of microscopic NRs on the contralateral kidney with increased risk of WT development. Limited publications have assessed the clinical course and the effect of management decisions on the outcome of children with NB. Most available data derive from small number of cases. In the current paper we discuss our experience on two cases of perilobar NB (PLNB) presented in our department with an interval of 20 years and we review challenging issues for the management of this rare condition.

2. Case Presentation

A 3.5-months-old girl was admitted to our department with right-sided hemihypertrophy. Screening with abdominal ultrasonography showed an enlarged right kidney with a large hypoechoic region presenting no corticomedullary differentiation as well as multifocal hypoechoic parenchymal foci bilaterally in both kidneys, suggesting PLNB. Magnetic Resonance Imaging (MRI) revealed multiple hypodense and nonenhancing cortical masses at both kidneys; the largest with a diameter of 2.65 cm was localized at the enlarged right kidney and presented reduced diffusion and faint enhancing tissue at periphery (Figures 1(a) and 1(b)). As all lesions were homogeneous without enhancement after contrast administration and a lenticular shape the diagnosis of PLNB was further suggested by the MRI findings. Spherical shape, heterogeneous, and enhancing nodules that would be suspicious for a WT were not present in the MRI. A second abdominal ultrasonography 2 months later showed enlargement of the already existing and new foci of NB bilaterally.

(a)

(b)

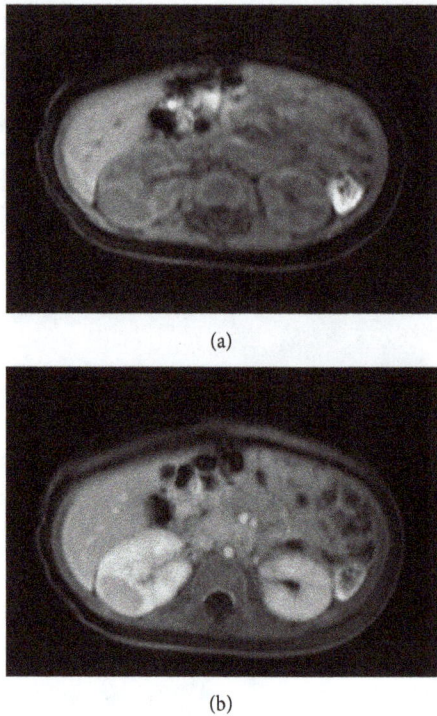

FIGURE 1: Noncontrast (a) and contrast enhanced (b) T1 weighted MR images show a large hypointense cortical mass at the right kidney and multiple smaller foci in both kidneys.

(a)

(b)

FIGURE 2: (a) Abdominal ultrasound showing an enlarged right kidney with a large hypoechoic region with no corticomedullary differentiation before chemotherapy treatment; (b) decrease of right kidney large hypoechoic lesion dimensions after 4 months of treatment.

Some years ago we presented the case of a 23-month-old boy, who did not received any treatment for the initial diagnosis of right NB and developed WTs 24 and 42 months later at the left and the right kidney, respectively, despite regression of initial lesions of NB [3]. Review of the literature on the management of NB revealed one large retrospective study and several case reports describing in most cases adverse outcome in nontreated patients. Thus, our female patient initiated chemotherapy according to SIOP Wilms Tumor/2001 protocol and received vincristine and actinomycin D for 4 weeks. Abdominal ultrasonography at 4 weeks showed decrease of lesion's size (shrinkage of the large right kidney mass volume from 7,56 cm^3 to 3,26 cm^3) and the patient received further cycles of vincristine and actinomycin D every 14 days for the next 3 months. Follow-up ultrasound at 4 months of treatment showed additional decrease of lesions dimensions (Figure 2). However, the follow-up period is currently too short to allow us to determine the response to treatment with confidence.

3. Discussion

In 1990 Beckwith et al. proposed the classification for NB into four categories: the perilobar (PLNB), intralobar (ILNB), combined, and universal [1]. All four categories have been associated with WT, PLNB with synchronous bilateral WTs, and ILNB with metachronous contralateral WTs. NRs and NB have been reported to have an increased frequency in several syndromes, including Beckwith-Wiedemann syndrome,

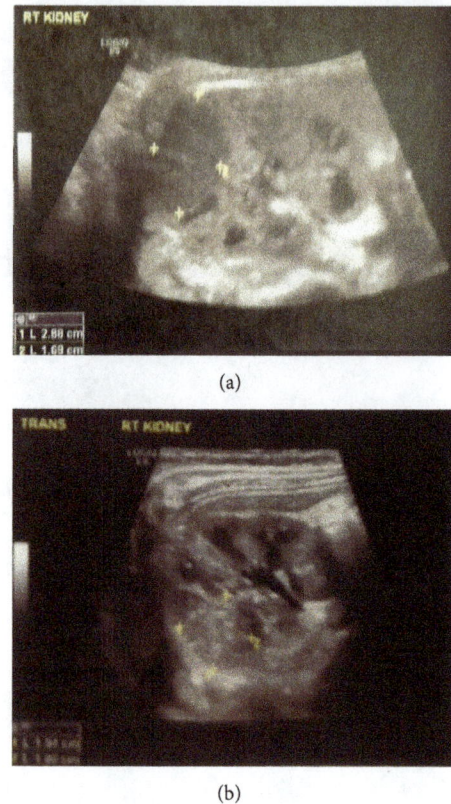

hemihypertrophy, Perlman syndrome, and trisomy 18 [1, 4]. Nodular appearance may be more frequent in association with the presence of the above syndromes although diffuse pattern has also been reported [4, 5]. Pediatric patients with Beckwith-Wiedemann syndrome and idiopathic hemihypertrophy also have an increased risk, reported about 4%–10%, for developing embryonic tumors [4]. The clinical course of PLNB presents large variation; some lesions may grow and expand or decrease or fade and relapse later in childhood. The risk of developing one or more WTs during the natural history of disease is increased, especially in cases with diffuse hyperplastic PLNB (DHPLNB) [5]. DHPLNB presents as massive kidney enlargement due to thick ride of nephroblastic tissue. DHPLNB has also been associated with increased incidence of anaplastic WTs [5, 6].

As nephroblastomatosis is a preneoplastic condition, administration of chemotherapy could be considered under the concept of decreasing the volume of lesions and reducing the number of cells with malignant potential and subsequently the risk of malignant transformation [5, 7]. Treatment of NB with vincristine and actinomycin D is currently recommended as for stage 1 WT. However, chemotherapy may not be effective or prevent malignant transformation. Moreover, there are currently limited data in the literature to assess this issue with confidence.

TABLE 1: Cases with initial diagnosis of NB (NB) without synchronous WT published since 1990.

Case	Reference	Age at diagnosis	Sex	Diagnosis	Clinical presentation at diagnosis	Congenital defects	Biopsy for NB	Ch for NB/ duration	Response to initial Ch	Srg For NB	Ra For NB	Development of WT	Outcome/ follow-up since initial diagnosis
1	Gaulier et al., Pediatr Pathol., 1993 [8]	Newborn		Unilateral universal NB	Cystic renal process discovered prenatally	Yes	Yes	No	—	Yes	No	No	Alive/1 yr
2	Regalado et al., Pediatr Pathol.,1994 [9]	Newborn	M	Bilateral universal NB	Potter's-like facies, hypoplastic lungs, ascites, and bilateral nephromegaly	Yes	Yes (postmortem)	No	—	No	No	No	Dead at age of 21 h
3	Verloes et al., Clin Genet., 1995 [10]	Newborn		Bilateral NB	Fetal overgrowth, macroglossia, and ambiguous genitalia	Yes/atypical Simpson-Golabi-Behmel and Beckwith-Wiedemann S	Yes (postmortem)	No	—	No	No	No	Dead at age of 2 days
4	Regalado et al., Pediatr Pathol Lab. Med., 1996 [11]	Newborn	M	Bilateral universal NB	Prenatally diagnosed nephromegaly and renal failure	No	Yes (postmortem)	NO	—	No	No	No	DOD at age of 3.5 mo
5	Henneveld et al., Am J Med Genet., 1999 [12]	8 mo	F	Unilateral NB	Nephromegaly FTH and other features of Perlman S	Yes/Perlman S	Yes (postmortem)	NO	—	No	No	No	Dead
6	Spranger et al., J Clin Dysmorphol., 2001 [13]	8 mo	M	Peri- and intralobar NB	Macrocephaly and short trunk	Yes/Ischiospinal dysostosis with rib gaps	Yes	NO	—	No	No	No	Alive/2 mo
7	Prasil et al., Med Pediatr Oncol., 2000 [7]	15 mo	M	Bilateral HPLN	Abdominal mass	No	Yes	5 course VCR-AMD/20 wks	Partial regression	No	No	Yes/5 yrs	Alive/5.5 yrs
8	Prasil et al., Med Pediatr Oncol., 2000 [7]	13 mo	M	Unilateral HPLN	Abdominal mass	No	Yes	3 course VCR-AMD/24 wks	Partial regression	No	No	Yes/28 mo	Alive/3.5 yrs
9	Prasil et al., Med Pediatr Oncol., 2000 [7]	3 yrs	F	Bilateral HPLN	Abdominal mass	No	Yes	2 course VCR-AMD/20 wks	Partial regression	NO	NO	Yes, multifocal with anaplasia/18 mo	NED/4 yrs
10	Günther et al., Pediatr Radiol., 2004 [14]	2 yrs	F	Bilateral DHPLN	NR	NR	No	NR	—	NO	NO	Yes/12 mo	NR
11	Cozzi et al., J Urol, 2004 [15]	12 mo	F	Bilateral HPLN	Abdominal mass	No	No	2-drug/	—	NO	NO	Yes/4 wks	NED/6 yrs
12	Cozzi et al., J Urol, 2004 [15]	13 mo	F	Unilateral HPLN	Abdominal mass/pain	No	No	2-drug/10 wks	Complete regression	NO	NO	Yes/14 wks	NED/32 mo
13	Hu et al., Nephrol Dial Transplant., 2004 [16]	21 mo	M	Bilateral NB	Hypoplastic genitalia, glomerulopathy, and renal failure	Yes/atypical Denys-Drash S and mutation of WT1 gene	Yes (nephrectomy at time of TN)	No	—	NO	NO	No	NR

TABLE 1: Continued.

Case	Reference	Age at diagnosis	Sex	Diagnosis	Clinical presentation at diagnosis	Congenital defects	Biopsy for NB	Ch for NB/duration	Response to initial Ch	Srg For NB	Ra For NB	Development of WT	Outcome/follow-up since initial diagnosis
14	Hu et al., Nephrol Dial Transplant., 2004 [16]	6 yrs	M	Bilateral NB	Pseudohermaphroditism, glomerulopathy, and renal failure	Yes/atypical Denys-drash S and mutation of WT1 gene	Yes (nephrectomy at time of TN)	No	—	NO	NO	NO	NR
15	Christiansen et al., Pediatr Dev Pathol., 2005 [17]	Newborn	F	Bilateral DHPLN	Congenital heart disease, and diaphragmatic hernia	Yes/mosaic duplication 1(q11q44)	Yes (postmortem)	No	—	NO	NO	NO	Dead at first day of life
16	Machmouchi et al., Pediatr Nephrol, 2005 [18]	8 mo	F	Bilateral HPLN	Abdominal distention/respiratory distress/macroscopic hematuria	No	Yes	VRC-AMD-DX/24 wks	Partial regression	NO	NO	NO	NED/1 yr
17 (sibl. of 18)	Gonzales et al., Am J Med Genet., 2005 [19]	Newborn	M	Bilateral NB	Lumbosacral meningocele, large cystic and dysplastic kidneys, and oligohydramnios	Yes/diaphanospondylodysostosis	Yes (postmortem)	No	—	NO	NO	No	Dead at first day of life
18 (sibl. of 17)	Gonzales et al., Am J Med Genet., 2005 [19]	Newborn	F	Bilateral NB	Oligohydramnios and cystic kidneys	Yes/diaphanospondylodysostosis	Yes (postmortem)	No	—	No	No	No	Dead at first day of life
19	Traub et al., Virchows Arch., 2006 [20]	Fetus 24 weeks	M	Bilateral diffuse peri- and intralobar NB		Yes/trisomy 13 and loss of WT1 expression	Yes (postmortem)	No	—	No	No	No	Dead at birth
20	Witt et al., J Pediatr Hematol Oncol, 2009 [21]	9 mo	F	Bilateral DHPLN	Abdominal distention/respiratory distress/acquired von Willebrand disease	Yes/hip dysplasia	Yes	VCR-AMD/122 wks 13-cis retinoic acid/9 wks VCR-AMD-DX/NR	Partial regression	No	No	Yes/31.5 mo	Alive/3.6 yrs
21	Vicens et al., Pediatr Dev Pathol, 2009 [22]	1 yr	M	Unilateral DHPLN	Abdominal mass	No	Yes	VCR-AMD/4 wks	Partial regression	Yes	No	No	NR
22 (sibl. of 22)	Katzman et al., Pediatr Dev Pathol, 2009 [23]	Newborn	F	Combined NB	Prenatally diagnosed nephromegaly	No	Yes (postmortem)	No	—	No	No	No	DOD at 6 day of life
23 (sibl. of 21)	Katzman et al., Pediatr Dev Pathol, 2009 [23]	Newborn	M	Intralobar universal NB	Prenatally diagnosed nephromegaly	No	Yes (postmortem)	No	—	No	No	No	DOD at 10th day of life
24	Borny et al., JBR-BTR, 2009 [24]	12 mo	F	Multifocal PLN	NR	Yes/Beckwith-Wiedemann S	NR	NR	NR	NR	NR	NR	NR

TABLE 1: Continued.

Case	Reference	Age at diagnosis	Sex	Diagnosis	Clinical presentation at diagnosis	Congenital defects	Biopsy for NB	Ch for NB/ duration	Response to initial Ch	Srg For NB	Ra For NB	Development of WT	Outcome/ follow-up since initial diagnosis
25	Sethi et al., Radiographics., 2010 [25]	6 mo	F	Bilateral DHPLN	Abdominal mass	No	No	No	—	No	No	Yes/12 mo	Alive/NR
26	Rauth et al., J Pediatr Surg., 2011 [26]	10 mo	F	Bilateral DHPLN	Urinary infection	No	No	2 courses of VCR-AMD/18 wks and 24 wks	Partial regression	No	No	Yes/3.5 yrs	NR

Abbreviations: NB: nephroblastomatosis, Ch: chemotherapy, Srg: surgery, Ra: radiation, WT: Wilms tumor, f: female, m: male, sibl: sibling, HPRN: hyperplastic perilobar NB, DHPRN: diffuse hyperplastic perilobar NB, VRC: Vincristine, AMD: dactinomycin, DX: doxorubicin, NR: not reported, DOD: dead of disease, NED: no evidence of disease, TN: transplantation.

Observation and close follow-up may be an option although epidemiologic evidence may not favor such decision. The main arguments in favor of nontreatment are the possible side effects of chemotherapy applied for nonmalignant condition, which has usually a favorable prognosis even when WT is developed. Moreover, chemotherapy may enhance the selection of resistant tumors [5, 7]. There are sporadic reported cases with spontaneous resolution of NB without treatment. However, the risk of developing WT seems to persist even years after initial diagnosis. Our male patient described above, who did not receive any treatment, presented spontaneous resolution of left kidney NB but developed new foci of NB and metachronous WT at the right kidney [3].

Forty-one individual cases have been published in the literature since 1978, of which 26 were after the classification from Beckwith et al. (Table 1) [7–25]. Observation of reported cases provides some evidence of the natural history of disease, but could not result in generalized conclusions about treatment decisions. Of nine with PLNB patients who received chemotherapy as initial treatment, seven developed WT at a mean of 29.9 months from diagnosis. Only one patient presented anaplastic pathology. All patients had a favorable outcome. Three patients did not receive any treatment; one of those suffering from PLNB developed WT, while the others have been followed up for a too short period. Ten cases of newborns with NB detected in postmortem biopsies were reported. The majority of these cases were associated with congenital abnormalities and died within the first days of life. In two cases, in which renal failure was a predominant feature, NB was found at biopsies performed after native nephrectomies during renal transplantation.

One large series of 52 patients provides data on patients with long-term survival of HPLNB [5]. The patients were followed up for at least 5 years. The lesions were bilateral in 49/52 cases, 45/52 had DHPLNB, and 8/52 patients had features of Beckwith-Wiedemann or other syndromes. Only three patients were observed without receiving chemotherapy at diagnosis. All three developed WT subsequently at 4 and 10 months later. Similar was the clinical course in our first case, as described earlier. Of the remaining 49 patients who received chemotherapy all presented an initial decrease in lesions volume. However, 55% of those that received only chemotherapy developed WT, while among patients who were treated with nephrectomy and chemotherapy 19% (three patients) developed WT. Chemotherapy seems to delay the occurrence of WT in patients with HPLNB. In the study by Perlman et al., the mean time from initial diagnosis of HPRNB to the appearance of WT was 35 months in treated pediatric patients (range of 12–60 months) compared to mean of 6.5 months in those who did not receive treatment. Similarly in cases in Table 1, WT developed in shorter time period if chemotherapy was administrated (35 months versus 12 months in the nontreated patients). Even if the patient develops WT during treatment the delay of appearance may allow nephron-sparing approaches.

Another interesting issue concerning the clinical course of PLNB is that the speed of the response to chemotherapy, which may suggest the duration of chemotherapy, presented significant variation among reported cases. In many cases prolonged chemotherapy is required to achieve regression of disease [5]. These observations may suggest that the duration of chemotherapy in children with PLNB needs to be continuously assessed during follow-up and treatment. DHPLNB may represent increased burden of disease. Moreover, in the cohort described by Perlman et al., children who presented relapses with new lesions during chemotherapy and children with genetic syndromes had an increased risk for WT. These children may need prolonged treatment. In the case of our female patient the cluster of unfavorable prognostic factors including hemihypertrophy and transient initial response to treatment reinforce the decision for chemotherapeutic treatment. Genetic analysis for mutations in WT1, WT2, and WTX genes may further guide the duration and the intensity of chemotherapeutic schemes. An ongoing trial on the effect of chemotherapy in preserving renal units in children with DHPLNB and preventing WT development may give guidance for the management of disease [6]. Patients will initially receive vincristine and actinomycin D and maybe partial nephrectomy after initial chemotherapy, especially if there is no response or if there is progression of disease or development of new lesions during therapy.

In conclusion, chemotherapy maybe the optimal treatment decision for pediatric patients with PLNB. Current evidence favor the individualization of treatment and close follow-up of the children with PLNB as suggested for individuals with increased risk for WT [6]. Patients should be followed up by imaging at a maximum interval of 3 months for a minimum of 7 years, as early detection of a WT may be critical for patient and kidney survival.

Conflict of Interests

The authors declare that there is no conflict of interests regarding the publication of this paper.

References

[1] J. B. Beckwith, N. B. Kiviat, and J. F. Bonadio, "Nephrogenic rests, nephroblastomatosis, and the pathogenesis of Wilms' tumor," *Pediatric Pathology*, vol. 10, no. 1-2, pp. 1–36, 1990.

[2] C. Bergeron, C. Iliescu, P. Thiesse et al., "Does nephroblastomatosis influence the natural history and relapse rate in Wilms' tumour? A single centre experience over 11 years," *European Journal of Cancer*, vol. 37, no. 3, pp. 385–391, 2001.

[3] F. Papadopoulou, S. C. Efremidis, N. Gombakis, J. Tsouris, and T. Kehagia, "Nephroblastomatosis: the whole spectrum of abnormalities in one case," *Pediatric Radiology*, vol. 22, no. 8, pp. 598–599, 1992.

[4] P. L. Choyke, M. J. Siegel, A. W. Craft et al., "Screening for Wilms tumor in children with Beckwith-Wiedemann syndrome or idiopathic hemihypertrophy," *Medical and Pediatric Oncology*, vol. 32, no. 3, pp. 196–200, 1999.

[5] E. J. Perlman, P. Faria, A. Soares et al., "Hyperplastic perilobar nephroblastomatosis: long-term survival of 52 patients," *Pediatric Blood and Cancer*, vol. 46, no. 2, pp. 203–221, 2006.

[6] E. J. Perlman, "Pediatric renal tumors: practical updates for the pathologist," *Pediatric and Developmental Pathology*, vol. 8, no. 3, pp. 320–338, 2005.

[7] P. Prasil, J. M. Laberge, M. Bond et al., "Management decisions in children with nephroblastomatosis," *Medical and Pediatric Oncology*, vol. 35, no. 4, pp. 429–432, 2000.

[8] A. Gaulier, L. Boccon-Gibod, P. Sabatier, and G. Lucas, "Panlobar nephroblastomatosis with cystic dysplasia: an unusual case with diffuse renal involvement studied by immunohistochemistry," *Pediatric Pathology*, vol. 13, no. 6, pp. 741–749, 1993.

[9] J. J. Regalado, M. M. Rodriguez, J. H. Bruce, and J. B. Beckwith, "Bilateral hyperplastic nephromegaly, nephroblastomatosis, and renal dysplasia in a newborn: a variety of universal nephroblastomatosis," *Pediatric Pathology*, vol. 14, no. 3, pp. 421–432, 1994.

[10] A. Verloes, B. Massart, I. Dehalleux, J. P. Langhendries, and L. Koulischer, "Clinical overlap of Beckwith-Wiedemann, Perlman and Simpson-Golabi-Behmel syndromes: a diagnostic pitfall," *Clinical Genetics*, vol. 47, no. 5, pp. 257–262, 1995.

[11] J. J. Regalado, M. M. Rodriguez, and J. B. Beckwith, "Multinodular hyperplastic pannephric nephroblastomatosis with tubular differentiation: a new morphologic variant," *Pediatric Pathology and Laboratory Medicine*, vol. 16, no. 6, pp. 961–972, 1996.

[12] H. T. Henneveld, R. A. van Lingen, B. C. Hamel, I. Stolte-Dijkstra, and A. J. van Essen, "Perlman syndrome: four additional cases and review," *American Journal of Medical Genetics*, vol. 86, no. 5, pp. 439–446, 1999.

[13] J. Spranger, S. Self, K. B. Clarkson, and G. S. Pai, "Ischiospinal dysostosis with rib gaps and nephroblastomatosis," *Clinical Dysmorphology*, vol. 10, no. 1, pp. 19–23, 2001.

[14] P. Günther, J. Tröger, N. Graf, K. L. Waag, and J. P. Schenk, "MR volumetric analysis of the course of nephroblastomatosis under chemotherapy in childhood," *Pediatric Radiology*, vol. 34, no. 8, pp. 660–664, 2004.

[15] F. Cozzi, A. Schiavetti, D. A. Cozzi et al., "Conservative management of hyperplastic and multicentric nephroblastomatosis," *Journal of Urology*, vol. 172, no. 3, pp. 1066–1069, 2004.

[16] M. Hu, G. Y. Zhang, S. Arbuckle et al., "Prophylactic bilateral nephrectomies in two paediatric patients with missense mutations in the WT1 gene," *Nephrology Dialysis Transplantation*, vol. 19, no. 1, pp. 223–226, 2004.

[17] L. R. Christiansen, J. M. Lage, D. J. Wolff, G. S. Pai, and R. A. Harley, "Mosaic duplication 1(q11q44) in an infant with nephroblastomatosis and mineralization of extraplacental membranes," *Pediatric and Developmental Pathology*, vol. 8, no. 1, pp. 115–123, 2005.

[18] M. Machmouchi, M. Bayoumi, I. Mamoun, K. Al-Ahmadi, and H. Kanaan, "Bilateral universal nephroblastomatosis in an 8-month-old infant treated with chemotherapy," *Pediatric Nephrology*, vol. 20, no. 7, pp. 1007–1010, 2005.

[19] M. Gonzales, A. Verloes, M. H. Saint Frison et al., "Diaphanospondylodysostosis (DSD): confirmation of a recessive disorder with abnormal vertebral ossification and nephroblastomatosis," *The American Journal of Medical Genetics*, vol. 136, no. 4, pp. 373–376, 2005.

[20] F. Traub, K. Sickmann, M. Tessema, L. Wilkens, H. H. Kreipe, and K. Kamino, "Nephroblastomatosis and loss of WT1 expression associated with trisomy 13," *Virchows Archiv*, vol. 448, no. 2, pp. 214–217, 2006.

[21] O. Witt, S. Hämmerling, C. Stockklausner et al., "13- cis retinoic acid treatment of a patient with chemotherapy refractory nephroblastomatosis," *Journal of Pediatric Hematology/Oncology*, vol. 31, no. 4, pp. 296–299, 2009.

[22] J. Vicens, A. Iotti, M. G. Lombardi, R. Iotti, and M. T. G. De Davila, "Diffuse hyperplastic perilobar nephroblastomatosis," *Pediatric and Developmental Pathology*, vol. 12, no. 3, pp. 237–238, 2009.

[23] P. J. Katzman, G. L. Arnold, E. C. Lagoe, and V. Huff, "Universal nephroblastomatosis with bilateral hyperplastic nephromegaly in siblings," *Pediatric and Developmental Pathology*, vol. 12, no. 1, pp. 47–52, 2009.

[24] E. Borny, B. Mortelé, and P. Seynaeve, "Multifocal nephroblastomatosis in beckwith-wiedemann syndrome," *JBR-BTR*, vol. 92, no. 3, pp. 144–145, 2009.

[25] A. T. Sethi, L. D. Narla, S. J. Fitch, and W. J. Frable, "Wilms tumor in the setting of bilateral nephroblastomatosis," *Radiographics*, vol. 30, no. 5, pp. 1421–1425, 2010.

[26] T. P. Rauth, J. Slone, G. Crane, H. Correa, D. L. Friedman, and H. N. Lovvorn III, "Laparoscopic nephron-sparing resection of synchronous Wilms tumors in a case of hyperplastic perilobar nephroblastomatosis," *Journal of Pediatric Surgery*, vol. 46, no. 5, pp. 983–988, 2011.

7

Neonatal Pulmonary Hemosiderosis

Boris Limme,[1] **Ramona Nicolescu,**[1] **and Jean-Paul Misson**[1,2]

[1] *Department of Pediatrics, General Hospital Citadelle, Boulevard du 12 ème de Ligne 1, 4000 Liège, Belgium*
[2] *Université de Liège, Place du 20 Août 7, 4000 Liège, Belgium*

Correspondence should be addressed to Ramona Nicolescu; rcnicolescu@yahoo.com

Academic Editor: Paul A. Rufo

Idiopathic pulmonary hemosiderosis (IPH) is a rare complex entity characterized clinically by acute or recurrent episodes of hemoptysis secondary to diffuse alveolar hemorrhage. The radiographic features are variable, including diffuse alveolar-type infiltrates, and interstitial reticular and micronodular patterns. We describe a 3-week-old infant presenting with hemoptysis and moderate respiratory distress. Idiopathic pulmonary hemosiderosis was the first working diagnosis at the Emergency Department and was confirmed, 2 weeks later, by histological studies (bronchoalveolar lavage). The immunosuppressive therapy by 1 mg/kg/d prednisone was immediately started, the baby returned home on steroid therapy at a dose of 0,5 mg/kg/d. The diagnosis of idiopathic pulmonary hemosiderosis should be evocated at any age, even in the neonate, when the clinical presentation (hemoptysis and abnormal radiological chest images) is strongly suggestive.

1. Introduction

Idiopathic pulmonary hemosiderosis, a rare condition in newborns, can have both a rapid and dramatic clinical beginning, with pulmonary hemorrhage. A combined clinical and radiological approach is necessary to rapid diagnosis and therapeutic intervention, particularly in very young children in whom the pulmonary hemorrhage could be fatal.

The idiopathic feature keeps its actuality during neonatal period because the immunological mechanisms, supposed to be responsible for the disease, are rarely identified.

The immunosuppressive treatment should be started once the diagnosis is histologically confirmed. A long-term clinic and immunological follow-up is required, trying to make an etiological diagnosis.

2. Case Presentation

A 3-week-old previously healthy full-term newborn was presented to our tertiary hospital, shortly (15 min) after an episode of hemoptysis. No symptoms were reported by parents preceding the hemorrhage. There was no nasal cleaning and no trauma history. The hemoptysis was mistaken for nose bleeding with secondary laryngospasm.

The baby had been born at full term by normal vaginal delivery. There were no problems during pregnancy, neither at delivery nor at perinatal period. He was born to no consanguineous parents of Belgium descent. He has 2 female siblings both of whom are well and there is no family history of notable diseases. He had been well before this current illness, with appropriate neonatal evolution.

The baby is breastfed exclusively. Prevention of early and late vitamin K deficiency bleeding was assured by parenteral administration of vitamin K, according to national policy.

At his arrival in the Pediatric Emergency Department, on his pyjama, there was a lot of red blood. We have also traced the blood on his face, around the nose and inside of his mouth. On admission time, he was pale and hypotonic with moderate tachycardia (170/min) and moderate tachypnea (46/min). There was no fever. Central cyanosis (around the mouth) was noted. Initial oxygen saturation was around 96%, with progressive deterioration over the time. The capillary refill time was normal. There was no actively hemorrhagic skin or mucous lesions. The cardiovascular exam is normal, without clinical signs of congenital cardiopathy.

The pulmonary auscultation was also normal, and no alveolar crackles are identified. The abdominal examination reveals no palpable mass. The neurological exam and the archaic reflexes are normal. The remaining part of the systemic examination was unremarkable.

During his stay in the Emergency Department, a moderate grunting becomes noticeable and pink frothy sputum is visible on the lips. The oxygen saturation gets impaired (86%), so the baby requires some oxygen supplementation (3 L/min).

Initial routine laboratory work-up included a septic, haemostatic, renal, hepatic, and metabolic profile. All laboratory investigations returned normal, with 2 exceptions: moderate anemia (Hb 10 g/dL) and metabolic acidosis (pH 7,20, pCO_2 44 mm Hg, and bicarbonate 10 mmol/L).

A bolus of 10 mL/kg of saline serum was given, followed by glucose 5% with electrolytes perfusion.

First chest radiograph showed bilateral diffuse alveolar infiltrates over upper, middle, and lower zones (Figure 1).

The rhinoscopy procedure has found some red blood in the nose. There were no active hemorrhagic lesions.

The baby was admitted to the Intensive Care Unit (24 hours) under triple antibiotic coverage (followed up for only 24 hours, the time necessary to have back all bacteriological results, which were all negative). A progressive clinical improvement was noted and the newborn was discharged into the Pediatric Unit, where the investigational work-up was completed. There was no melenic stool. No other hemorrhagic episodes were noted during hospitalization.

Two thoracic scanners were performed and they were completely normal.

An immunological work-up (anti-DNA, antineutrophil cytoplasmic, and antiglomerular basement membranes and antinuclear antibodies) was performed and it was negative. Cow-milk allergy was ruled out.

Following the dynamic of siderophages generation in pulmonary alveoli (6, 7), a bronchoscopic alveolar lavage was performed on the 10th day in the evolution. Haemosiderin-laden macrophages (siderophages) > 98% were demonstrated in the bronchoalveolar lavage fluid (Golde score at 244). No vasculitis (interstitial neutrophilic predominant infiltration, fibrinoid necrosis of the alveolar and capillary walls, and leukocytoclasis) was described on histological result.

The immunosupressive therapy by 1 mg/kg/d prednisone was immediately started with a steroid taper to 0,5 mg/kg/d and the baby returned home on steroid therapy at a dose of 0,5 mg/kg/d.

The baby is regularly seen in external consultation and he is doing very well. Actually, the diagnosis is idiopathic/primary pulmonary hemosiderosis, but the infant's immunological profile will be regularly monitored over a long period for the early detection of any immunological abnormalities. A new, more extensive, immune check-up will be done at the age of 12 months.

3. Discussion

Idiopathic pulmonary hemosiderosis is an association of 3 key elements including recurrent episodes of hemoptysis, secondary, refractory iron deficiency anemia, diffuse alveolar infiltrates or opacities, and abnormal accumulation/presence of haemosiderin in the alveolar macrophages.

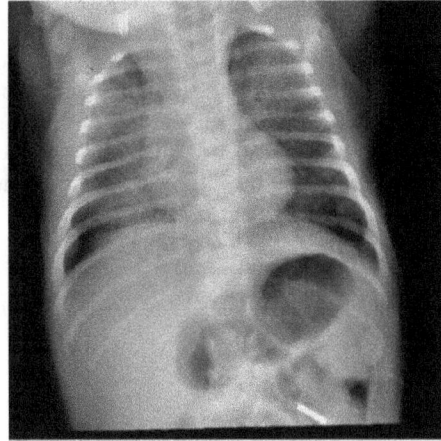

FIGURE 1

The incidence and prevalence of the disease in the pediatric population are still difficult to evaluate. To date there are around 500 cases reported in the literature [1].

The etiology and physiopathology remain also not well explained. Some etiologic hypotheses are debated, and for the pediatric age, the most cited are the allergic or autoimmune theories [1].

Age at the diagnosis is variable, with many cases presenting before the age of 10 [1, 2]. The evolution and therapeutic response are also individual characteristics.

The most frequent and classically described onset in childhood seems to be insidious, with recurrent hemoptysis secondary to diffuse or focal alveolar bleeding.

Secondarily, an extensive work-up for an unexplained, persistent iron deficiency anemia with typical chest radiographs, can also permit discovering a pulmonary hemosiderosis.

Less frequently, but much more dramatically, the first symptom is a moderate or massive pulmonary hemorrhage, potentially fatal [3].

The cause of IPH remains unknown, but an immunological origin has been suggested [2, 4]. Alveolar hemorrhage may be the first manifestation occurring long time (months to years) before the development of immunological disorders.

It was reported that some infants and young children with pulmonary haemosiderosis have plasma antibodies against cow milk proteins, and these patients dramatically improved on a cows-milk-free diet (Heiner's syndrome) [5].

Confirmatory diagnosis of IPH implies evidence of diffuse alveolar hemorrhage together with exclusion of other causes of pulmonary bleeding. In children of any age, some possible immune and nonimmune causes should be investigated and ruled out [5].

In acute hemorrhagic episodes, supportive management includes blood transfusions, oxygen therapy, high-dose corticosteroid therapy, or mechanical ventilation.

The long-term pharmaceutical therapy includes corticosteroids and when ineffective, other immune therapies should be envisaged.

4. Conclusion

We described here a case of neonatal pulmonary hemosiderosis, expressed clinically by an acute pulmonary hemorrhage with typical bilateral diffuse alveolar infiltrates and confirmed by the abundance of hemosiderin-laden macrophages in the bronchoalveolar lavage on the 10th day of the evolution.

Conflict of Interests

The authors declare that there is no conflict of interests regarding the publication of this paper.

References

[1] O. C. Ioachimescu, S. Sieber, and A. Kotch, "Idiopathic pulmonary haemosiderosis revisited," *European Respiratory Journal*, vol. 24, no. 1, pp. 162–170, 2004.

[2] L. Le Clainche, M. Le Bourgeois, B. Fauroux et al., "Long-term outcome of idiopathic pulmonary hemosiderosis in children," *Medicine*, vol. 79, no. 5, pp. 318–326, 2000.

[3] M. M. Saeed, M. S. Woo, E. F. MacLaughlin, M. F. Margetis, and T. G. Keens, "Prognosis in pediatric idiopathic pulmonary hemosiderosis," *Chest*, vol. 116, no. 3, pp. 721–725, 1999.

[4] N. Milman and F. M. Pedersen, "Idiopathic pulmonary haemosiderosis. Epidemiology, pathogenic aspects and diagnosis," *Respiratory Medicine*, vol. 92, no. 7, pp. 902–907, 1998.

[5] D. C. Heiner, "Pulmonary haemosiderosis," in *Disorders of the Respiratory Tract in Children*, V. Chernick and E. L. Kendig Jr., Eds., pp. 498–509, WB Saunders, Philadelphia, Pa, USA, 1990.

8

Orthosis Effects on the Gait of a Child with Infantile Tibia Vara

Serap Alsancak and Senem Guner

Department of Orthopedic Prosthetics and Orthotics, Vocational School of Health Services, Ankara University,
Fatih Street 197/A Gazino, Kecioren, 06280 Ankara, Turkey

Correspondence should be addressed to Senem Guner; sguner@ankara.edu.tr

Academic Editor: Anibh Martin Das

Infantile tibia vara (ITV) is an acquired form of tibial deformity associated with tibial varus and internal torsion. As there is currently insufficient data available on the effects of orthotics on gait parameters, this study aimed to document the influence of orthosis on walking. A male infant with bilateral tibia vara used orthoses for five months. Gait evaluations were performed pre- and posttreatment for both legs. The kinematic parameters were collected by using a motion analysis system. The orthotic design principle was used to correct the femur and tibia. Posttreatment gait parameters were improved compared to pretreatment parameters. After 5 months, there was remarkable change in the stance-phase degrees of frontal plane hip joint abduction and knee joint varus. We found that orthoses were an effective treatment for the infantile tibia vara gait characteristics in this patient. Full-time use of single, upright knee-ankle-foot orthosis with a drop lock knee joint and application of corrective forces at five points along the full length of the limb were effective.

1. Introduction

Studies on surgical correction, orthotic applications, and spontaneous healing of infantile tibia vara (ITV) have been performed since the 1960s [1–9]. Most of them were radiographic evaluations describing metaphyseal-diaphyseal proximal tibial angles and the progression of distal femoral deformity [2, 10, 11]. Body weight and early walking were found to be factors that contributed to the development of the condition, which is not seen in nonambulatory patients. Ligamentous laxity and the lateral thrust of the knee in the stance phase of gait have been cited as determining factors [1, 12] and abnormally increased knee internal rotation and hip external rotation moments have been observed [13].

Nonsurgical treatment of ITV has been somewhat controversial. However, recent studies have reported success when knee-ankle-foot orthosis (KAFO) was used nearly full-time to improve biomechanics in patients under 4 years of age [14–16]. The effectiveness of orthoses with corrective forces and/or distraction systems is related to their ability to relieve weight bearing stresses on the medial physeal region of the proximal tibia. Alsancak et al. reported that a single upright KAFO with a drop lock knee joint was effective for the treatment of ITV in 22 children of about 31 months of age [14]. The duration of treatment in that study was nearly 6 months. A case report by Whiteside of two children with an approximate age of 46 months showed that double solid upright KAFOs with free knee motion significantly improved ITV after 17 months of treatment [15]. Orthotic management of ITV with drop lock or unlocked knee joints, single or double upright KAFOs applying four or five corrective forces or a distraction system or variations of these devices have been reported. However, none of the studies evaluated patient gait parameters after orthotic treatment.

The aim of this report was to evaluate the effect of treatment with a single upright KAFO with a drop lock knee joint on hip and knee walking kinematics in an ITV patient.

2. Case Description and Methods

A male ITV patient with an age of 2.5 years, a weight of 14 kg, and a height of 90 cm was referred to the clinic at our university by an orthopedic surgeon. The radiographic classification of the patient was Langenskiöld Stage II, and the deformity was judged not to be due to traumatic, congenital,

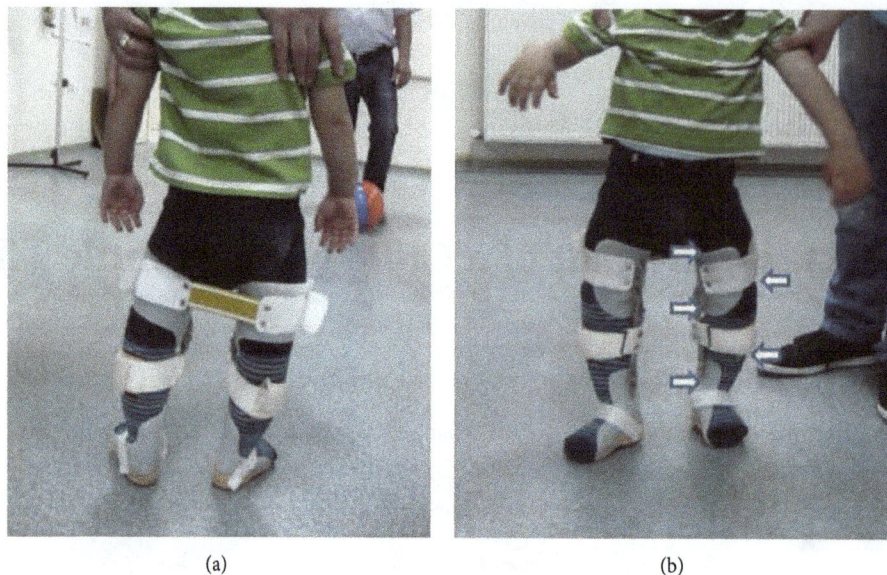

FIGURE 1: Anterior and posterior view of KAFOs application with flexible posterior strap (a) and mediolateral forces (b).

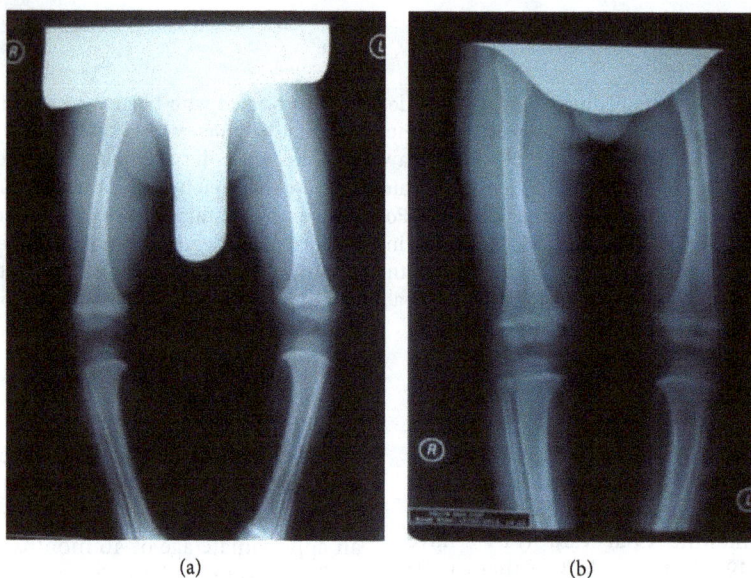

FIGURE 2: Anteroposterior radiographs of lower extremity: (a) pretreatment, (b) posttreatment.

metabolic, or infectious causes. The study was approved by the Ethics Committee of Ankara University.

The child was fitted with bilateral single medial metal upright KAFOs with drop lock knee joints. The orthoses applied five constant corrective forces to the femur and proximal tibia, and the lateral corrective band applied across the tibia produced a rigid column (Figure 1) [14]. The orthosis was used full-time until the first follow-up visit at 3 months after application. The orthosis was removed for 3 hours every day from beginning of treatment and evaluation after 3 months. The child was subjected to clinical examinations and radiologic evaluations before treatment and at 3- and 5-month follow-up visits (Figure 2). Stretching exercises directed at the tensor fascia lata and strengthening exercises

for the knee flexor and extensors and abdominal and back muscles were taught to the families. A classic massage for the lower extremities was also taught to the families during this process.

Three dimensional gait analysis was conducted in a gait laboratory using a Vicon motion analysis system (Vicon Nexus, Oxford Metrics, Oxford, UK) with six infrared cameras at 240 Hz. Before data collection, each camera and force plate was calibrated. Data was collected after several practice trials. The average of five trials for each barefoot walking condition was calculated. The patient walked a distance of 10 m at a self-selected speed in the gait laboratory before treatment and at each follow-up visit. We used Helen Hayes marker protocol in gait analysis.

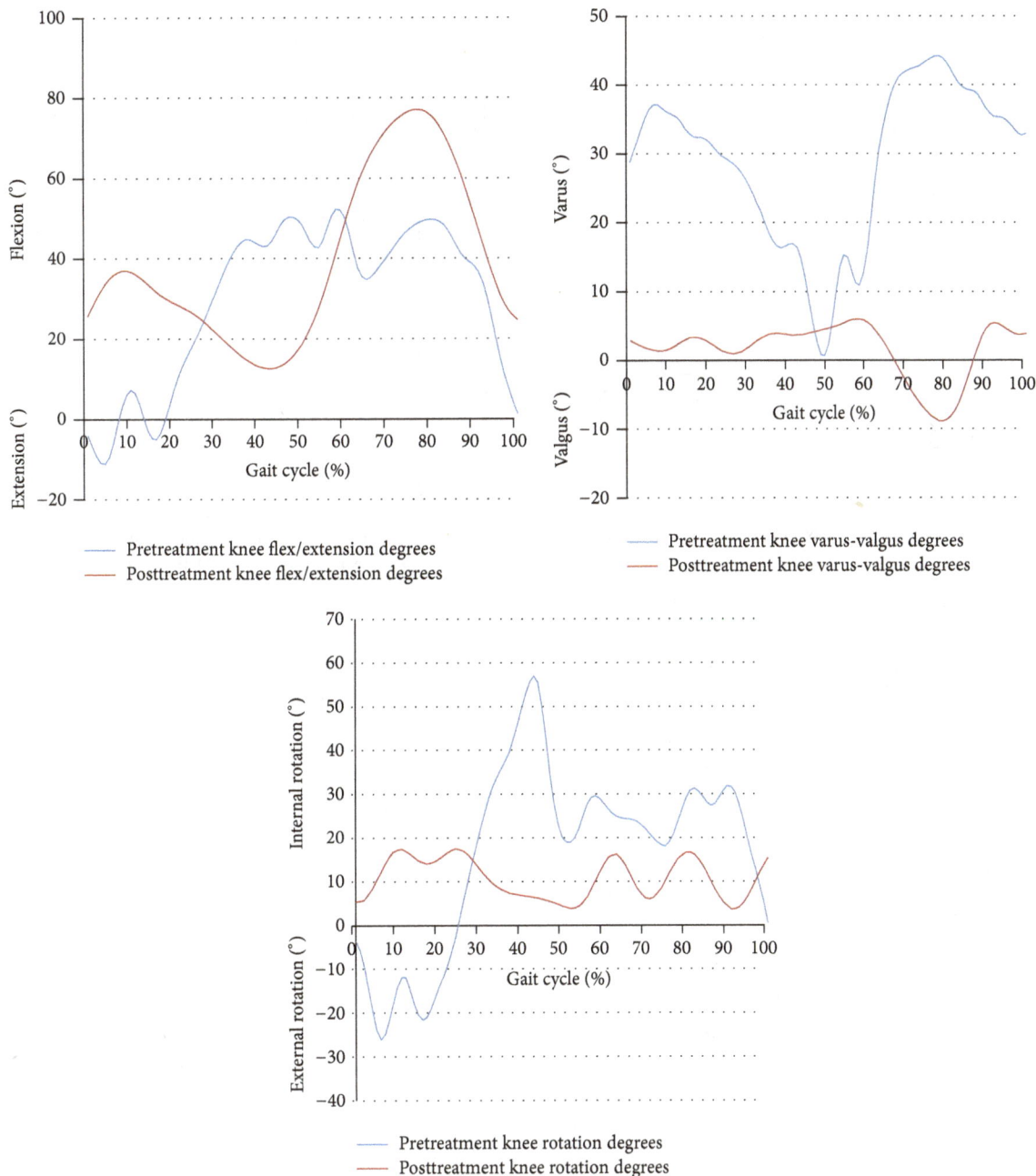

FIGURE 3: Knee joint kinematic degrees.

3. Findings and Discussion

The results of the kinematic analysis of the hip and knee joint walking parameters are shown in Tables 1 and 2. The mean pre- and posttreatment values of flexion-extension excursion of the hip and knee joints were different. Before treatment, the lower extremity kinematic assessments indicated knee hyperextension and insufficient knee flexion during the early stance phase, with external knee rotation, knee flexion, and increased internal rotation during the late stance phase. Knee varus degree and degrees of hip flexion-extension and abduction were increased during both the early and late

stance phases. After 5 months of orthotic treatment, the knee-flexion wave occurring in the early stance phase and knee extension during the late stance phase had increased, and knee flexion was closer to the normal curve. By 2 years of age, we observed a more clearly defined knee-flexion wave, an increased hip adduction in stance, and a decreased external rotation of the hip [17]. The primary change in the knee-flexion-extension curve by age showed gradual development of an initial knee-flexion wave. It should be noted that the term initial knee-flexion wave describes the flexion of the knee during a loading response and a subsequent extension during midstance. The abduction-adduction excursion of

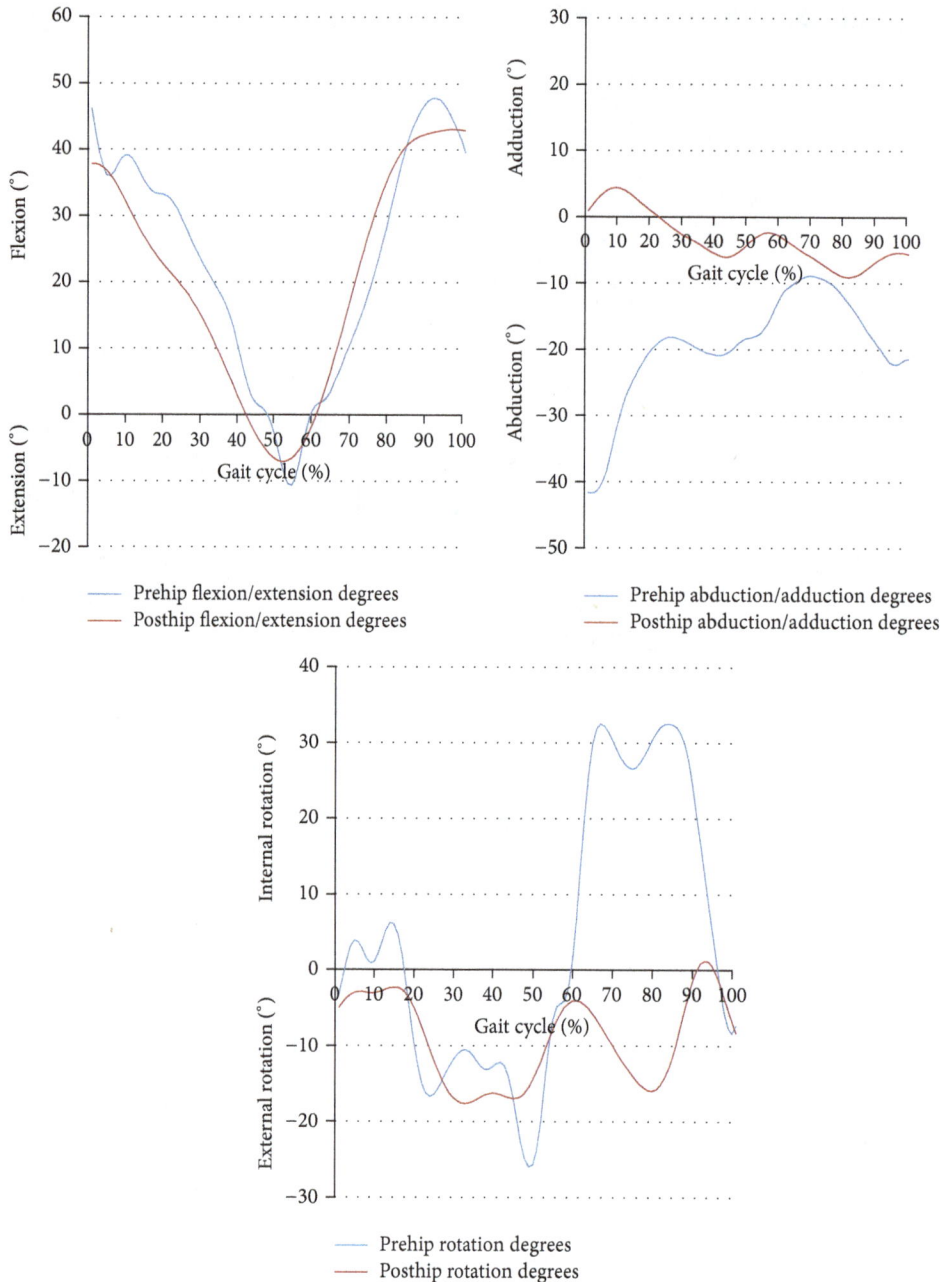

FIGURE 4: Hip joint kinematic degrees.

the hip and varus/valgus excursion of knee joint decreased significantly with treatment. Degrees of knee varus and hip abduction decreased significantly. Knee varus decreased nearly 30° during the early stance phases and 20° during the late stance phases (Figures 3 and 4). The excursion of the hip and knee joint rotation degrees in the sagittal plane observed after treatment were significantly different from those observed before treatment. Degrees of knee internal rotation and hip external rotation declined during late stance. Kinematic joint angles were within the closed normal curve for a child of 2 years of age. We think that the flexible posterior strap had a positive impact on the degrees of hip and knee

external rotation in the horizontal plane. Application of the single upright KAFO with drop lock knees did not have any adverse effects on knee motion in the sagittal plane at the end of treatment.

To our knowledge there have been no studies reporting the influence of orthotic treatment on gait performance in ITV patients. The results of this evaluation showed significant improvement in the kinematic gait pattern of the hip and knee joints after KAFO treatment (Figures 2 and 5).

Most specialist evaluations indicate that a mature gait is present in normal children by age 5. However, in an evaluation of 309 normal children, Sutherland concluded

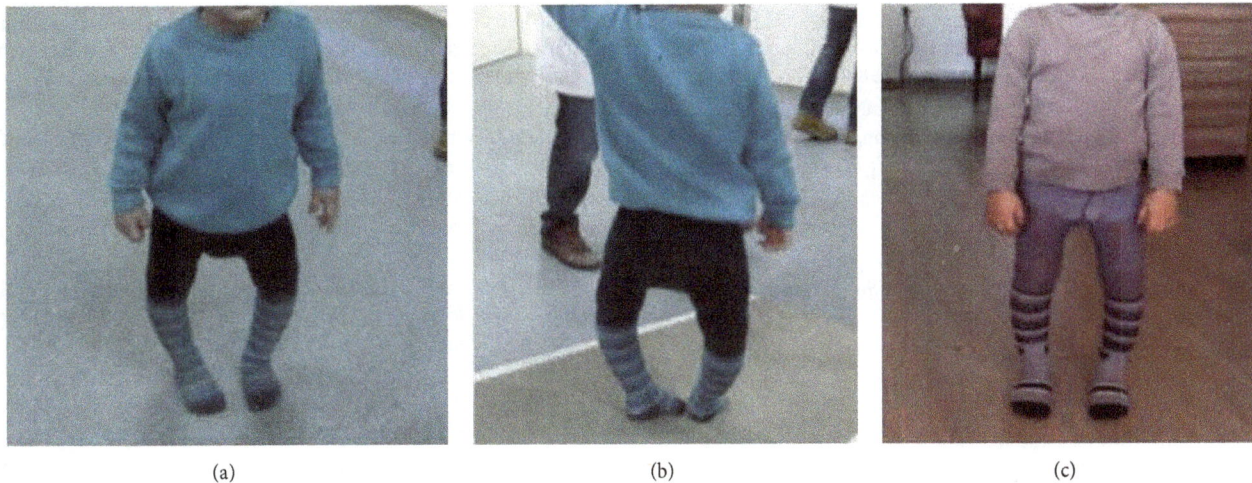

(a)   (b)   (c)

FIGURE 5: Before treatment (a, b) and after treatment (c).

TABLE 1: The kinematics of the hip and knee joints total excursion degree during pre- and posttreatment in ITV.

Parameters	Knee joint			Hip joint		
	Flexion-extension (°)	Abduction-adduction (°)	Rotation (°)	Flexion-extension (°)	Abduction-adduction (°)	Rotation (°)
Pretreatment	63 ± 33	44 ± 75	82 ± 80	58 ± 40	50 ± 60	58 ± 53
Posttreatment	65 ± 25	14 ± 84	20 ± 96	50 ± 11	13 ± 52	18 ± 83

TABLE 2: The kinematics of the hip and knee joints maximum degree during pre- and posttreatment in ITV.

Parameters	Knee joint			Hip joint		
	Max knee flexion (°)	Max knee abduction (°)	Max knee internal rotation (°)	Max hip flexion (°)	Max hip abduction (°)	Max hip external rotation (°)
Pretreatment	52.22	44.14	56.78	47.83	−41.68	−25.89
Posttreatment	77.04	5.97	17.36	43.05	−9.14	−17.64

that a mature gait pattern is established in most children by age 4 [18]. Hillman et al. reported temporal and distance parameters in normal children that supported a normal walk ratio and stride length as an idiosyncratic feature of gait from the age of 7–11 years [19]. Many authors believe that treatment by orthosis is effective in the early stages of ITV [20–28]. Our study showed successful orthotic treatment at 2.5 years of age. Alsancak et al. advised that KAFO was effective in children between 1.5 and 3.5 years of age. Bilateral orthotic treatment duration is longer than unilateral treatment of patients with ITV. Blount advised that his bowleg brace was used at night in patients younger than 2 years of age [29]. Loder and Johnston reported successful outcomes in 12 of 23 extremities in patients with Stage I-II disease, but the success rate was only 50% with orthotic treatment [30]. They concluded that orthoses were indicated only for children between 1.5 and 2.5 years of age. Full-time use of the orthosis at the beginning of treatment was important in our study.

Improved gait parameters revealed that use of a KAFO was a very effective treatment for ITV in this child. Future research should incorporate larger patient and control groups to further evaluate the effectiveness of orthosis treatment.

Conflict of Interests

The authors declare there is no conflict of interests regarding the publication of this paper.

References

[1] S. T. Canale, "Tibia Vara; osteochondrosis or epiphysitis and other miscellaneous affections," in Campbells Operative Orthopaedics, A. H. Crenshaws, Ed., vol. 3, pp. 1981–1988, Mosby Year Book, St Louis, Miss, USA, 8th edition, 1992.

[2] A. Langenskiöld and E. B. Riska, "Tibia varus (Osteocondrosis deformans tibiae): a survey of 23 cases," The Journal of Bone & Joint Surgery—American Volume, vol. 46, pp. 1405–1420, 1964.

[3] P. Salenius and E. Vankka, "The development of the tibiofemoral angle in children," The Journal of Bone and Joint Surgery—American Volume, vol. 57, no. 2, pp. 259–261, 1975.

[4] E. I. Mitchell, S. M. K. Chung, M. M. Dask, and J. R. Greg, "A new radiographic grading system for Blount's disease," *Orthopaedic Review*, vol. 9, pp. 27–33, 1980.

[5] A. Langenskiöld, "Tibia vara (A critical review)," *Clinical Orthopaedics and Related Research*, no. 246, pp. 195–207, 1989.

[6] A. H. Crawford, R. Ayyangar, and G. L. Durrett, "Congenital and acquired disorders," in *Atlas of Orthoses Assistive Devices*, B. Goldberg and J. D. Hsu, Eds., pp. 493–495, Mosby Year Book, St Louis, Mo, USA, 3rd edition, 1997.

[7] C. E. Johnston II, "İnfantil tibia vara," *Clinical Orthopaedics and Related Research*, no. 255, pp. 13–23, 1990.

[8] J. O. Tavares and K. Molinero, "Elevation of medial tibial condyle for severe tibia vara," *Journal of Pediatric Orthopaedics Part B*, vol. 15, no. 5, pp. 362–369, 2006.

[9] M. Rang, "Bowlegs and knock knees," in *The Art and Practice of Children's Orthopedics*, D. R. Wenger and M. Rang, Eds., pp. 201–219, Roven Press, New York, NY, USA, 1993.

[10] R. E. Bowen, F. J. Dorey, and C. F. Moseley, "Relative tibial and femoral varus as a predictor of progression of varus deformities of the lower limbs in young children," *Journal of Pediatric Orthopaedics*, vol. 22, no. 1, pp. 105–111, 2002.

[11] M. D. Feldman and P. L. Schoenecker, "Use of the metaphyseal-diaphyseal angle in the evaluation of bowed legs," *The Journal of Bone and Joint Surgery—American Volume*, vol. 75, no. 11, pp. 1602–1609, 1993.

[12] K. Gabrial, "Congenital and acquired disorders," in *AAOS Atlas of Orthoses and Assistive Devices*, J. Hsu and J. R. Michael, Eds., pp. 460–464, Mosby Elsevier, 4th edition, 2008.

[13] F. Stief, H. Böhm, A. Schwirtz, C. U. Dussa, and L. Döderlein, "Dynamic loading of the knee and hip joint and compensatory strategies in children and adolescents with varus malalignment," *Gait and Posture*, vol. 33, no. 3, pp. 490–495, 2011.

[14] S. Alsancak, S. Guner, and H. Kinik, "Orthotic variations in the management of infantile tibia vara and the results of treatment," *Prosthetics and Orthotics International*, vol. 37, no. 5, pp. 375–383, 2013.

[15] J. W. Whiteside, "Successful outcomes using a new free motion KAFO for treatment of infantile tibia vara," *Journal of the Association of Children's Prosthetic & Orthotic Clinics*, vol. 17, pp. 26–29, 2011.

[16] J. G. Marshall, *Orthotic Treatment of the Toddler with Bowed Legs*, O&P Business News, 2010.

[17] G. L. Smidt, "Gait in rehabilitation," in *Gait in Children*, M. Patten, Ed., pp. 157–184, Churchill Livingstone, Philadelphia, Pa, USA, 1990.

[18] D. H. Sutherland, R. A. Olshen, E. N. Biden, and M. P. Wyatt, *The Development of Mature Walking*, Blackwell Scientific Publications, Oxford, UK, 1988.

[19] S. J. Hillman, B. W. Stansfield, A. M. Richardson, and J. E. Robb, "Development of temporal and distance parameters of gait in normal children," *Gait and Posture*, vol. 29, no. 1, pp. 81–85, 2009.

[20] P. L. Schoenecker, W. C. Meade, R. L. Pierron, J. J. Sheridan, and A. M. Capelli, "Blount's disease: a retrospective review and recommendations for treatment," *Journal of Pediatric Orthopaedics*, vol. 5, no. 2, pp. 181–186, 1985.

[21] A. Langenskiold, "Tibia vara: osteochondrosis deformans tibiae. Blount's disease," *Clinical Orthopaedics and Related Research*, vol. 158, pp. 77–82, 1981.

[22] W. B. Greene, "Infantile tibia vara," *The Journal of Bone and Joint Surgery—American Volume*, vol. 75, no. 1, pp. 130–143, 1993.

[23] A. M. Levine and J. C. Drennan, "Physiological bowing and tibia vara. The metaphyseal-diaphyseal angle in the measurement of bowleg deformities," *The Journal of Bone & Joint Surgery—American Volume*, vol. 64, no. 8, pp. 1158–1163, 1982.

[24] T. J. Supan and J. M. Mazur, "Orthotic correction of Blount's diseas," *Clinical Orthotics and Prosthetics*, vol. 9, pp. 3–6, 1985.

[25] B. S. Richards, D. E. Katz, and J. B. Sims, "Effectiveness of brace treatment in early infantile Blount's disease," *Journal of Pediatric Orthopaedics*, vol. 18, no. 3, pp. 374–380, 1998.

[26] L. E. Zionts and C. J. Shean, "Brace treatment of early infantile tibia vara," *Journal of Pediatric Orthopaedics*, vol. 18, no. 1, pp. 102–109, 1998.

[27] E. M. Raney, T. A. Topoleski, R. Yaghoubian, K. J. Guidera, and J. G. Marshall, "Orthotic treatment of infantile tibia vara," *Journal of Pediatric Orthopaedics*, vol. 18, no. 5, pp. 670–674, 1998.

[28] S. J. Kumar, C. Barron, and G. D. MacEwen, "Brace treatment of Blount disease," *Orthopaedic Transactions*, vol. 9, p. 501, 1985.

[29] W. P. Blount, "Tibia vara: osteochondrosis deformans tibiae," in *Current Practice in Orthopaedic Surgery*, J. P. Adams, Ed., vol. 3, pp. 141–156, Mosby, St Louis, Mo, USA, 1966.

[30] R. T. Loder and C. E. Johnston, "Infantile tibia vara," *Journal of Pediatric Orthopaedics*, vol. 7, no. 6, pp. 639–646, 1987.

9

Septic Bursitis in an 8-Year-Old Boy

Panagiotis Kratimenos,[1,2] **Ioannis Koutroulis,**[3] **Dante Marconi,**[2]
Jennifer Ding,[2] **Christos Plakas,**[2] **and Margaret Fisher**[2]

[1] *Neonatal-Perinatal Medicine, St. Christopher's Hospital for Children, Drexel University College of Medicine, Philadelphia, PA, USA*
[2] *Department of Pediatrics, The Unterberg Children's Hospital at Monmouth Medical Center, Drexel University College of Medicine, Long Branch, NJ, USA*
[3] *Department of Emergency Medicine, St. Christopher's Hospital for Children, Drexel University College of Medicine, Philadelphia, PA, USA*

Correspondence should be addressed to Panagiotis Kratimenos; pkratimenos@drexelmed.edu

Academic Editor: Nan-Chang Chiu

Background. The prepatellar bursa can become inflamed owing to repeated trauma. Prepatellar bursitis is extremely rare in children. *Methods.* We report the case of an 8-year-old boy who was treated for an erythematous, swollen, and severely painful right knee, fever, inability to bear weight on the leg, and purulent material draining from a puncture wound. We describe the differential diagnosis for tender swollen knee, including infection, gout, rheumatoid arthritis, and osteoarthritis. If untreated, prepatellar bursitis can progress to patellar osteomyelitis. *Results.* Wound cultures grew *Streptococcus pyogenes*, with the infection resolving with amoxicillin. *Conclusions.* A high index of suspicion is necessary in children presenting with prepatellar bursitis to prevent potentially devastating sequelae of infection of the septic joint.

1. Introduction

A bursa is a synovium-like cellular membrane overlying bony prominences such as subdeltoid, olecranon, ischial, trochanteric, semimembranosus-gastrocnemius, and prepatellar. The prepatellar bursa is located between the patella and the overlying skin and commonly becomes inflamed due to repeated trauma, such as kneeling on hard surfaces, causing bursitis. Prepatellar bursitis often occurs in adults who work in an occupation that requires frequent kneeling, for example, cleaning floors. In fact, prepatellar bursitis has nicknames such as "housemaid's knee" due to this common etiology. Patients with prepatellar bursitis normally have preserved range of motion [1, 2].

2. Case Report

An 8-year-old boy, with no significant medical history, presented to the emergency department reporting an erythematous, swollen, and severely painful right knee. Two days prior to his presentation to the emergency department, he was in his usual state of health when he fell off his scooter and scraped his knee on the pavement. He sustained a puncture wound but did not recall any foreign object lodging in his knee. Over the next 2 days, his knee became progressively red, swollen, and tender. He developed a tactile temperature that was not recorded. On the day of admission, he was unable to bear weight on the leg, and purulent material was draining from the wound. As per his mother, this was the child's first trauma and hospitalization.

On admission his vital signs were as follows: temperature 102.3°F, heart rate 102 beats/minute, respiratory rate 38 breaths/minute, blood pressure 102/58 mm Hg, and oxygen saturation 100% in room air. His weight was 52 kg (100th percentile), height was 132 cm (100th percentile), and body mass index was 17.4 (79th percentile).

Physical examination findings were significant for a midline 8 × 10 mm puncture wound on the anterior aspect of the right knee. Purulent material was actively draining from the wound. The knee was erythematous, swollen, and severely

TABLE 1: Comparison of bursitis, septic arthritis, and osteomyelitis [11–19].

	Clinical	Labs	Microbiology	Imaging
Bursitis	(i) Localized tenderness over area of infection (ii) Decreased range of motion of affected joint or pain with movement (iii) Erythema or edema (iv) History of repetitive movement of involved joint	**Noninfectious** Joint fluid analysis: <2000/μL—predominantly mononuclear cells **Septic** (i) Leukocyte count: mildly to moderately elevated (ii) ESR*: mildly to moderately elevated (iii) Joint fluid analysis: predominantly polymorphonuclear cells (iv) WBC count: 5,000–20,000 μL (possibly >70,000 μL) usually less than septic arthritis (v) Increased protein (vi) Decreased glucose	(i) S. aureus most common (>80%) (ii) Streptococcus (5–20%)	(i) Plain radiograph and bone scans are not sensitive for bursitis (ii) MRI, if needed, is very sensitive for bursitis
Septic Arthritis	(i) Red, warm, and immobile joint (ii) Often has palpable effusion (iii) Chills and fever occur secondary to bacteremia	(i) Joint fluid; yellow-green color (ii) WBC count >50,000 μL (>75% polymorphonuclear cells) (iii) ESR: elevated	(i) Staphylococcus (40%) (ii) Streptococcus (30%) (iii) Gram-negative rods (20%)	(i) Plain radiograph: periarticular soft-tissue swelling is most common finding, linear deposition of calcium pyrophosphate (ii) US: used to dx effusions in chronically distorted joints
Osteomyelitis	(i) Swelling, warmth, and erythema over area of infection or affected bone (ii) Painful range of motion of affected joint (iii) Pain in area of infection (iv) Fevers or chills	(i) WBC count: usually does not exceed 15,000 μL and can be normal in chronic osteomyelitis (ii) ESR and CRP** usually increased	(i) Blood cultures positive in only 50% (ii) Most common cause; Staphylococcus aureus	(i) Plain radiograph: periosteal thickening or elevation; cortical thickening, sclerosis or irregularity; osteolysis; new bone formation (ii) CT: useful for guiding needle biopsy in closed infections (iii) MRI: gold standard; shows localized marrow abnormalities (iv) US: fluid next to bone without soft-tissue in between usually suggests osteomyelitis (v) Nuclear medicine: 3-phase bone scan helpful for acute stages and shows increased metabolic activity

*ESR (normal values): males (0–15 mm/hr), females (0–20 mm/hr); **CRP (normal value): 0–10 mg/dL.

tender to palpation. The erythema extended up to the mid femur. There was marked swelling of the lateral and anterior thigh. Joint effusion was not appreciated. The right lower leg and ankle were also edematous. There was mild active and passive movement approximately 10° to 25° in total. Other physical examination findings were unremarkable.

Complete blood count values were as follows: white blood cell count 27.6 K/mm^3, red blood cell count 4.62 M/mm^3, hemoglobin 12.3 g/dL, hematocrit 37.3%, platelets 325 K/mm^3, neutrophils 63%, lymphocytes 14, bands 18, erythrocyte sedimentation rate 68 mm/h, and C-reactive protein 228 mg/L.

Because infectious arthritis was high in the differential diagnosis, wound and blood cultures were obtained and antimicrobial treatment was initiated with intravenous vancomycin and clindamycin and the patient was admitted to the hospital. An orthopedic surgery consult was obtained and explorative arthroscopy was undertaken.

In the operating department, the puncture wound was extended about a centimeter in both directions. Pus was expressed with manual manipulation. There was a moderate amount of pus still under the skin. Sterile cotton swabs were used to break up any adhesions under the skin and to make sure there were no pockets of pus or anything walled off such as an abscess or phlegmon; cultures were sent and the joint was irrigated with approximately 3 L of saline. The capsule was inspected and there was no communication into the joint but some necrotic tissue was excised. A Penrose drain was placed in the bursa and the skin was closed loosely around it.

The patient improved rapidly after surgery. Active and passive movement increased to a total of 90°. Wound cultures grew *Streptococcus pyogenes* sensitive to ampicillin. The vancomycin and clindamycin were discontinued and intravenous ampicillin was started.

The tenderness gradually resolved, range of motion in the joint improved, and the fever resolved. On day 4 of admission, the child was discharged home on amoxicillin with instructions to follow up with pediatric orthopedics in 2 weeks.

3. Discussion

The differential diagnosis for a tender swollen knee includes infection and arthritic conditions such as gout, rheumatoid arthritis, and osteoarthritis. Therefore, thorough workup must be performed to make this diagnosis. Bursitis can be differentiated from septic arthritis and osteomyelitis with a history of more focal tenderness and/or swelling (Table 1). To rule out an infection, joint aspiration is necessary. A synovial fluid white blood cell count greater than 1000/μL suggests infection, rheumatoid arthritis, or gout. Septic arthritis is defined as a white blood cell count greater than 50,000/μL. Once the diagnosis is established, initial management of prepatellar bursitis consists of rest and avoidance of the aggravating factors. Nonsteroidal anti-inflammatory drugs are used to alleviate the inflammation of the bursa. In patients who cannot tolerate nonsteroidal agents, local glucocorticoid injections may be appropriate.

A common consequence of untreated prepatellar bursitis is patellar osteomyelitis. Osteomyelitis is considered a disease of childhood [3]. Because it presents in various ways, diagnosis is often delayed [3]. Osteomyelitis frequently has an unclear course, typically beginning as largely cartilaginous prior to ossification [3]. It is important to prevent bursitis from progressing to osteomyelitis, which can lead to further bony destruction [3]. As a result, a high index of suspicion is necessary in children presenting with prepatellar bursitis initially. Diagnostic tests such as high-quality radiography should be used [3]. Haine et al. [4] explained the importance of magnetic resonance imaging in aiding in the diagnosis as well.

Freys [5] reported a prevalence of septic bursitis as high as three of 1000 patients. In their report the two most frequently infected bursae were the olecranon and the prepatellar. Patients with prepatellar septic bursitis were more likely to be hospitalized than patients with olecranon septic bursitis. The most common organism seen in septic bursitis is *Staphylococcus aureus*, thought to occur in about two-thirds of cases. Other causal organisms include streptococcal species (most commonly group A β-hemolytic *Streptococcus*), Gramnegative organisms, and *Mycobacterium marinum*. Raddatz et al. [6] reported that cellulitis adjacent to bursitis occurred in 89% of cases and was often extensive. Also, they found profound edema in 11% of affected extremities. Ten case reports of septic bursitis in children studied over a 25-year period showed a balance between male and female. Eighty percent involved the prepatellar bursa, 80% occurred during the summer months, and 70% required incision and drainage [7]. Temperature, humidity, and local factors as well as bacterial components may favor skin penetration and invasion of superficial bursitis [7]. If the aspiration shows only serous content, then conservative treatment is appropriate with compression, immobilization, antiphlogistics medications (or agents that reduce inflammation, for example, nonsteroidal anti-inflammatory medications), and/or corticosteroids [5]. Typically, patients with a purulent aspiration respond to antibiotics to the targeted organism(s) and to aspirations of the effusions. However, incision and drainage may be necessary if the bursitis does not respond to at least one aspiration [8].

Prepatellar bursitis is extremely rare in children. Searching in PubMed using the words "prepatellar bursitis in children" revealed only two case reports published in 1982. In children, the limited intra-articular joint space and the devastating sequelae of infection of the septic joint decrease our threshold for performing arthrocentesis and sometimes explorative arthroscopy [9, 10].

Disclosure

None.

Conflict of Interests

The authors declare that they have no conflict of interests regarding the publication of this paper.

Acknowledgments

The authors thank Diana Winters, Academic Publishing Services, and Drexel University College of Medicine, for editing the paper.

References

[1] C. A. Langford and B. C. Gilliland, "Periarticular disorders of the extremities," in *Harrison's Principles of Internal Medicine*, A. S. Fauci, E. Braunwald, D. L. Kasper et al., Eds., pp. 2184–2186, McGraw-Hill Medical, New York, NY, USA, 17th edition, 2008.

[2] D. B. Hellmann and J. B. Imboden Jr., "Musculoskeletal and immunologic disorders," in *Current Medical Diagnosis & Treatment*, S. J. McPhee and M. A. Papadakis, Eds., pp. 2056–2061, McGraw-Hill Lange, 2010.

[3] H.-R. Choi, "Patellar osteomyelitis presenting as prepatellar bursitis," *Knee*, vol. 14, no. 4, pp. 333–335, 2007.

[4] S. E. Haine, V. J. Reenaers, J. F. van Offel et al., "Recurrent arthritis as presenting symptom of osteomyelitis," *Clinical Rheumatology*, vol. 22, no. 3, pp. 237–239, 2003.

[5] S. M. Freys, "Olecranon and pre-patellar bursitis," *Langenbecks Archiv für Chirurgie. Supplement. Kongressband*, vol. 114, pp. 493–496, 1997 (German).

[6] D. A. Raddatz, G. S. Hoffman, and W. A. Franck, "Septic bursitis: presentation, treatment and prognosis," *Journal of Rheumatology*, vol. 14, no. 6, pp. 1160–1163, 1987.

[7] J. C. Cea-Pereiro, J. Garcia-Meijide, A. Mera-Varela, and J. J. Gomez-Reino, "A comparison between septic bursitis caused by Staphylococcus aureus and those caused by other organisms," *Clinical Rheumatology*, vol. 20, no. 1, pp. 10–14, 2001.

[8] F. D. Pien, D. Ching, and E. Kim, "Septic bursitis: experience in a community practice," *Orthopedics*, vol. 14, no. 9, pp. 981–984, 1991.

[9] A. J. Alario, E. Y. Su, and G. Ho Jr., "Septic prepatellar bursitis in a child," *Rhode Island Medical Journal*, vol. 65, no. 7, pp. 279–281, 1982.

[10] J. W. Paisley, "Septic bursitis in childhood," *Journal of Pediatric Orthopaedics*, vol. 2, no. 1, pp. 57–61, 1982.

[11] T. Gross, A. H. Kaim, P. Regazzoni, and A. F. Widmer, "Current concepts in posttraumatic osteomyelitis: a diagnostic challenge with new imaging options," *Journal of Trauma*, vol. 52, no. 6, pp. 1210–1219, 2002.

[12] S. A. Paluska, "Osteomyelitis," *Clinics in Family Practice*, vol. 6, no. 1, pp. 127–156, 2004.

[13] L. Bernard, A. Lübbeke, R. Stern et al., "Value of preoperative investigations in diagnosing prosthetic joint infection: retrospective cohort study and literature review," *Scandinavian Journal of Infectious Diseases*, vol. 36, no. 6-7, pp. 410–416, 2004.

[14] M. J. Spangehl, B. A. Masri, J. X. O'Connell, and C. P. Duncan, "Prospective analysis of preoperative and intraoperative investigations for the diagnosis of infection at the sites of two hundred and two revision total hip arthroplasties," *Journal of Bone and Joint Surgery. American*, vol. 81, no. 5, pp. 672–683, 1999.

[15] J. H. Calhoun and M. M. Manring, "Adult osteomyelitis," *Infectious Disease Clinics of North America*, vol. 19, no. 4, pp. 765–786, 2005.

[16] J. W. Smith and E. A. Piercy, "Infectious arthritis," *Clinical Infectious Diseases*, vol. 20, no. 2, pp. 225–231, 1995.

[17] C. J. E. Kaandorp, P. Krijnen, H. J. Bernelot Moens, J. D. F. Habbema, and D. Van Schaardenburg, "The outcome of bacterial arthritis: a prospective community-based study," *Arthritis and Rheumatism*, vol. 40, no. 5, pp. 884–892, 1997.

[18] M. L. Wilson and W. Winn, "Laboratory diagnosis of bone, joint, soft-tissue, and skin infections," *Clinical Infectious Diseases*, vol. 46, no. 3, pp. 453–457, 2008.

[19] Z. Hirji, J. S. Hunjun, and H. N. Choudur, "Imaging of the bursae," *Journal of Clinical Imaging Science*, vol. 1, p. 22, 2011.

10

Metastatic Malignant Ectomesenchymoma Initially Presenting as a Pelvic Mass: Report of a Case and Review of Literature

A. Nael,[1] P. Siaghani,[1] W. W. Wu,[2] K. Nael,[3] Lisa Shane,[4] and S. G. Romansky[4]

[1] Department of Pathology and Laboratory Medicine, University of California Irvine Medical Center, 101 The City Drive, Orange, CA 92868, USA

[2] Department of Pathology and Laboratory Medicine, Memorial Sloan Kettering Cancer Center, 1275 York Avenue, New York, NY 10065, USA

[3] Department of Medical Imaging, University of Arizona Medical Center, 1501 N. Campbell Avenue, P.O. Box 245067, Tucson, AZ 85724-5067, USA

[4] University of California Irvine, Long Beach Memorial Care Health System, 2801 Atlantic Avenue, Long Beach, CA 908068, USA

Correspondence should be addressed to A. Nael; anaelamz@hs.uci.edu

Academic Editor: Amalia Schiavetti

Pediatric soft tissue sarcomas account for approximately 10% of all pediatric malignancies. Malignant ectomesenchymoma is rare biphasic sarcomas consisting of both mesenchymal and neuroectodermal elements. Approximately 64 cases have been reported in the literature and are believed to arise from pluripotent embryologic migratory neural crest cells. We report a 4-year-old boy who initially presented with a pelvic mass and inguinal lymphadenopathy at 6 months of age. Inguinal lymph node biopsy revealed a distinct biphasic tumor with microscopic and immunophenotypic characteristics diagnostic for both alveolar rhabdomyosarcoma and poorly differentiated neuroblastoma. The patient received national protocol chemotherapy against rhabdomyosarcoma with good response and presented with a cerebellar mass 21 months later. The metastatic tumor revealed sheets of primitive tumor cells and diagnostic areas of rhabdomyosarcoma and neuroblastoma were identified only by immunohistochemistry. Cytogenetic analysis of metastatic tumor demonstrated complex karyotype with multiple chromosomal deletions and duplications. The patient received national protocol chemotherapy against neuroblastoma and adjuvant radiotherapy after surgical resection of the cerebellar tumor with good response. He is currently off from any treatment for 18 months with no evidence of tumor recurrence or metastasis.

1. Introduction

Pediatric soft tissue sarcomas account for approximately 10% of all pediatric malignancies and are considered the fifth most common pediatric soft tissue neoplasm following leukemia/lymphoma, central nervous system tumor, neuroblastoma, and Wilms' tumor [1]. Malignant ectomesenchymoma (MEM) is a rare soft tissue sarcoma with a biphasic morphology consisting of both mesenchymal and neuroectodermal elements such as rhabdomyosarcoma (RMS) and ganglioneuroblastoma. MEMs are believed to arise from pluripotent embryologic migratory neural crest cells able to form both mesenchymal and neuroectodermal tissues [2]. Because these cells are widely distributed throughout the body, MEMs may arise in diverse sites but the most

common reported location is perineal/pelvic area [3]. These tumors are exceedingly rare and approximately 64 cases have been reported in English literature in all age groups with preponderance in the first decade of life [3]. Due to the rare incidence of MEM, our knowledge of tumor genetics, biological behavior, treatment, outcome, and prognosis is limited.

2. Case Report

Our patient is a 4-year-old Hispanic boy. He first presented at 6 months old to the Emergency Room with a chief complaint of left leg swelling and pain for a month. Further work-up including pelvic and thigh magnetic resonance imaging (MRI) revealed a heterogeneous partially cystic enhancing bilobed mass at the left side of the pelvis, measuring 5.7 × 4.3 × 4.0 cm (Figure 1). The left external iliac artery and vein coursed between the two lobes of the mass. In addition, multiple enlarged left inguinal lymph nodes were identified with solid and cystic appearance, suggestive of tumor metastasis. Diagnostic excisional inguinal lymph node biopsy was done. Sections revealed a distinct biphasic appearance by light microscopy (Figures 2 and 3) and immunohistochemical analysis (Figure 4) demonstrated both alveolar rhabdomyosarcoma-like (ARMS-like) and poorly differentiated neuroblastoma components. No evidence of residual lymph node was identified. The RMS component was composed of prominent spaces separated by fibrovascular septa (Figure 2(a)). The septa were lined by loosely cohesive primitive cells with hyperchromatic nuclei and variable amount of scant cytoplasm, imparting an alveolar pattern (Figure 2(b)). However, there were foci where tumor cells demonstrated nesting pattern within the fibrovascular septa with pleomorphic nuclei (Figure 2(c)). The neuroblastoma component showed schwannian stroma poor tumor with more primitive neuroblasts and scant amount of neuropil in a nodular growth pattern (Figures 3(a) and 3(b)). Moreover, the neuroblastic tumor cells showed speckled salt and pepper nuclei, inconspicuous nucleoli, and little nuclear pleomorphism with a variable amount of scant cytoplasm. The mitotic-karyorrhectic index (MKI) was low (<2%) (Figure 3(c)). The RMS component was strongly positive for myogenin (Figure 4(b)) and desmin by immunohistochemical staining, while the neuroblastoma component was stained with neural markers such as PGP9.5 and tyrosine-hydroxylase (Figures 4(c) and 4(d)), CD56, synaptophysin, and S100. Whole body work-up including MRI, positron emission tomography scan (PET scan), and bone marrow biopsy did not show any evidence of tumor involvement in other areas of the body including the central nervous system. Due to the extensive lymphadenopathy in the pelvic and inguinal area, the patient's tumor was considered to be metastatic and treated against RMS as it was the more aggressive component of the tumor. He received and completed national protocol chemotherapy for ARMS (COG-ARST08P1 protocol [22]), with significant reduction in his tumor burden. He was doing well and had been off of chemotherapy for about four months, when he became less active and showed ataxic gait with episodes of vomiting, 21 months after first presentation. MRI of the brain showed a 5.6 × 5.1 × 4.2 cm left cerebellar cystic mass with thick peripheral enhancement and some hemorrhage, consistent with metastasis (Figure 5). The tumor showed significant mass effect on the fourth ventricle and brain stem. There was no evidence of tumor recurrence or metastasis in other sites. Due to the location of the tumor, mass effect, and tumor size reduction, excisional surgery was done. The metastatic tumor displayed a more homogenous microscopic appearance with sheets of primitive tumor cells resembling a primary medulloblastoma (Figure 6(a)). Diagnostic areas of RMS and neuroblastoma were only identified by immunohistochemistry demonstrating strong positivity for myogenin, CD56, and tyrosine hydroxylase (Figures 6(b)–6(d)). However, neuroblastoma was the predominant component. Peripheral blood chromosome analysis revealed a normal male chromosome complement (46, XY) with no abnormalities. Molecular analysis utilizing reverse transcription polymerase chain reaction (RT-PCR) was performed on the cerebellar tumor and showed no evidence of a PAX3-FOXO1 t(2;13) (q35;q14) or a PAX7-FOXO1 t(1;13) (p36;q14) chromosomal translocation. Although fluorescence in situ hybridization (FISH) studies revealed FOXO1 (FKHR) gain on chromosome 13q14.11 in 75% of the tumor cells, there was no PAX-FOXO1 translocation. Tumor chromosome analysis showed complex karyotype with near-triploid cell line (71, XYY) and multiple chromosomal deletions (chromosomes 3 and 4) and duplications (chromosomes 5, 7, 19, and 22). After surgical resection, he received national chemotherapy protocol against the neuroblastoma component (COG-ANBL0532 protocol [23]), which was the most prominent component of the metastatic tumor. In addition, he received adjuvant local radiation therapy. He completed his chemoradiation therapy with excellent tumor response. Currently he is not receiving any additional treatments for about 18 months and his most recent follow-up MRI and PET scan did not show any evidence of residual or metastatic tumor. We report another MEM case with cytogenetic analysis, as there are only 5 reported cases in the literature with these data. Moreover our case emphasizes the importance of multimodality treatment approach in prognosis, even in nonresectable primary tumors.

3. Discussion

Across all ages with MEM, the mesenchymal component is generally RMS with predominantly embryonal subtype [2, 3, 7, 24–27] but pleomorphic sarcoma, undifferentiated sarcoma, chondrosarcoma, liposarcoma, and gliosarcoma have been reported [3, 11, 21]. The neuroectodermal component can be highly variable ranging from clustered ganglion cells to immature primitive neural elements only identified by immunohistochemical staining [2, 11, 24–27]. Freitas et al. have reported 40 MEM cases from 1946 to 1998 with related data regarding the sex, age, primary site, histology pattern, treatment, and survival from the time of presentation. After reviewing the English literature from 1998 to the present, we found additional 24 MEM cases, which have both microscopic and immunophenotype characteristics of MEM (Table 1). Combining data from the Freitas et al. study and our observation revealed RMS and ganglioneuroma/ganglioneuroblastoma with clustered or scattered ganglion cells are the most common histological patterns seen in MEM cases (Figure 7(a)). Moreover, the most common site of presentation is the perineal/pelvic area, followed by head and neck, intracranial, limbs, intra-abdominal, and retroperitoneal (Figure 7(b)). While some reports support the idea of MEM having male predilection and occurring typically in infancy [2, 7, 24, 26], other studies do not show this predilection [3, 13, 27]. Our observation shows these tumors to have a slightly male predominance (male to female ratio of 1.4) and most commonly present in the first decade of life (82%) (Figure 8). Our case showed RMS as mesenchymal component but with alveolar pattern and poorly

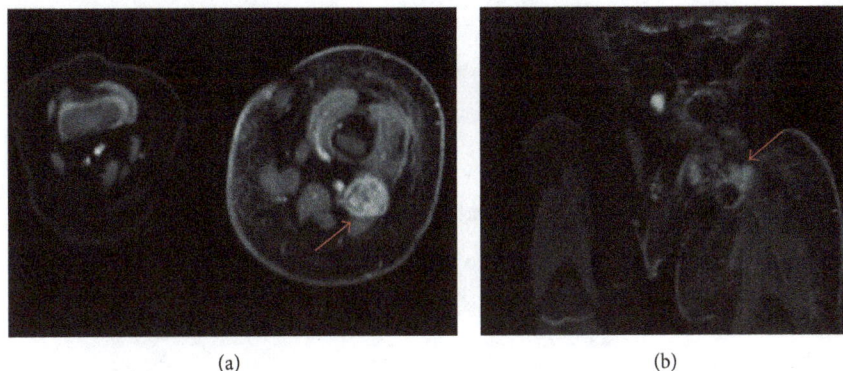

(a) (b)

FIGURE 1: Axial (a) and coronal (b) T1-contrast-enahnced MR images through the thighs are shown. There is a heterogeneously enhancing mass in the posterior thigh involving the adductor compartment (arrow in (a)). There are also several enlarged external iliac lymph nodes: some with cystic and necrotic changes (arrow in (b)). Note the enlargement of the left lower extremity and significant soft-tissue edema and fat stranding.

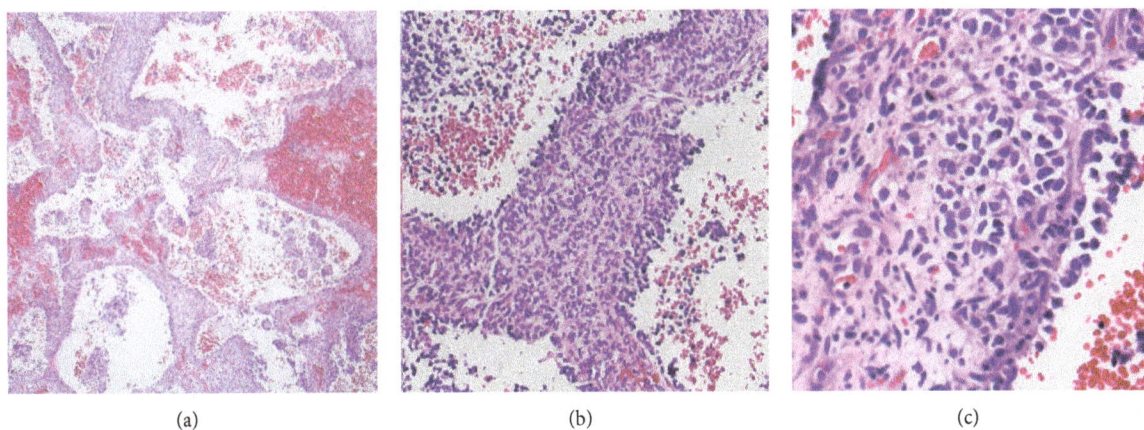

(a) (b) (c)

FIGURE 2: Histologic features of tumor in the left inguinal lymph node. (a) The RMS-like component showed variably sized cystic spaces separated by fibrovascular septa. (b) Cystic spaces lined by loosely cohesive primitive cells floating into spaces, imparting an alveolar pattern. (c) The tumor cells demonstrated nesting pattern within the fibrovascular septa (hematoxylin-eosin, original magnification ×40 (a); original magnification ×200 (b); original magnification ×400 (c)).

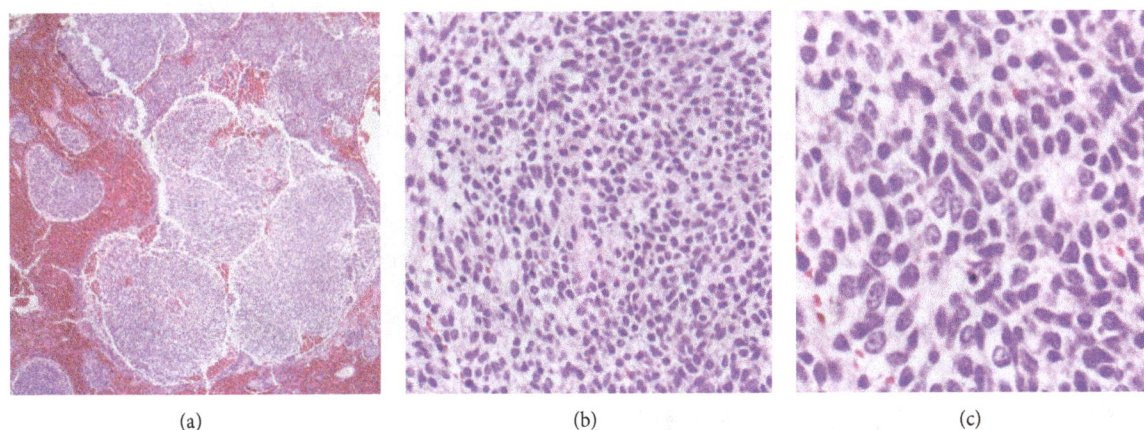

(a) (b) (c)

FIGURE 3: Histologic features of tumor in the left inguinal lymph node. (a) Neuroblastoma component with nodular growth pattern. (b) Each nodule is composed of primitive neuroblasts with scant amount of neuropil. (c) Neuroblasts with salt and peppery nuclei and low MKI (hematoxylin-eosin, original magnification ×40 (a); original magnification ×200 (b); original magnification ×400 (c)).

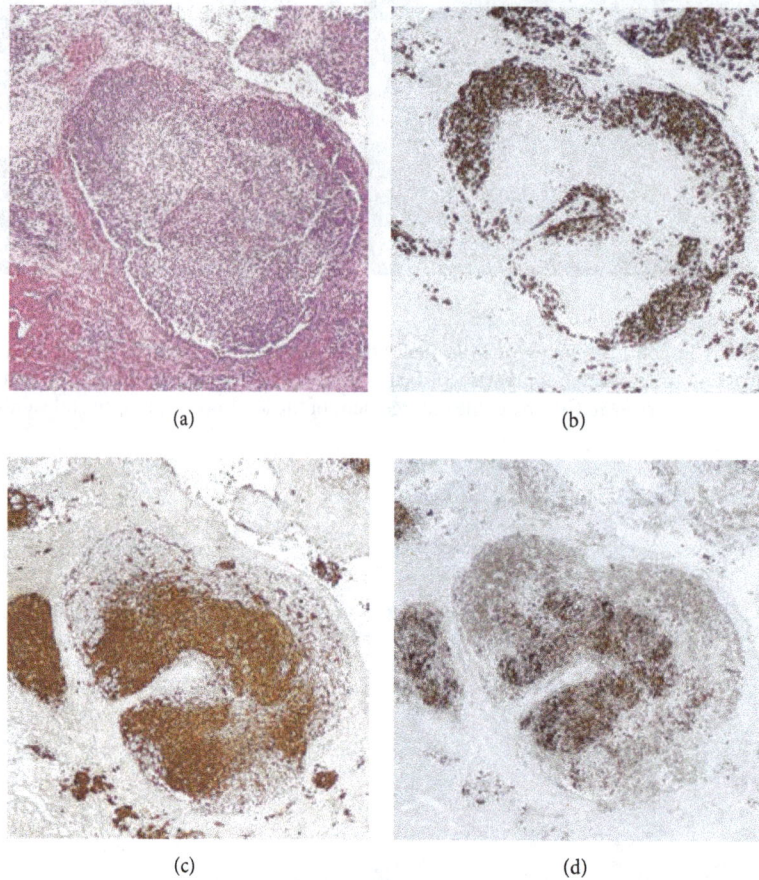

FIGURE 4: Immunohistochemical features of tumor in the left inguinal lymph node. (a) Microscopic photographs from left inguinal lymph node biopsy reveal primitive tumor cells with nodular growth pattern. The tumor cells demonstrate immunohistochemical reactivity for (b) myogenin, (c) PGP9.5, and (d) tyrosine-hydroxylase to show both myogenic and neural differentiation (original magnification ×200 (a–d)).

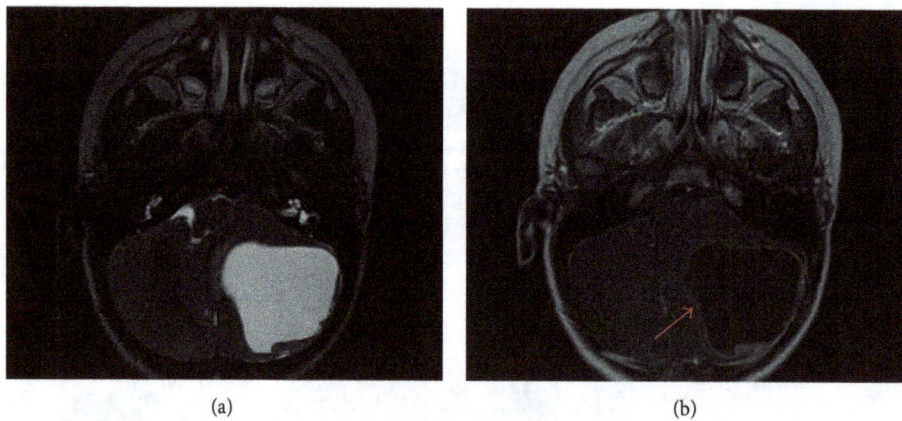

FIGURE 5: Axial T2 (a) and T1-contrast-enhanced (b) MR images of brain. There is a 5.6 × 5.1 cm largely cystic mass with peripheral nodular enhancement (arrow in (b)) involving the left cerebellar hemisphere. There is mass effect with compression of the 4th ventricle and effacement of the left premedullary cistern.

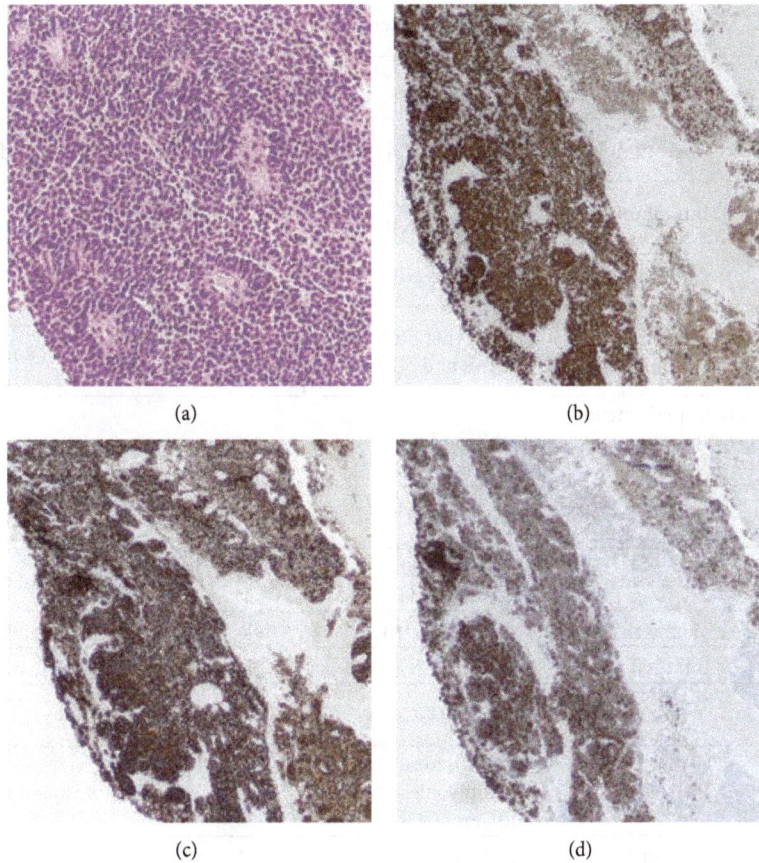

(a)

(b)

(c)

(d)

FIGURE 6: Histologic and immunohistochemical features of tumor in the left cerebellum. (a) Microscopic photographs from left cerebellar resection show sheets of primitive tumor cells with neuroblastic rosettes resembling a primary medulloblastoma. The tumor cells demonstrate immunohistochemical reactivity for (b) myogenin, (c) CD56, and (d) tyrosine-hydroxylase to show both myogenic and neural differentiation (original magnification × 200 (a–d)).

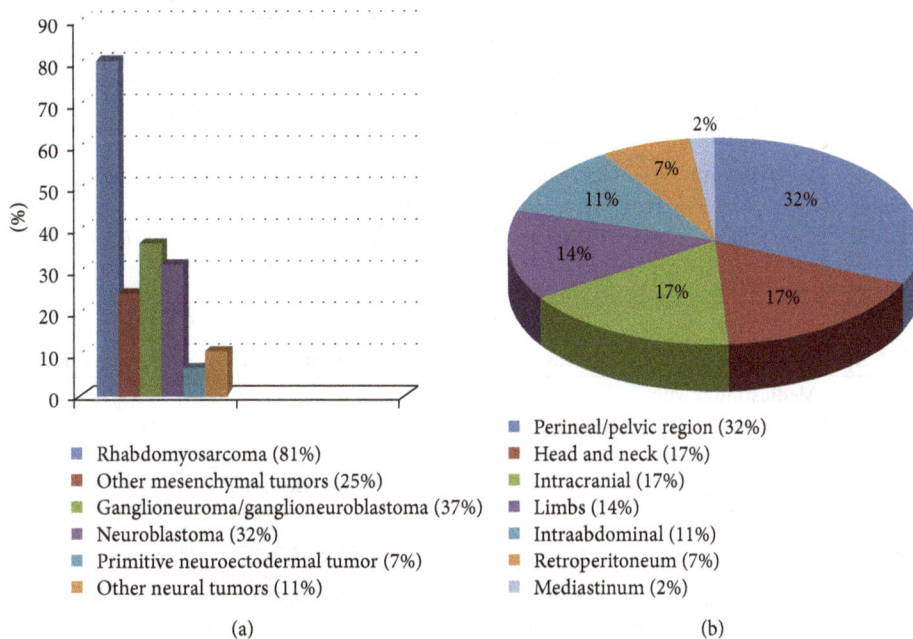

■ Rhabdomyosarcoma (81%)
■ Other mesenchymal tumors (25%)
■ Ganglioneuroma/ganglioneuroblastoma (37%)
■ Neuroblastoma (32%)
■ Primitive neuroectodermal tumor (7%)
■ Other neural tumors (11%)

(a)

■ Perineal/pelvic region (32%)
■ Head and neck (17%)
■ Intracranial (17%)
■ Limbs (14%)
■ Intraabdominal (11%)
■ Retroperitoneum (7%)
■ Mediastinum (2%)

(b)

FIGURE 7: Charts to show (a) histological features and (b) primary anatomical sites of involvement of malignant ectomesenchymoma.

TABLE 1: Review of malignant ectomesenchymoma cases reported after 1998.

Case number	Age[a]	Sex	Primary site	Histology[b]	Recurrence or metastasis[a]	Treatment[c]	Follow-up[a]
1 [4]	13 yr.	M	Scrotum	ERMS and GCs	Retroperitoneum Met. after 2 yr.	DS, CT, and RT	NA
2 [5]	10 yr.	F	Intracranial	US with rhabdoid features and NB	Local Rec. after 5 wk.	TSR	NED after 12 mo.
3 [6]	19 mo.	M	Pelvic	ERMS and NB	Local Rec. and BM Met. after 8 yr.	TSR and CT	NED for 8 yr., NA after Met.
4 [7]	11 mo.	M	Intra-abdomen	US with rhabdoid features and NB	Liver, lung, and BM Met. at the time of presentation	DS, CT, and RT	DOD after 9 mo.
5 [8]	61 yr.	M	Retroperitoneum with invasion to vertebral bone	ERMS and GN	No	DS and RT	DOD after 14 mo.
6 [9]	1.5 yr.	M	Upper lip	ERMS and GCs	Local Rec. after 1 yr.	TSR and CT	NED for 1 year, NA after Rec.
7 [10]	4 mo.	M	Pelvic	ERMS, GCs, and schwannoma	NA	TSR and CT	NA
8 [11]	17 mo.	M	Left wrist	RMS, CRS, GNB	No	TSR and CT	NED after 4 yr.
9 [12]	10 yr.	F	Intracranial	ERMS and NB	No	TSR, CT, and RT	NED after 6 yr.
10 [13]	10 d.	F	Face	RMS and GCs	No	Biopsy and CT	DOD, after a few days
11 [14]	4 yr.	F	Intracranial	US with focal rhabdomyoblastic diff. and GCs	Lung Met. at the time of presentation	TSR and CT	DOD after 10 wk.
12 [15]	8 mo.	M	Scrotum	ERMS and GC	NA	TSR and CT	NA
13 [16]	10 yr.	M	Intracranial	US and GCs	No	TSR, CT, and RT	NED after 20 mo.
14 [17]	36 yr.	F	Ethmoid sinus and orbit	RMS and NB	No	Biopsy, CT, and RT	NED after 28 mo.
15 [18]	6 mo.	F	Vagina	ERMS and GCs	Abdomen-pelvic Met. after 4 mo.	DS and CT	DOD after 15 mo.
16 [19]	43 yr.	F	Nasal cavity	RMB and NB	No	Biopsy, CT, and RT	NED after 10 mo.
17 [20]	6 yr.	M	Intracranial, frontal lobe	US and GCs	No	TSR, CT, and RT	NED after 2 years
18 [2]	4 yr.	F	Orbit	ERMS and NB	No	TSR, CT, and RT	NED after 12.9 years
19 [2]	2.5 mo.	F	Upper arm	ARMS and pPNET	No	TSR and CT	NED after 13.7 years
20 [2]	13.5 yr.	M	Buttock	ARMS and NB	Local Rec. and lungs Met. after 1.1 yr.	DS, CT, and RT	DOD after 1.3 years
21 [2]	1 yr.	M	Groin	ERMS and NB	No	TSR and CT	NED after 5 years
22 [2]	7 mo.	F	Sole	ERMS and NB	Local Rec. after 5 mo.	TSR and CT	NED after 2.3 years
23 [2]	8 mo.	M	Intra-abdomen	ERMS and NB	Local Rec. after 1.4 yr.	TSR and CT	NED after 2.1 years
24 [21]	5 mo.	M	Mediastinum with invasion into lung and SVC	RMS and pPNET	No	DS and CT	DOD after 11 mo.
25 (Our case)	6 mo.	M	Inguinal and pelvic	ARMS and NB	Cerebellum Met. after 21 mo.	Biopsy, CT, and RT	NED after 3 yr.

ARMS, alveolar rhabdomyosarcoma; BM, bone marrow; CRS, chondrosarcoma; CT, chemotherapy; diff., differentiation; DOD, dead due to disease; DS, debulking surgery; ERMS, embryonal rhabdomyosarcoma; F, female; GC, ganglion cell; GN, ganglioneuroma; GNB, ganglioneuroblastoma; M, male; Met., metastasis; mo., month(s); NA, no data available; NB, neuroblastoma; NED, no evidence of disease; pPNET, peripheral primitive neuroectodermal tumor; Rec., recurrence; RMB, rhabdomyoblastoma; RMS, rhabdomyosarcoma; RT, radiation therapy; SVC, superior vena cava; TSR, total surgical resection; US, undifferentiated sarcoma; wk, week(s); yr., year(s); [a]age, recurrence/metastasis and follow-up since first diagnosis; [b]itdescribes which tumor components were present in respect to diagnosis of MEM; [c]itdescribes type of treatment on the primary tumor.

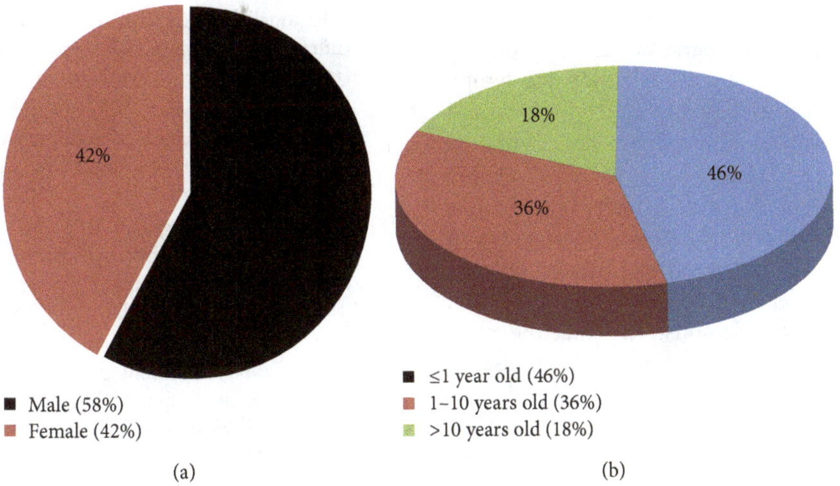

FIGURE 8: Charts to show (a) incidence according to sex and (b) incidence according to age of malignant ectomesenchymoma.

differentiated neuroblastoma as neuroectodermal component. The area resembling RMS has both histological and immunohistochemical staining pattern typical of alveolar type RMS. FISH analysis failed to detect any of the two recurrent chromosomal translocations commonly seen in alveolar rhabdomyosarcoma (ARMS) such as t(2;13)(q35;q14), seen in 55% of the cases, or t(1;13)(p36;q14), seen in 22% of cases [28, 29]. In addition to our case, there are five reports of MEM in the literature with cytogenetic analysis. Karyotyping analysis of malignant ectomesenchymoma cases is shown as follows.

Case 1. A 5-month-old girl with pelvic mass [25]:

49,XY, +8, +8, +11/49,XY, +2, +11, +11/46,XX.

Case 2. A 16-month-old boy with abdominal mass [30]:

53,XY, +2, add(6)(p24), +8, +8, +9, +10, +11, t(12;15)(p12;q24), +20.

Case 3. An 8-month-old boy with scrotal mass [15]:

49,XY, +2, −6, +11, +20, +mar(chromosome 6 material by florescent in situ hybridization).

Case 4. A 4-year-old girl with intracranial mass [14]:

84–87, XXX, −X, −1, der(2)t(1;2)(q12;q14.1), −4, −5, −5,

der(5)t(5;?;5)(p15;?;q13)x2, −9, −9, del(11)(q22)x2, −17, −19, −21,

der(21)t(17;21)(q21;q22), −22, −22, +r, +mar1, +mar2, mar3[cp10].

Case 5. A 6-month-old girl with protruding vaginal mass [18]:

46,XX,der(1)t(1;12)(p32;p13)inv(1)(p13q25), del(5)(q13q22),

der(12)t(1;12)(p32;p13)[9]/46,XX [3].

Case 6. A 6-month-old boy with pelvic mass (our case):

71, XYY, add(1)(p13), −3, −4, +5, +7, +19, +22.

Four of these cases had complex karyotypes. Trisomies 2, 8, and 11 were the most commonly reported genetic abnormalities [14, 15, 25, 30]. One case demonstrated a t(1;12) translocation without ETV6 rearrangement as seen in congenital cellular mesoblastic nephroma [18]. In our case the tumor chromosome analysis revealed a complex karyotype with near-triploid cell line and multiple chromosomal deletions and duplications (71⟨3n⟩, XYY, add (1) (p13), −3, −4, +5, +7, +19, +22), none of which were tumor specific (Table 1). Since MEM is a biphasic tumor with variable differentiation and percentage of its components, it can be in the differential diagnosis of well differentiated to poorly differentiated mesenchymal sarcomas or neuroectodermal tumors such as embryonal rhabdomyosarcoma (ERMS), ARMS, pleomorphic sarcoma, chondrosarcoma, undifferentiated sarcoma, ganglioneuroma, neuroblastoma, peripheral primitive neuroectodermal tumor (pPNET), and malignant schwannoma [2, 21]. However, to diagnose MEM, there must be both mesenchymal and neural elements with immunohistochemical reactivity for myogenin and/or desmin, CD56, PGP9.5, synaptophysin, chromogranin, and tyrosine hydroxylase [2, 27]. Due to the rarity of MEM, data regarding treatment and prognosis is limited. Most investigators suggest a multimodality treatment approach including surgery, chemotherapy, and radiation therapy as these tumors almost will act and have the same prognosis as RMS-like soft tissue sarcomas [2, 31]. In fact, when the predominant mesenchymal element in MEM is RMS, the overall outcome and prognosis are similar to RMS; thus, underdiagnoses may not have a major impact on clinical treatment [27]. In such cases, the International Rhabdomyosarcoma Study Group-IV (IRS-IV) recommends that risk stratification and treatment planning should be done based on age, pretreatment stage (including tumor size, tumor site, regional lymph node status, and disseminated disease), and postoperative clinical grouping depending on completeness of disease resection and lymph node status [2, 7, 27, 32]. Based on this study, for localized disease surgical resection with clear margins and additional chemotherapy is favored [32]. However, for disseminated disease chemotherapy is preferred and tumor debulking is not recommended. Instead, a biopsy should be provided to confirm the diagnosis [33]. Moreover, consideration of additional radiation therapy depends on postoperative clinical grouping. Some studies have demonstrated that the most important independent prognostic factor in MEM cases is tumor resectability as most patients who have died of disease had an unresectable primary tumor or metastasis at the time of presentation [11, 12]. Similar to chemotherapy for other biphasic tumors, in cases where chemotherapy is the mainstay option, agents targeting the most aggressive component are chosen, which is RMS in MEM cases [2]. However, initial reports have shown MEM to have a poor prognosis [7, 24]. Case reviews [34] from 2005 and 2013 revealed MEM to have the same prognosis as other pediatric chemotherapy-sensitive soft tissue sarcomas, with 71% (15/21) and 83% (5/6) of children with MEM surviving following multimodality treatment approach, respectively [2, 11]. Finally, as these tumors have different morphology and genetics from other soft tissue sarcomas, further investigation is necessary to better understand the tumor biology and behavior with the hope of improving treatment protocols and ultimately patient prognosis.

Conflict of Interests

The authors declare that there is no conflict of interests regarding the publication of this paper and that there have been no significant financial contributions for this work that could have influenced its outcome.

References

[1] V. Jairam, K. B. Roberts, and J. B. Yu, "Historical trends in the use of radiation therapy for pediatric cancers: 1973–2008," *International Journal of Radiation Oncology, Biology, Physics*, vol. 85, no. 3, pp. e151–e155, 2013.

[2] T. M. Dantonello, I. Leuschner, C. Vokuhl et al., "Malignant ectomesenchymoma in children and adolescents: report from the Cooperative Weichteilsarkom Studiengruppe (CWS)," *Pediatric Blood & Cancer*, vol. 60, no. 2, pp. 224–229, 2013.

[3] A. B. R. Freitas, P. H. Aguiar, F. K. Miura et al., "Malignant ectomesenchymoma. Case report and review of the literature," *Pediatric Neurosurgery*, vol. 30, no. 6, pp. 320–330, 1999.

[4] V. Edwards, G. Tse, J. Doucet, R. Pearl, and M. J. Phillips, "Rhabdomyosarcoma metastasizing as a malignant ectomesenchymoma," *Ultrastructural Pathology*, vol. 23, no. 4, pp. 267–273, 1999.

[5] M. Papós, A. Pekrun, J. W. Herms et al., "Somatostatin receptor scintigraphy in the management of cerebral malignant ectomesenchymoma: a case report," *Pediatric Radiology*, vol. 31, no. 3, pp. 169–172, 2001.

[6] O. Paramelle, A. Croué, F. Dupré, X. Rialland, and J.-P. Saint-André, "Pelvic malignant ectomesenchymoma: a case report," *Annales de Pathologie*, vol. 21, no. 4, pp. 344–347, 2001.

[7] H. L. Müller, A. Marx, M. Trusen, P. Schneider, and J. Kühl, "Disseminated malignant ectomesenchymoma (MEM): case report and review of the literature," *Pediatric Hematology and Oncology*, vol. 19, no. 1, pp. 9–17, 2002.

[8] S. Kimura, S. Kawaguchi, T. Wada, S. Nagoya, T. Yamashita, and K. Kikuchi, "Rhabdomyosarcoma arising from a dormant dumbbell ganglioneuroma of the lumbar spine: a case report.," *Spine*, vol. 27, no. 23, pp. E513–517, 2002.

[9] N. J. Sebire, A. D. Ramsay, M. Malone, and R. A. Risdon, "Extensive posttreatment ganglioneuromatous differentiation of rhabdomyosarcoma: Malignant ectomesenchymoma in an infant," *Pediatric and Developmental Pathology*, vol. 6, no. 1, pp. 94–96, 2003.

[10] M. Kösem, I. Ibiloğlu, V. Bakan, and B. Köseoğlu, "Ectomesenchymoma: case report and review of the literature," *The Turkish Journal of Pediatrics*, vol. 46, no. 1, pp. 82–87, 2004.

[11] O. Oppenheimer, E. Athanasian, P. Meyers, C. R. Antonescu, and R. Gorlick, "Malignant ectomesenchymoma in the wrist of a child: case report and review of the literature," *International Journal of Surgical Pathology*, vol. 13, no. 1, pp. 113–116, 2005.

[12] E. Weiss, C. F. Albrecht, J. Herms et al., "Malignant ectomesenchymoma of the cerebrum. Case report and discussion of therapeutic options," *European Journal of Pediatrics*, vol. 164, no. 6, pp. 345–349, 2005.

[13] I. Bayram, G. Leblebisatan, H. Yildizdaş et al., "A neonate with malignant ectomesenchymoma," *The Turkish Journal of Pediatrics*, vol. 47, no. 4, pp. 382–384, 2005.

[14] B. K. Kleinschmidt-DeMasters, M. A. Lovell, A. M. Donson et al., "Molecular array analyses of 51 pediatric tumors shows overlap between malignant intracranial ectomesenchymoma and MPNST but not medulloblastoma or atypical teratoid rhabdoid tumor," *Acta Neuropathologica*, vol. 113, no. 6, pp. 695–703, 2007.

[15] G. Floris, M. Debiec-Rychter, A. Wozniak et al., "Malignant ectomesenchymoma: genetic profile reflects rhabdomyosarcomatous differentiation," *Diagnostic Molecular Pathology*, vol. 16, no. 4, pp. 243–248, 2007.

[16] D. L. Altenburger, A. S. Wagner, D. E. Esl In, G. S. Pearl, and J. V. Pattisapu, "A rare case of malignant pediatric ectomesenchymoma arising from the falx cerebri," *Journal of Neurosurgery: Pediatrics*, vol. 7, no. 1, pp. 94–97, 2011.

[17] A.-S. Vinck, B. Lerut, R. Hermans, S. Nuyts, R. Sciot, and M. Jorissen, "Malignant ectomesenchymoma of the paranasal sinuses with proptosis," *B-ENT*, vol. 7, no. 3, pp. 201–204, 2011.

[18] S. Howley, D. Stack, T. Morris et al., "Ectomesenchymoma with t(1;12)(p32;p13) evolving from embryonal rhabdomyosarcoma shows no rearrangement of ETV6," *Human Pathology*, vol. 43, no. 2, pp. 299–302, 2012.

[19] C. N. Patil, S. Cyriac, U. Majhi, R. Rajendranath, and T. G. Sagar, "Malignant ectomesenchymoma of the nasal cavity," *Indian Journal of Medical and Paediatric Oncology*, vol. 32, no. 4, pp. 242–243, 2011.

[20] A. Ito, T. Kumabe, R. Saito et al., "Malignant pediatric brain tumor of primitive small round cell proliferation with bland-looking mesenchymal spindle cell elements," *Brain Tumor Pathology*, vol. 30, no. 2, pp. 109–116, 2013.

[21] M. E. Yohe, E. D. Girard, F. S. Balarezo et al., "A novel case of pediatric thoracic malignant ectomesenchymoma in an infant,"

Journal of Pediatric Surgery Case Reports, vol. 1, no. 2, pp. 20–22, 2013.

[22] Children's Oncology Group, *Temozolomide, Cixutumumab, and Combination Chemotherapy in Treating Patients*, National Library of Medicine (US), Bethesda, Md, USA, 2010, http://clinicaltrials.gov/show/NCT01055314%20NLM%20Identifier: NCT01055314.

[23] Children's Oncology Group, *Comparing Two Different Myeloablation Therapies in Treating Young Patients Who Are Undergoing a Stem Cell Transplant for High-Risk Neuroblastoma*, ClinicalTrials.gov, National Library of Medicine (US), Bethesda, Md, USA, 2007, http://clinicaltrials.gov/ct/show/NCT00567567.

[24] E. H. Kawamoto, N. Weidner, R. M. Agostini Jr., and R. Jaffe, "Malignant ectomesenchymoma of soft tissue. Report of two cases and review of the literature," *Cancer*, vol. 59, no. 10, pp. 1791–1802, 1987.

[25] C. A. Hajivassiliou, R. Carachi, E. Simpson, W. J. A. Patrick, and D. G. Young, "Ectomesenchymoma: one or two tumors? Case report and review of the literature," *Journal of Pediatric Surgery*, vol. 32, no. 9, pp. 1351–1355, 1997.

[26] S. C. E. Mouton, H. S. Rosenberg, M. C. Cohen, R. Drut, and M. Emms, "Malignant ectomesenchymoma in childhood," *Pediatric Pathology & Laboratory Medicine*, vol. 16, no. 4, pp. 607–624, 1996.

[27] D. R. Boué, D. M. Parham, B. Webber, W. M. Crist, and S. J. Qualman, "Clinicopathologic study of ectomesenchymomas from intergroup rhabdomyosarcoma study groups III and IV," *Pediatric and Developmental Pathology*, vol. 3, no. 3, pp. 290–300, 2000.

[28] P. H. Sorensen, J. C. Lynch, S. J. Qualman et al., "PAX3-FKHR and PAX7-FKHR gene fusions are prognostic indicators in alveolar rhabdomyosarcoma: a report from the Children's Oncology Group," *Journal of Clinical Oncology*, vol. 20, no. 11, pp. 2672–2679, 2002.

[29] D. M. Loeb, K. Thornton, and O. Shokek, "Pediatric soft tissue sarcomas," *Surgical Clinics of North America*, vol. 88, no. 3, pp. 615–627, 2008.

[30] R. E. Goldsby, C. S. Bruggers, A. R. Brothman, P. H. B. Sorensen, J. B. Beckwith, and T. J. Pysher, "Spindle cell sarcoma of the kidney with ganglionic elements (malignant ectomesenchymoma) associated with chromosomal abnormalities and a review of the literature," *Journal of Pediatric Hematology/Oncology*, vol. 20, no. 2, pp. 160–164, 1998.

[31] E. Koscielniak, D. Harms, G. Henze et al., "Results of treatment for soft tissue sarcoma in childhood and adolescence: a final report of the German cooperative soft tissue sarcoma study CWS-86," *Journal of Clinical Oncology*, vol. 17, no. 12, pp. 3706–3719, 1999.

[32] C. Leaphart and D. Rodeberg, "Pediatric surgical oncology: management of rhabdomyosarcoma," *Surgical Oncology*, vol. 16, no. 3, pp. 173–185, 2007.

[33] G. Cecchetto, G. Bisogno, F. de Corti et al., "Biopsy or debulking surgery as initial surgery for locally advanced rhabdomyosarcomas in children? The experience of the Italian Cooperative Group studies," *Cancer*, vol. 110, no. 11, pp. 2561–2567, 2007.

[34] A. I. Al-Dabbagh and S. A. R. Salih, "Primary lymphoma of Meckle diverticulum: a case report," *Journal of Surgical Oncology*, vol. 28, no. 1, pp. 19–20, 1985.

11

Acute Brachial Artery Thrombosis in a Neonate Caused by a Peripheral Venous Catheter

Simon Berzel,[1] Emilia Stegemann,[2,3] Hans-Joerg Hertfelder,[4]
Katja Schneider,[1] and Nico Hepping[1]

[1] Department of Neonatology, GFO-Hospitals Bonn, St Mary's Hospital, Robert-Koch Street 1, 53115 Bonn, Germany
[2] Department of Vascular Surgery, GFO-Hospitals Bonn, St Mary's Hospital, Bonn, Germany
[3] Department of Cardiology, Pulmonology and Angiology, University Medical Centre, Dusseldorf, Germany
[4] Department of Experimental Hematology and Transfusion Medicine, University Medical Centre, Bonn, Germany

Correspondence should be addressed to Nico Hepping; nico.hepping@marien-hospital-bonn.de

Academic Editor: Francois Cachat

This case describes the diagnostic testing and management of an acute thrombosis of the brachial artery in a female neonate. On day seven of life, clinical signs of acutely decreased peripheral perfusion indicated an occlusion of the brachial artery, which was confirmed by high-resolution Doppler ultrasound. Imaging also showed early stages of collateralization so that surgical treatment options could be avoided. Unfractionated heparin was used initially and then replaced by low-molecular-weight heparin while coagulation parameters were monitored closely. Within several days, brachial artery perfusion was completely restored. Acetylsalicylic acid was given for additional six weeks to minimize the risk of recurring thrombosis. If inadequately fixated in a high-risk location, a peripheral venous catheter can damage adjacent structures and thus ultimately cause arterial complications.

1. Introduction

Occlusion of venous and arterial vessels in childhood is a rare but serious complication. The incidence of neonatal thrombosis is 0.5 per 10,000 live births [1]. The in-hospital incidence of venous or arterial thrombosis is approximately 5.3 per 10,000 children, with increased risk in the neonatal and adolescent period [2].

As per definition, spontaneous thrombotic events are vascular occlusions without an underlying cause, whereas acquired thrombotic events require the presence of a predisposing disease or occur after a therapeutic or diagnostic vascular intervention.

Prothrombotic risk factors in neonates are congenital coagulation defects, maternal gestational diabetes, diabetic fetopathy, neonatal sepsis, necrotizing enterocolitis, asphyxia, polycythemia, and various metabolic diseases [3].

However, the majority of thrombotic events are caused by vascular catheters—more than 90% in neonates are associated with umbilical venous and/or arterial catheters as well as other central venous lines. An acute arterial thrombosis caused by a peripheral venous catheter is extremely rare and quite challenging to manage in a multidisciplinary approach.

2. Case

At 40 + 1/7 weeks of gestational age, a female neonate was born with a birth weight of 4,350 gm via spontaneous vaginal delivery. The pregnancy was uneventful except for a maternal insulin-dependent diabetes. The family history did not reveal any risk factors for hypercoagulability or thrombotic events. As the mother's vaginal smear was GBS-positive, she received a single dose of an antibiotic given intravenously during labor.

The newborn girl did well initially (APGAR 10/10/10; umbilical-artery pH 7,22) but developed hypoglycemia with a blood glucose level of 21 mg/dL after one hour of life, which prompted her transfer to the neonatal intensive care unit. She received glucose intravenously. As elevated inflammatory markers (IL-6 was 146 pg/mL) suggested a neonatal infection, antibiotic therapy (Ampicillin/Sulbactam and Tobramycin) was initiated.

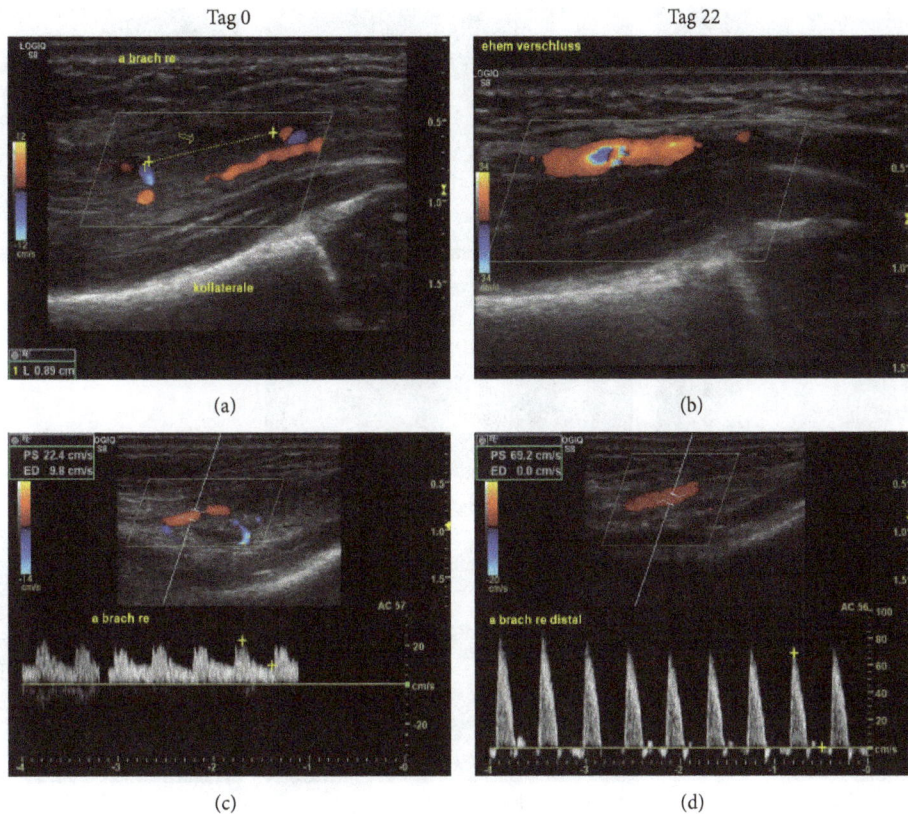

FIGURE 1: (a) Thrombosis of the right brachial artery at the time of diagnosis. (c) Corresponding severely diminished Doppler velocities distal to the site of occlusion (day 0). (b) Restored patency of the brachial artery (day 22). (d) Corresponding normalized Doppler pattern (day 22).

On day two of life, the newborn's blood glucose levels normalized, so glucose infusion was stopped. She received antibiotics for a total of seven days. On day five of treatment, a new peripheral venous catheter (24G Abbocath) was placed at the right antecubital fossa. Approximately 48 hours later, her right hand and forearm showed acute signs of significantly decreased perfusion: pallor, capillary refill of greater than ten seconds, hypothermia, and no detectable radial or ulnar pulses. The PIV was immediately removed.

High-resolution Doppler ultrasound (GE S8, 18 MHz linear hockey stick transducer L8-18i) demonstrated complete occlusion of the distal brachial artery of 8.9 mm in length. Collateral vessels distal from the occlusion site showed a postocclusive, minimally pulsatile Doppler pattern (see Figure 1).

One hour after clinical signs had occurred, the fingertips of the right thumb and index finger developed a livid discoloration due to the predominating ulnar artery, and the remaining fingers continued to have a markedly prolonged capillary refill.

It was felt that the ultrasound images provided all the essential information needed for management decisions so that other imaging modalities such as phlebography or MRI angiography were not pursued, given that they carry significant inherent risks and potential negative side effects for neonates.

Early stages of collateralization and clinical improvement were reassuring, so neonatologists, angiologists, vascular surgeons, and hematology experts agreed on a conservative approach as there was no acute danger of limb loss.

Unfractionated heparin was intravenously given and adjusted to a maximum of 400 IU/kg/d while monitoring activated partial thromboplastin time (aPTT; 65 sec on second day of treatment; target aPTT 60–80 sec) and platelet count. Three days later, it was replaced by subcutaneous Enoxaparin (Clexane). An antifactor Xa level of 0.3 IU/mL was reached with a dose of 3 mg/kg/d on day five of treatment. Although the level was below the therapeutic target range, the dose was not increased further due to clinical improvement. The livid discoloration disappeared on day three of treatment; the capillary refill continued to improve and eventually normalized.

Daily follow-up ultrasound imaging showed progressing recanalization of the brachial artery (illustrated in Figure 2 on day seven after diagnosis). Clinically, radial and ulnar pulses were equally strong on both arms.

Platelet counts remained within the normal range for age and did not suggest heparin-induced thrombocytopenia (HIT). D-dimers showed an initial rise of up to 2.1 mg/L and quickly normalized under therapy. The girl was discharged home on day 18 of life. At that time, her right brachial artery was completely recanalized with unobstructed flow (see Figure 2).

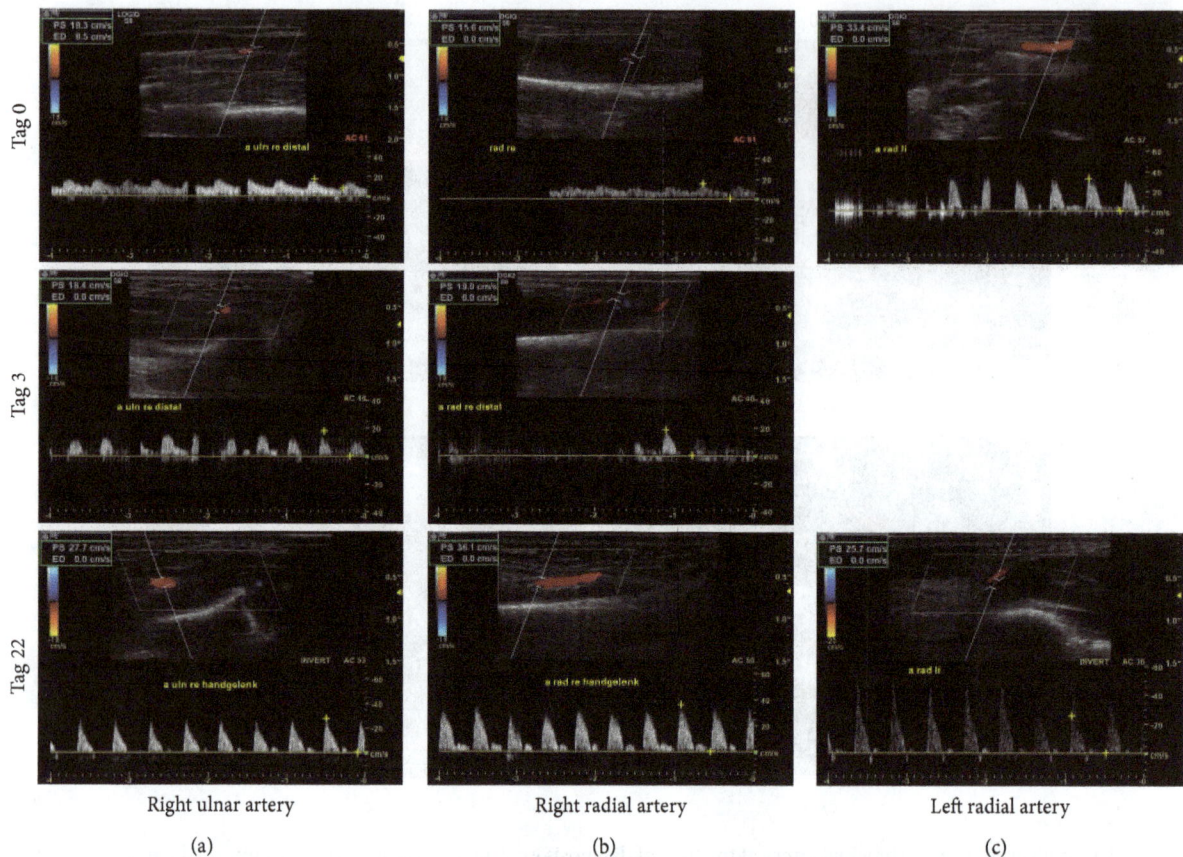

Right ulnar artery	Right radial artery	Left radial artery
(a)	(b)	(c)

FIGURE 2: Velocities of the right radial and ulnar arteries (on day 0 and day 3 and after recanalization on day 22), compared to the left radial artery on days 0 and 22.

Enoxaparin was given subcutaneously until day 20 of treatment; acetylsalicylic acid (ASA) was given in a dose of 3 mg/kg/d for six weeks to minimize the risk of recurring thrombosis. Extensive diagnostic testing (3 days after the thrombotic event) did not reveal any risk factors for hypercoagulability (e.g., deficiency of proteins C and S, antiphospholipid syndrome, and APC resistance).

The brachial artery remained patent beyond the end of therapy. Further clinical observation was done by the pediatrician in the routine preventive examinations.

3. Discussion

Children and adolescents tend to have thrombotic events much less often than adults. The highest risk occurs during the neonatal period, mainly in association with an umbilical venous or arterial catheter or other central venous lines [4]. Thromboembolism caused by a peripheral venous catheter is rare; however, placement can damage both the vein and adjacent tissues such as arteries or nerves.

The case above illustrates the serious complication of brachial artery thrombosis two days after placement of a peripheral venous catheter with subsequent acute ischemia of forearm and hand. It is thought that, because of the time interval between placement and clinical presentation, the peripheral venous catheter was properly placed initially but affected the adjacent artery with repetitive movements of the cubital joint. Unfortunately, at this time, the patient's joint was not stabilized as required. In order to minimize the risk of movement-related complications, arm boards are considered standard of care [5].

Early diagnosis, that is, recognizing the clinical presentation quickly and confirming the suspicion of acute thrombosis with imaging, is crucial for successful treatment and long-term prognosis. One can choose between ultrasounds with color Doppler, venous or arterial angiography, magnetic resonance angiography (MRA), or computed tomography angiography (CTA). With the exception of ultrasound, all other modalities are invasive and carry significant inherent risks and potential negative side effects, particularly for neonates.

Color Doppler ultrasound confirmed the diagnosis and provided all the information necessary for treatment, including clear visualization of collateral vessels. The chance of successful and complete recanalization is highest in the first few days of life in comparison to other age groups, making invasive treatment options for neonates extremely rare. Management should be aimed at reducing thrombus growth, with recanalization of the affected artery being the ultimate treatment goal.

The most recent practice guidelines for pediatric patients are based on adapted treatment regiments for adults. Unfractionated heparin (UFH) is highly recommended as first choice in acute situations [6].

Activated partial thromboplastin time (aPTT) is the most important parameter for monitoring, provided the antithrombin (AT) level is within normal range for age. Therapeutic intravascular lysis or surgical procedures are considered high risk and are therefore only indicated if there is acute danger of limb loss or potential hemodynamic compromise.

The use of UFH is usually followed by LMWH (monitored by antifactor Xa-levels), the subcutaneous application of which can be continued as outpatient therapy. Other advantages include reducing the risk for heparin-induced thrombocytopenia and not requiring any venous catheter for its application.

Moreover, any arterial thrombosis warrants an interdisciplinary discussion about the prophylactic use of antiplatelet medications such as ASA for the individual patient. The duration of ASA therapy for 6 weeks was a clinical decision made in this individual case in the absence of risk factors.

4. Conclusions

Ultrasound is an essential imaging modality used in neonatal intensive care medicine. Our case illustrates how high-resolution color Doppler ultrasound served as a noninvasive diagnostic tool in a seriously sick newborn and as a monitoring device for successful treatment progress.

Anticoagulation with low-molecular-weight heparin should be adjusted based on antifactor Xa-levels. D-dimers are used as an indicator of successful resolution of thrombotic material [7].

Conflict of Interests

The authors declare that there is no conflict of interests regarding the publication of this paper.

References

[1] G. Kenet and U. Nowak-Göttl, "Bleeding and thrombosis issues in pediatric patients: current approach to diagnosis and treatment," *Acta Haematologica*, vol. 115, no. 3-4, pp. 137–140, 2006.

[2] S. Revel-Vilk and A. K. C. Chan, "Anticoagulation therapy in children," *Seminars in Thrombosis and Hemostasis*, vol. 29, no. 4, pp. 425–432, 2003.

[3] Y. I. G. Vladimir Tichelaar, H. J. C. Kluin-Nelemans, and K. Meijer, "Infections and inflammatory diseases as risk factors for venous thrombosis: a systematic review," *Thrombosis and Haemostasis*, vol. 107, no. 5, pp. 827–837, 2012.

[4] B. Schmidt and M. Andrew, "Neonatal thrombosis: Report of a prospective Canadian and international registry," *Pediatrics*, vol. 96, no. 5 I, pp. 939–943, 1995.

[5] J. Pettit, "Assessment of the infant with a peripheral intravenous device," *Advances in Neonatal Care*, vol. 3, no. 5, pp. 230–240, 2003.

[6] P. Monagle, A. K. Chan, N. A. Goldenberg et al., "Antithrombotic therapy in neonates and children: antithrombotic therapy and prevention of thrombosis, 9th ed: American college of chest physicians evidence-based clinical practice guidelines," *Chest*, vol. 141, supplement 2, pp. e737S–e801S, 2012.

[7] J. H. Payne, "Aspects of anticoagulation in children," *British Journal of Haematology*, vol. 150, no. 3, pp. 259–277, 2010.

12

A Rare Case of Esophageal Dysphagia in Children: Aberrant Right Subclavian Artery

Claudia Barone, Nicolina Stefania Carucci, and Claudio Romano

Pediatric Department, University of Messina, Italy

Correspondence should be addressed to Claudio Romano; romanoc@unime.it

Academic Editor: Bernhard Resch

Dysphagia is an impairment of swallowing that may involve any structures from the mouth to the stomach. Esophageal dysphagia presents with the sensation of food sticking, pain with swallowing, substernal pressure, or chronic heartburn. There are many causes of esophageal dysphagia, such as motility disorders and mechanical and inflammatory diseases. Infrequently dysphagia arises from extrinsic compression of the esophagus from any vascular anomaly of the aortic arch. The most common embryologic abnormality of the aortic arch is aberrant right subclavian artery, clinically known as *arteria lusoria*. This abnormality is usually silent. Here, we report a case of six-year-old child presenting to us with a history of progressive dysphagia without respiratory symptoms. A barium esophagogram showed an increase of the physiological esophageal narrowing at the level of aortic arch, while at esophagogastroduodenoscopy there was an extrinsic pulsatile compression of the posterior portion of the esophagus suggesting an extrinsic compression by an aberrant vessel. Angio-CT (computed tomography) scan confirmed the presence of an aberrant right subclavian artery.

1. Introduction

Swallowing is an important function in maintaining optimal nutritional status [1]. It occurs in three phases: oral, pharyngeal, and esophageal. Dysphagia is any disturbance in swallowing, often described by the patients as a "perception" that there is an impediment to the normal passage of the swallowed material [2]. Oropharyngeal dysphagia involves the initial two phases and is rather common in patients with neurological impairment; esophageal dysphagia occurs at the third phase and is most commonly due to functional causes or anatomic abnormalities affecting the esophagus [3, 4]. Early detection of dysphagia in infants and children is important to prevent or minimize complications because if not diagnosed this medical condition can lead to failure to thrive, aspiration pneumonia, gastroesophageal reflux, and/or the inability to establish and maintain proper nutrition and hydration [5]. A variety of medical conditions cause swallowing disorders in pediatric patients [6]. Aberrant right subclavian artery (ARSA) is a rare cause of dysphagia, but it must be taken into account in the differential diagnosis [7]. The majority of patients with this abnormality remain asymptomatic. In other cases ARSA may cause respiratory symptoms in children and dysphagia, cough, and chest pain in adults [7–10]. We report a rare case of six-year-old child presenting to us with a history of progressive dysphagia.

2. Case Report

A six-year-old child presented to our hospital with a progressive history of dysphagia, chest pain, and slow feeding. He did not have respiratory symptoms. His examination was normal with weight and length at the 90th percentile for age. His blood tests were normal. There were no abnormalities on ECG or echocardiography. A barium esophagogram showed an increase of the physiological esophageal narrowing at the level of aortic arch, being suggestive of extrinsic compression. At esophagogastroduodenoscopy, the esophageal mucosa was normal in appearance; biopsy examinations confirmed normal mucosa. About 15 cm from the buccal rhyme there was an extrinsic compression of the posterior portion of the esophagus that was pulsatile, suggestive of an aberrant vessel. Angio-CT (computed tomography) scan confirmed an aberrant right subclavian artery compressing the posterior middle third of the thoracic esophagus (Figure 1). This

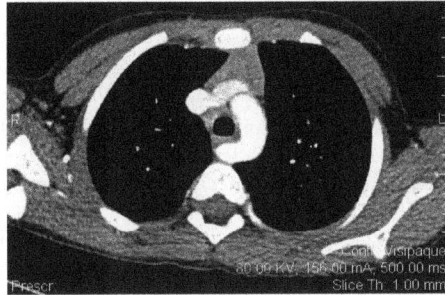

FIGURE 1: *Angio-computed tomography*: demonstrating the aberrant right subclavian artery compressing the esophagus.

artery originated from an aneurismal dilatation (11 mm), Kommerell's diverticulum. An additional finding was the common origin of the right and left carotid arteries from the aortic arch. The patient's discomfort indicated operative repair of this condition. A vascular clamp was applied to the right subclavian artery at its origin from the aortic arch. This artery was divided and the distal portion was trimmed; then an end-to-side anastomosis was made with the right common carotid artery. Our patient reported complete resolution of his symptoms and tolerated a regular diet without dysphagia.

3. Discussion

Dysphagia is defined as difficulty in swallowing food (semisolid or solid), liquid, or both [11]. During normal swallowing, the bolus is propelled from the oral cavity through the pharynx and down the esophagus. Dysphagia occurs when there is a problem with bolus containment and/or propulsion and may occur at the oral, pharyngeal, and/or esophageal phases of swallowing [5, 11–13]. Esophageal dysphagia can arise from a variety of causes such as motility disorders and mechanical and inflammatory diseases [14] shown below.

Causes of esophageal dysphagia in children are as follows

GERD.

Eosinophilic esophagitis.

Tracheoesophageal fistula and esophageal atresia.

Ingestional injuries:

> Caustic.
> Foreign body.

Congenital diaphragmatic hernia.

Cicatricial stenosis.

Esophageal diverticulae.

Motor disorders:

> Achalasia.
> Diffuse esophageal spasm.
> Nutcracker esophagus.
> Hypertensive lower esophageal sphincter.

Extraesophageal compression:

> Mediastinal masses (lymphoma, lymph nodes, and thyromegaly).
> Vascular compression (dysphagia lusoria, dysphagia aortica, and cardiomegaly).

Systemic diseases:

> Crohn's disease.
> Leiomyomatosis.

Iatrogenic complications:

> Radiotherapy.
> Drugs.
> Postsurgical complications.

It is rarely caused by extrinsic compression of the esophagus from any vascular anomaly of the aortic arch [15]. ARSA is the most common congenital anomaly of the aortic arch and has a prevalence ranging from 0.5% to 1.8% in the general population [7, 16, 17]. Although most cases of this anomaly are asymptomatic, symptoms may appear when a "ring" completely encircles the trachea or the esophagus. Extrinsic compression of the esophagus may lead to dysphagia [18, 19]. Symptoms, when present, occur at the two extremes of life. In infants, the trachea is compressible; therefore, the typical signs and symptoms of the compression by arteria lusoria are respiratory, such as wheezing, stridor, recurrent pneumonia, and cyanosis. Dysphagia mostly occurs in adults, in whom respiratory symptoms are rare [8, 20]; adequate management of dysphagia includes a detailed history, evaluation with barium radiography, upper endoscopy, and manometry [14]. The best initial diagnosis would be a barium swallow that will allow for visualization of the esophagus via contrast radiography to determine if there is any evidence of a narrowing due to a stricture, an intraluminal mass, or extraluminal compression [4]. In ARSA, barium esophagogram is often suggestive, showing oblique compression of the esophagus at the level of the third and the fourth thoracic vertebrae [16, 21]. Upper gastrointestinal endoscopy may show prominent aortic pulsation but it is not necessary for the diagnosis. CT or MRI (magnetic resonance imaging) angiography has replaced conventional angiography and is considered the gold standard for the diagnosis. It not only does confirm the diagnosis but also helps to plan the operation and to exclude aneurysm of the aorta or presence of other associated anomalies [17]. Echocardiography has the advantage of a comprehensive assessment of intracardiac anatomy and function. In the presence of respiratory symptoms, the evaluation normally begins with chest radiography [22]. When noisy breathing, stridor, or brassy cough is evident flexible airway endoscopy is the procedure of choice. Despite the accuracy of both MRI and CT in evaluating the nature of the vascular compression of the airways, current techniques do not reliably distinguish between dynamic and static airway narrowing, and coexisting (laryngo) tracheo- or bronchomalacia or tracheal rings can be differentiated with flexible bronchoscopy [23]. Manometry cannot be used to diagnose the condition nor has it been of any assistance in distinguishing which patients may benefit from surgery [21]. The treatment depends on the symptoms, age comorbidity, and concomitant vascular abnormalities of each patient [7]. Surgical approach is indicated when ARSA is symptomatic or has evidence of aneurysm [9]. Various surgical approaches can be used, each with its own advantages and limitations [24]. A symptomatic ARSA can be safely repaired through minimally invasive surgery and endovascular techniques, although symptoms do not always regress. Aggressive treatment of an aneurysmal lusorian artery should be proposed, given the rapid natural evolution towards rupture and high mortality of this complication, despite high operative mortality associated with this elective procedure. Endovascular exclusion is an option in patients who are not good surgical candidates [19].

Summarizing, dysphagia is any disturbance in swallowing that may involve oropharyngeal or esophageal phase. Esophageal dysphagia can arise from a variety of disorders and it is rarely caused by arteria lusoria. Symptoms of ARSA are usually different according to age: children predominantly have respiratory symptoms while dysphagia, cough, and chest pain occur mostly in adults. On the contrary, our patient presented with a long history of dysphagia, associated with chest pain and slow feeding. In conclusion, ARSA is a rare cause of dysphagia but it should be taken into account in the differential diagnosis. It is important to be aware of its existence and features to allow an early diagnosis and avoid unnecessary therapeutic interventions. Only an early detection can prevent or minimize complications: unlike adults, children have rapidly developing body systems and even short-term dysphagia can have a detrimental effect on dietary intake. As a result, swallowing difficulties can interrupt physical growth and cognitive development and cause serious long-term sequelae. For all these reasons, it is imperative to accurately identify and appropriately manage dysphagia in pediatric population.

Abbreviation

ARSA: Aberrant right subclavian artery.

Disclaimer

All the authors approved the final paper as submitted and agree to be accountable for all aspects of the work.

Conflict of Interests

The authors declare that there is no conflict of interests regarding the publication of this paper.

Authors' Contribution

Claudia Barone, Nicolina Stefania Carucci, and Claudio Romano were involved directly in patient care, conducted a literature search of the topic, drafted the initial paper, and approved the final paper as submitted.

References

[1] B. P. Garg, "Dysphagia in children: an overview," *Seminars in Pediatric Neurology*, vol. 10, no. 4, pp. 252–254, 2003.

[2] A. N. Khan, K. Said, M. Ahmad, K. Ali, R. Hidayat, and H. Latif, "Endoscopic findings in patients presenting with oesophageal dysphagia," *Journal of Ayub Medical College Abbottabad*, vol. 26, no. 2, pp. 216–220, 2014.

[3] E. Vaquero-Sosa, L. Francisco-Gonzalez, A. Bodas-Pinedo et al., "Oropharyngeal dysphagia, and underestimated disorder in pediatrics," *Revista Espanola de Enfermedades Digestivas*, vol. 107, pp. 113–115, 2015.

[4] A. B. Grossman and J. Markowitz, "A 12-year-old boy with progressive dysphagia," *The Medscape Journal of Medicine*, vol. 10, no. 10, p. 248, 2008.

[5] J. E. Prasse and G. E. Kikano, "An overview of pediatric dysphagia," *Clinical Pediatrics (Philadelphia)*, vol. 48, no. 3, pp. 247–251, 2009.

[6] L. A. Newman, "Optimal care patterns in pediatric patients with dysphagia," *Seminars in Speech and Language*, vol. 21, no. 4, pp. 281–291, 2000.

[7] M. González-Sánchez, J. L. Pardal-Refoyo, and A. Martín-Sánchez, "The aberrant right subclavian artery and dysphagia lusoria," *Acta Otorrinolaringologica Espanola*, vol. 64, no. 3, pp. 244–245, 2013.

[8] M. Polguj, Ł. Chrzanowski, J. D. Kasprzak, L. Stefańczyk, M. Topol, and A. Majos, "The aberrant right subclavian artery (arteria lusoria): the morphological and clinical aspects of one of the most important variations—a systematic study of 141 reports," *The Scientific World Journal*, vol. 2014, Article ID 292734, 6 pages, 2014.

[9] G. De Araújo, J. W. Junqueira Bizzi, J. Muller, and L. T. Cavazzola, "'Dysphagia lusoria'—right subclavian retroesophageal artery causing intermittent esophageal compression and eventual dysphagia—a case report and literature review," *International Journal of Surgery Case Reports*, vol. 10, pp. 32–34, 2015.

[10] S. Fukuhara, B. Patton, J. Yun, and T. Bernik, "A novel method for the treatment of dysphagia lusoria due to aberrant right subclavian artery," *Interactive Cardiovascular and Thoracic Surgery*, vol. 16, no. 3, pp. 408–410, 2013.

[11] A. Wieseke, D. Bantz, L. Siktberg, and N. Dillard, "Assessment and early diagnosis of dysphagia," *Geriatric Nursing*, vol. 29, no. 6, pp. 376–383, 2008.

[12] P. Dodrill, "Feeding problems and oropharyngeal dysphagia in children," *Journal of Gastroenterology and Hepatology Research*, vol. 3, no. 5, pp. 1055–1060, 2014.

[13] P. Dodrill and M. M. Gosa, "Pediatric dysphagia: physiology, assessment, and management," *Annals of Nutrition and Metabolism*, vol. 66, no. 5, pp. 24–31, 2015.

[14] A. Lawal and R. Shaker, "Esophageal dysphagia," *Physical Medicine and Rehabilitation Clinics of North America*, vol. 19, no. 4, pp. 729–745, 2008.

[15] C. Erami, A. Charaf-Eddine, A. Aggarwal, A. L. Rivard, H. W. Giles, and M. J. Nowicki, "Dysphagia lusoria in an infant," *The Journal of Pediatrics*, vol. 162, no. 6, pp. 1289–1290, 2013.

[16] P. A. Hart and P. S. Kamath, "Dysphagia lusoria," *Mayo Clinic Proceedings*, vol. 87, no. 3, p. e17, 2012.

[17] V. Abraham, A. Mathew, V. Cherian, S. Chandran, and G. Mathew, "Aberrant subclavian artery: anatomical curiosity or clinical entity," *International Journal of Surgery*, vol. 7, no. 2, pp. 106–109, 2009.

[18] R. R. Venugopal, J. P. Kolwalkar, S. P. Krishnajirao, and M. Narayan, "A novel approach for the treatment of dysphagia lusoria," *European Journal of Cardio-Thoracic Surgery*, vol. 43, no. 2, Article ID ezs498, pp. 434–436, 2013.

[19] P. O. Myers, J. H. D. Fasel, A. Kalangos, and P. Gailloud, "Arteria lusoria: developmental anatomy, clinical, radiological and surgical aspects," *Annales de Cardiologie et d'Angeiologie*, vol. 59, no. 3, pp. 147–154, 2010.

[20] S. K. Puri, S. Ghuman, P. Narang, A. Sharma, and S. Singh, "CT and MR angiography in dysphagia lusoria in adults," *Indian Journal of Radiology and Imaging*, vol. 15, no. 4, pp. 497–501, 2005.

[21] A. D. Rogers, M. Nel, E. P. Eloff, and N. G. Naidoo, "Dysphagia lusoria: a case of an aberrant right subclavian artery and a bicarotid trunk," *ISRN Surgery*, vol. 2011, Article ID 819295, 6 pages, 2011.

[22] A. Licari, E. Manca, G. A. Rispoli, S. Mannarino, G. Pelizzo, and G. L. Marseglia, "Congenital vascular rings: a clinical challenge for the pediatrician," *Pediatric Pulmonology*, vol. 50, no. 5, pp. 511–524, 2015.

[23] O. Sacco, S. Panigada, N. Solari et al., "Vascular malformations," in *ERS Handbook, Paediatric Respiratory Medicine*, E. Eber and F. Midulla, Eds., pp. 452–460, European Respiratory Society, Sheffield, UK, 2013.

[24] R. Rathnakar, S. Agarwal, V. Datt, and D. Satsangi, "Dysphagia lusoria with atrial septal defect: simultaneous repair through midline," *Annals of Pediatric Cardiology*, vol. 7, no. 1, pp. 58–60, 2014.

13

Can Attention Deficits Predict a Genotype? Isolate Attention Difficulties in a Boy with Klinefelter Syndrome Effectively Treated with Methylphenidate

Antonella Gagliano,[1] Eva Germanò,[1] Loredana Benedetto,[2] and Gabriele Masi[3]

[1] Division of Child Neurology and Psychiatry, Department of Pediatrics, University of Messina, Via Consolare Valeria, 98125 Messina, Italy

[2] Division of Psychology, Department of Humanities and Social Sciences, University of Messina, Via Concezione, No. 6/8, 98100 Messina, Italy

[3] IRCCS Stella Maris, Scientific Institute Child Neurology and Psychiatry, Viale del Tirreno, No. 331, 56018 Calambrone, Pisa, Italy

Correspondence should be addressed to Antonella Gagliano; agagliano@unime.it

Academic Editor: Karen Kowal

This paper describes a 17-year-old boy who was diagnosed with Klinefelter syndrome (KS) (XXY) at the age of 16 years. Although cognitive level was absolutely normal, he showed attentional difficulties that negatively affected school adjustment. He was successfully treated with methylphenidate. A significant improvement was observed in the ADHD Rating Scale IV and in the inattention subscale score of the Conners Scales. The CGI-S score improved from 3 to 1, and the CGI-I score at the end point was 1 (very much improved). Also attention measures, particularly forward and backward digit span, improved with MPH treatment. Given the widely variable and often aspecific features, KS may run undiagnosed in a large majority of affected patients. A close attention to the cognitive phenotype may favour a correct diagnosis, and a timely treatment.

1. Introduction

Klinefelter syndrome (KS) (47, XXY) is a sex chromosome aneuploidy associated with speech and language deficits, socioemotional difficulties, motor dysfunction, and frontal lobe deficits including attention, planning, and organization, possibly in response to the pubertal hormonal abnormalities. It is the most common chromosome abnormality in humans (1:500 to 1:1000 males), but due to the widely variable and often aspecific features, only one out of four cases are recognized [1]. Some studies hypothesize that supernumerary X chromosome and/or congenital hypogonadism can favour structural alterations in the subcortical pathways involved in language processing, thus providing a neurobiological substrate for cognitive deficits in KS. The phenotype might be due to overexpression of genes on the extra X chromosome. Examination of X-linked differentially expressed genes, such as GTPBP6, TAF9L, and CXORF21, suggesting

verbal cognition-gene expression correlations, may establish a causal link between these genes, neurodevelopment, and language function [2]. In order to explain the linguistic impairment, the neurexin-neuroligin hypothesis has been recently proposed [3]. Neuroligin genes, on both X and Y chromosomes, are involved in the same synaptic networks as neurexin genes, with common variants associated with increased risk for language impairment and autism. The effect of a triple dose of neuroligin gene product is particularly detrimental when associated with specific variants of neurexin genes on other chromosomes. Structural brain abnormalities have been also described by MRI, such as a decreased brain volume, particularly in frontal lobe, temporal lobe, and superior temporal gyrus were observed bilaterally in a sample of XXY men [4]. Cognitive phenotype is extremely etherogeneous. Youths with KS may present deficits in language skills, verbal processing speed, verbal and nonverbal executive abilities, motor dexterity, and in reading and spelling [5]. Early motor and speech disturbances are the earlier presentation of the central nervous system dysfunction associated with androgen deficiency that is influential in brain organization, neurobehavioral development, temperament, and mood [6]. Neuropsychological deficits have been also reported in tasks exploring executive functions (EF). Recent findings suggest that executive dysfunctions associated with KS can be selectively identified, and they are particularly evident in the inhibitory subcomponent [7]. The attention and behavioural features reported in KS boys, namely, the attentional deficits, are often consistent with a cooccurring diagnosis of attention deficit/hyperactivity disorder (ADHD) [8]. Behavioral features are not homogeneous, including attention disorders, impaired social skills, autism spectrum symptoms, and other psychiatric disturbance [9]. There is also a strong variability among affected individuals, from minimal to significant cognitive and behavioral disorders [10]. When patients with KS have a normal IQ, the attention deficit could be a strong indicator of a genotype that may be otherwise unrecognized. Moreover, during prepubertal age, pathognomonic clinical features of KS are often lacking, but a characteristic cognitive and behavioral pattern is usually evident [11]. Early detection and immediate starting of educational supports is crucial to ameliorate the outcome and to reduce the psychopathological risk. This paper describes and comments the case of a KS boy with normal cognitive abilities and selective attentional deficits, successfully treated with methylphenidate (MPH).

2. Case Presentation

L. is a 17-year-old boy who was diagnosed with KS (XXY) at the age of 16 years. His physical characteristics included tall stature, hypogonadism, and fertility problems. After an uneventful full-term birth, he had normal cognitive and motor development and only mild language delay, with rapid spontaneous normalization. During primary school, modest academic difficulties, but no academic failures, are reported. Emotional and social development was normal, with mild, not impairing social anxiety, subthreshold obsessive-compulsive symptoms and a mild weakening in self-esteem. Although cognitive level, assessed by Wechsler Intelligence Scale for Children (WISC-III) at 12 years old, was absolutely normal (Verbal IQ 108; Performance IQ 115; Full IQ 110); he showed attentional difficulties that negatively affected school adjustment. However, he was able to attend secondary school with no help. But, during his third level of junior high school, his difficulties grew and he failed a grade. Given the persisting attentional difficulties during the fourth year of junior high school, parents agreed to start treatment with methylphenidate immediate release (MPH). At that time L. was drug naïve and not treated with testosterone. MPH was started at a dose of 10 mg/day b.i.d. (0.3 mg/kg/day; weight 66 kg) (morning and early afternoon), with weekly increments with flexible dosing strategy of 5 mg for each administration, up to 40 mg/day b.i.d. (0.6 mg/kg/day). The followup was performed at baseline and at the end point of the 3rd month after the start of MPH. Behavioural

assessment was performed according to parent- and self-report scales and was performed by attentional tasks. The primary measure of effectiveness was the ADHD-RS-IV [12], with 18 items, rated on a scale from 0 (never/rarely) to 3 (very often). Secondary outcome measures were Conners Rating Scale-Revised, Short Form for Parents (CPRS), Teachers (CTRS), and Youth (CY-self-report) [13] and Clinical Global Impressions-Severity (CGI-S) and Improvement (CGI-I) [14]. The CPRS is an assessment tool that provides valuable information about the child's behavior. This instrument is helpful when a diagnosis of ADHD is being considered and when follow-up measures are required. It consists of four distinct subscales: (1) oppositional (this subscale indicates an individual with a tendency to break rules and to have problems with persons in authority); (2) inattention (it specifies problems organizing own work, completing tasks on schoolwork, or concentrating on tasks that require sustained mental effort); (3) hyperactivity (this subscale indicates a subject having difficulty sitting still or remaining at the same task for very long; (4) ADHD index consists of the single best set of items for differentiating children/adolescents with attention problems from those without attention problems.

Emotional symptoms were evaluated using a self-report scale for depressive symptoms (Children's Depression Inventory, CDI) [15] and a self-report Multidimensional Anxiety Scale for Children (MASC) [16]. Diagnostic assessment included also electroencephalogram (EEG) and magnetic resonance imaging (MRI), that were both normal. We used the "Di Nuovo" attention test (DNAT) as assessment instrument to measure the attentive subdomains [17], a neurophysiological measure of attention, based on a computerized series of tasks that assess the responses to either visual or auditory stimuli. The DNAT indices include both visual and auditory information processing, omission and commission errors, and reaction times. Furthermore a short term memory task (forward and backward digit span), encompassed in DNAT, was assessed. All attention measures were assessed between the 2nd and the 3rd hour after the administration of the MPH. Response to treatment was evaluated according to changes from the baseline (pretreatment) to the end point at week 12 (posttreatment). Weight, height, blood pressure and pulse were evaluated at each visit. The study was approved by the local Ethics Committee.

A significant improvement was observed in the primary outcome measure (ADHD Rating Scale IV). The total score (rated and scored by investigators based on parent reports; ADHD-RS-IV-Parent:Inv) changed from 21 ($M = 2.22$, SD = 0.97) to 9 ($M = 1.00$, SD = 0.71), paired-sample $t(8) = 5.50$; $P < .001$, one-tail, and Cohen's $d = 1.43$ (Figure 1).

The CGI-S score improved as well from 3 to 1, and the CGI-I score at the end point was 1 (very much improved).

According to the secondary measures, the CPRS Inattention subscale of parents and teachers significantly improved as well as boy's ratings of CY-self-report. Pairwise differences calculation has been performed between pretreatment (M_{pre}) and posttreatment scores (M_{post}). These scores corresponded to the mean values between parents, teachers, and self-report scores at CPRS, calculated for all four subscales: (1) oppositional, (2) inattentive, (3) hyperactive, and (4) ADHD

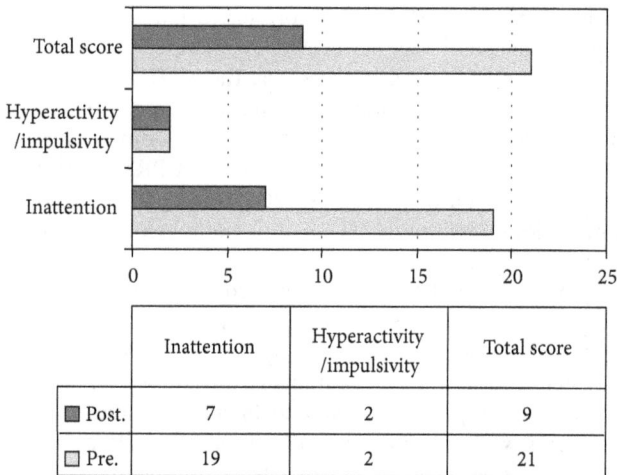

	Inattention	Hyperactivity /impulsivity	Total score
■ Post.	7	2	9
□ Pre.	19	2	21

FIGURE 1: ADHD-RS-IV-Parent:Inv: raw scores in baseline (pre-treatment) and with MPH treatment (posttreatment). The total score improved from 21 ($M = 2.22$, SD = 0.97) to 9 ($M = 1.00$, SD = 0.71), paired-sample $t(8) = 5.50$; $P < .001$, one-tail, and Cohen's $d = 1.43$.

index; $M_{pre} = 73.00$ ($SD_{pre} = 2.65$) versus $M_{post} = 48.67$ ($SD_{post} = 6.81$), paired-sample $t(2) = 8.54$; $P < .01$, one-tail, and Cohen's $d = 4.71$ (Figure 2).

The attention tests (DNAT) at the baseline showed scores below the average in two attentional tasks (task 2: multiple choice of visual stimuli; task 3B: visual selective attention). All attentional scores significantly improved after MPH treatment. A comparison between the mean value of all nine subscores pretreatment (M_{pre}) and the mean value of all nine subscores posttreatment (M_{post}) was performed: $M_{pre} = 2.78$ ($SD_{pre} = 3.42$) versus $M_{post} = 0.89$ ($SD_{post} = 1.05$); nonparametric Wilcoxon test $z = -2.26$; $P < .05$, one-tail (Figure 3). All measures significantly improved.

The DNAT forward and backward digit span improved with MPH treatment (Figure 4).

In addition, over a three-month MPH treatment, parents and teachers reported strong improvement in academic performances, with upgrading of the evaluations in all the domains. At the baseline, no significant self-reported depressive symptoms (CDI score 11, below the cutoff score 19) were reported, but subtle anxiety symptoms were detected. At the baseline MASC, subtle anxiety symptoms were detected. After the treatment, basal MASC global score decreased from 54 to 45 and anxiety disorder index from 56 to 48, with the main effect in social anxiety dimension score. Neither adverse effects nor medication-related problems were reported.

3. Discussion

Compared to other genetic syndromes deriving from chromosomal trisomy, cognitive abilities in KS may be apparently normal, although a specific assessment may evidence more subtle cognitive and behavioral impairments affecting social, emotional, and academic functioning. This case report focuses on cognitive features in a boy with KS and comorbid ADHD, inattentive subtype. Comorbid ADHD in

		Paired-sample t				
Subscales		Pairwise differences	t	df	P	d
		M SD				
(1)	Oppositional, pretreatment Oppositional, posttreatment	2.67 3.05	1.51	2	0.270	0.60
(2)	Inattentive, pretreatment Inattentive, posttreatment	24.33 4.93	8.54	2	0.013	4.71
(3)	Hyperactive, pretreatment Hyperactive, posttreatment	4.00 3.46	2.00	2	0.184	0.74
(4)	ADHD index, pretreatment ADHD index, posttreatment	19.67 1.15	29.50	2	0.001	3.51

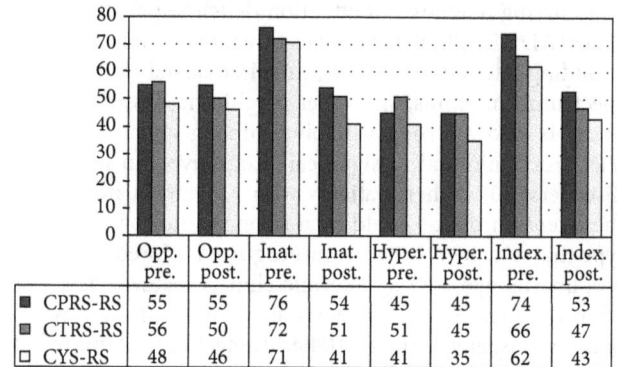

	Opp. pre.	Opp. post.	Inat. pre.	Inat. post.	Hyper. pre.	Hyper. post.	Index. pre.	Index. post.
■ CPRS-RS	55	55	76	54	45	45	74	53
■ CTRS-RS	56	50	72	51	51	45	66	47
□ CYS-RS	48	46	71	41	41	35	62	43

FIGURE 2: Conners Rating Scale for Parents (CPRS-RS), Teachers (CTRS-RS), and Boy (Conners Youth Self-report Rating Scale, CYS-RS); T scores in baseline (pretreatment) and with MPH treatment (posttreatment). Pairwise differences calculation has been performed between pre- and posttreatment scores. These scores corresponded to the mean values between parents, teachers, and self-report scores at CPRS, calculated for all four subscales: (1) oppositional, (2) inattentive, (3) hyperactive, and (4) ADHD index.

males with XXY is frequent, and it may be strongly related to poorer EF skills [18]. More in general, deficits in the ability to sustain attention with or without impulsivity are frequently reported in young boys with KS, and they can represent a component of the KS cognitive phenotype [5]. Nevertheless, there is a lack of data in the literature on ADHD treatment in KS. A recent paper of Tartaglia and colleagues [8] shows that psychopharmacologic treatment of ADHD with stimulants was effective in 73% of XXY, with a relatively low rate of significant side effects. Moreover, KS increased vulnerability to psychiatric disorders, such as ADHD, and to difficulties in language skills and social interactions can reveal important insights into genotype-phenotype associations [19]. Persisting school difficulties are usual, even in patients with normal IQ, with special needs of educational support. An analysis of these associations can yield more insight into genotype-phenotype associations [19], with implications on treatment. Our patient shows scores below the average in two attentional tasks regarding visual multiple choice and divided-attention tasks. Both neuropsychological deficits and scholastic difficulties dramatically improved during MPH treatment. Both visual multiple choice and divided-attention tasks improved, and MPH was effective as in patients without KS. The improvement of his divided-attention ability with MPH treatment is consistent with the behavioural

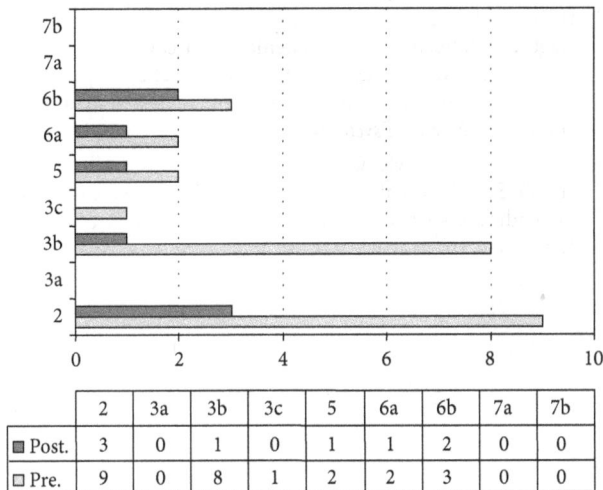

	2	3a	3b	3c	5	6a	6b	7a	7b
■ Post.	3	0	1	0	1	1	2	0	0
□ Pre.	9	0	8	1	2	2	3	0	0

FIGURE 3: "Di Nuovo" attention test is the number of commission errors on nine attention tasks in baseline (pretreatment) and with MPH treatment (posttreatment). The mean value of all nine subscores pretreatment (M_{pre}) was compared to the mean value of all nine subscores posttreatment (M_{post}). M_{pre} = 2.78 (SD_{pre} = 3.42) versus M_{post} = 0.89 (SD_{post} = 1.05); nonparametric Wilcoxon test $z = -2.26$; $P < .05$, one-tail. Description of tasks is as follows: 2: multiple choice (visual stimuli); 3A: selective attention (auditory stimuli); 3B: selective attention (visual stimuli); 3C: barrage (visual stimuli); 5: divided attention; 6A: Stroop task-trial A; 6B: Stroop task-trial B; 7A: multiple barrage (auditory stimuli); 7B: multiple barrage (visual stimuli).

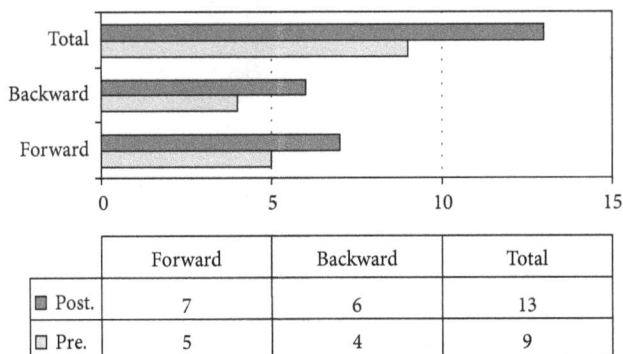

	Forward	Backward	Total
■ Post.	7	6	13
□ Pre.	5	4	9

FIGURE 4: Digit span: number of forward and backward digits in baseline (pretreatment) and with MPH treatment (posttreatment).

measures of attention capacities. Actually, improvement in visual attention can lead to a variety of changes in behavior, from more efficient information processing, to a large extent, what information about the environment is perceived. These abilities are conceptually related to working memory. Working memory span tasks may also measure interference proneness and suggests that resistance to interference may affect performance on many cognitive tasks. In our patient, the verbal working memory, as measured by performance on the backward digit span task, seems to be improved by MPH treatment. This evidence is consistent with a recent meta-analysis on effects of MPH on cognitive functions in children and adolescents with ADHD [20]. Furthermore,

MPH appeared helpful for anxious symptoms in our KS boy, as a consequence of positive changes in academic and social performances. This new condition could have positively influenced the emotional state, ameliorating his emotional symptoms and, subsequently, his enthusiasm and motivation to achieve scholastic contents. Our report, next to others that document psychiatric and social difficulties in KS patients, underlines that adaptive functioning is not only dependent on particular cognitive ability level, but also on the capability to use every skills effectively in order to get used to the social and work demands of everyday life. Given the pivotal role of attention in typically developing children in driving early developmental changes and outcomes and also more generally in shaping the broader sociocognitive landscape, some authors strongly suggest to extend the research to atypical populations, focusing on neurodevelopmental disorders with a clearly defined genetic origin [21]. Given the widely variable and often aspecific features, KS may run undiagnosed in a large majority of affected patients. A close attention to the cognitive phenotype may favour a correct diagnosis and a timely treatment. Psychiatric comorbidity in KS can be neglected as well. Symptoms of ADHD, and particularly attentional deficits, may be an important component of cognitive phenotype, even in patients with normal IQ. Thus it seems of paramount importance to explore how attention and other behavioral difficulties may constrain learning and sociocognitive outcomes across genetic neurodevelopmental disorders. When correctly diagnosed, ADHD in KS can be effectively treated with MPH across developmental time, even in late adolescence, and attentional deficits may strongly improve, with positive effects on academic performances and on emotional and social functioning.

Consent

Written informed consent was obtained from the parent of this patient for publication of this case report. The parents have discussed the consent with the authors of this paper and they have been guaranteed that the name will not be published and as far as possible all identifying features will be removed.

Conflict of Interests

The authors declare that there is no conflict of interests regarding the publication of this paper.

References

[1] J. C. Giltay and M. C. Maiburg, "Klinefelter syndrome: clinical and molecular aspects," *Expert Review of Molecular Diagnostics*, vol. 10, no. 6, pp. 765–776, 2010.

[2] M. P. Vawter, P. D. Harvey, and L. E. DeLisi, "Dysregulation of X-linked gene expression in Klinefelter's syndrome and association with verbal cognition," *American Journal Medical Genetics B*, vol. 144, no. 6, pp. 728–734, 2007.

[3] D. V. Bishop and G. Scerif, "Klinefelter syndrome as a window on the aetiology of language and communication impairments

in children: the neuroligin-neurexin hypothesis," *Acta Paedi-atrica, International Journal of Paediatrics*, vol. 100, no. 6, pp. 903–907, 2011.

[4] J. N. Giedd, L. S. Clasen, G. L. Wallace et al., "XXY (Klinefelter syndrome): a pediatric quantitative brain magnetic resonance imaging case-control study," *Pediatrics*, vol. 119, no. 1, pp. e232–e240, 2007.

[5] J. L. Ross, D. P. Roeltgen, G. Stefanatos et al., "Cognitive and motor development during childhood in boys with Klinefelter syndrome," *American Journal of Medical Genetics A*, vol. 146, no. 6, pp. 708–719, 2008.

[6] C. Samango-Sprouse, "Expansion of the phenotypic profile of the young child with XXY," *Pediatric Endocrinology Reviews*, vol. 8, supplement 1, pp. 160–168, 2010.

[7] K. Kompus, R. Westerhausen, L.-G. Nilsson et al., "Deficits in inhibitory executive functions in Klinefelter (47, XXY) syndrome," *Psychiatry Research*, vol. 189, no. 1, pp. 135–140, 2011.

[8] N. R. Tartaglia, N. Ayari, C. Hutaff-Lee, and R. Boada, "Attention-deficit hyperactivity disorder symptoms in children and adolescents with sex chromosome aneuploidy: XXY, XXX, XYY, and XXYY," *Journal of Developmental and Behavioral Pediatrics*, vol. 33, no. 4, pp. 309–318, 2012.

[9] D. V. M. Bishop, P. A. Jacobs, K. Lachlan et al., "Autism, language and communication in children with sex chromosome trisomies," *Archives of Disease in Childhood*, vol. 96, no. 10, pp. 954–959, 2011.

[10] N. Tartaglia, L. Cordeiro, S. Howell, R. Wilson, and J. Janusz, "The spectrum of the behavioral phenotype in boys and adolescents 47,XXY (Klinefelter syndrome)," *Pediatric Endocrinology Reviews*, vol. 8, pp. 151–159, 2010.

[11] M. F. Messina, D. L. Sgrò, T. Aversa, M. Pecoraro, M. Valenzise, and F. de Luca, "A characteristic cognitive and behavioral pattern as a clue to suspect Klinefelter syndrome in prepubertal age," *The Journal of the American Board of Family Medicine*, vol. 25, no. 5, pp. 745–749, 2012.

[12] G. J. DuPaul, T. J. Power, A. D. Anastopoulos, and R. Reid, *ADHD Rating Scale—IV: Checklists, Norms, and Clinical Inter-pretations*, The Guilford Press, New York, NY, USA, 1998.

[13] C. K. Conners, *Conners Rating Scales: Revised Technical Manual*, Multi-Health Systems, North Tonawanda, NY, USA, 1997.

[14] W. Guy, *ECDEU Assessment Manual for Psychopharmacology, Revised*, Publication ADM 76-338, U.S. Department of Health, Education, and Welfare, Bethesda, Md, USA, 1976.

[15] M. Kovacs, "Rating scales to assess depression in school-aged children," *Acta Paedopsychiatrica*, vol. 46, no. 5-6, pp. 305–315, 1981.

[16] J. S. March, J. D. Parker, K. Sullivan, P. Stallings, and K. Conners, "The multidimensional anxiety scale for children (MASC)," *Journal of the American Academy of Child & Adolescent Psychiatry*, vol. 36, pp. 554–565, 1997.

[17] S. Di Nuovo, "Attenzione e concentrazione. 7 test e 12 training di potenziamento," Ed Erikson, Trento, Italy, 2000.

[18] N. R. Lee, G. L. Wallace, L. S. Clasen et al., "Executive function in young males with Klinefelter (XXY) syndrome with and without comorbid attention-deficit/hyperactivity disorder," *Journal of the International Neuropsychological Society*, vol. 22, pp. 1–9, 2011.

[19] D. H. Geschwind, K. B. Boone, B. L. Miller, and R. S. Swerdloff, "Neurobehavioral phenotype of Klinefelter syndrome," *Mental Retardation and Developmental Disabilities Research Reviews*, vol. 6, no. 2, pp. 107–116, 2000.

[20] D. R. Coghill, S. Seth, S. Pedroso, T. Usala, J. Currie, and A. Gagliano, "Effects of methylphenidate on cognitive functions in children and adolescents with attention-deficit/hyperactivity disorder: evidence from a systematic review and a meta-analysis," *Biological Psychiatry*, 2013.

[21] K. Cornish, A. Steele, C. R. C. Monteiro, A. Karmiloff-Smith, and G. Scerif, "Attention deficits predict phenotypic outcomes in syndrome-specific and domain-specific ways," *Frontiers in Psychology*, vol. 3, article 227, 2012.

14

Multiple Cardiac Rhabdomyomas, Wolff-Parkinson-White Syndrome, and Tuberous Sclerosis: An Infrequent Combination

Elena Castilla Cabanes[1,2] **and Isaac Lacambra Blasco**[1]

[1] *Echocardiography Section, Department of Cardiology, Hospital Clínico Universitario de Zaragoza, Avenida San Juan Bosco 15, 50009 Zaragoza, Spain*
[2] *Department of Cardiology, Hospital General Universitario de Elche, Camí de L'Almassera 11, Alicante, 03023 Elche, Spain*

Correspondence should be addressed to Elena Castilla Cabanes; elena_castilla@hotmail.com

Academic Editor: Maria Moschovi

Cardiac rhabdomyomas are benign cardiac tumours and are often associated with tuberous sclerosis. They are often asymptomatic with spontaneus regresion but can cause heart failure, arrhythmias, and obstruction. There have also been a few isolated reports of Wolff-Parkinson-White syndrome occurring in association with tuberous sclerosis and the great majority has been detected in patients with concomitant rhabdomyomas. We report a 12-day-old infant girl with tuberous sclerosis who presented with intraparietal and intracavitary rhabdomyomas with a Wolff-Parkinson-White syndrome (WPW). She represents one of the few published cases of WPW syndrome and tuberous sclerosis and particularly interesting because of intramural rhabdomyomas regression with persistent intracavitary rhabdomyomas after two years of followup.

1. Introduction

Cardiac rhabdomyomas are benign cardiac tumours and are often associated with tuberous sclerosis [1]. They must be investigated by echocardiography in this setting. They are often asymptomatic but can cause heart failure, arrhythmias, and obstruction. In these cases, they must be operated upon. In other cases—and because of their tendency to regress spontaneously—these tumours are simply monitored by echocardiography and Holter recording, in addition to usual clinical examinations. There have also been a few isolated reports of Wolff-Parkinson-White syndrome occurring in association with tuberous sclerosis and the great majority has been detected in patients with concomitant rhabdomyomas; however its prevalence in this syndrome is unknown.

2. Case Report

We report a 12-day-old infant girl who presented with a supraventricular tachycardia at a rate of 250 beats/min and tachypnea. She was admitted to hospital and electrocardiogram showed supraventricular tachycardia with delta wave and diagnosis of Wolff-Parkinson-White (WPW) syndrome was made. Physical and radiological examination showed pulmonary congestion. She was treated with 0,07 mg/6 hours of intravenous propranolol and 6 mg/day of intravenous furosemide and had a satisfactory evolution. A transthoracic echocardiography was made to look for a possible structural cardiopathy that showed multiple rounded, homogeneous, and echo-dense intracavitary masses in interventricular septum, free lateral wall of left ventricle, free wall of right atrium, mitral valve, and septal tricuspid leaflet that conditioned moderate tricuspid regurgitation; all fit in with multiple congenital cardiac rhabdomyomas (Figure 1). No neurological deficit was detected at the time of diagnosis.

Therefore tuberous sclerosis was thought to be a possible concomitant disease with both WPW syndrome and cardiac rhabdomyomas. A second stigma of tuberous sclerosis was found in cranial magnetic resonance, a subependymal tumour, that allowed achieving the final diagnosis. Thoracic-abdominal-pelvic computed tomography and electroencephalogram were normal. Molecular genetic test for tuberous sclerosis showed mutation of *TSC1* gen.

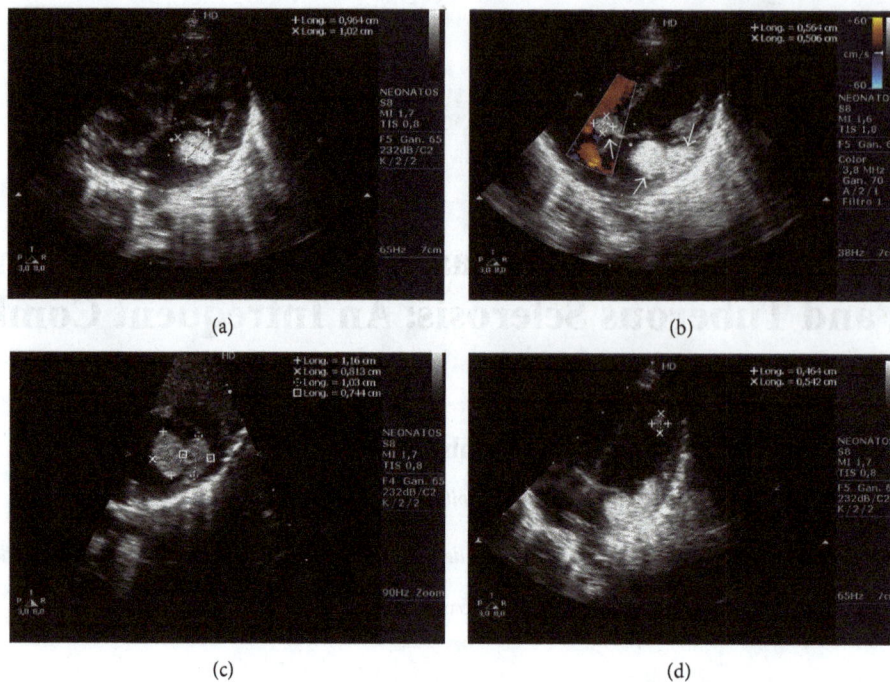

FIGURE 1: Views of different sizes and localisations of rhabdomyomas at the time of diagnosis. (a) Four-chamber view with intracavitary masses in mitral valve of 0,9 × 1 cm. (b) Four-chamber doppler-colour view of intracavitary mass of 0,5 × 0,5 cm in tricuspid valve, one intracavitary mass in mitral valve and one intraparietal mass in lateral wall of left atrium (arrows). (c) Subcostal view of left ventricule. One intracavitary mass and one intraparietal mass in lateral face of left ventricule. (d) Four-chamber view of intraparietal tumour in left ventricule apex.

Twenty-eight months after followup, the girl remained asymptomatic with propranolol 0,5 mg/mL, with only small skin lesions, suggestive of cutaneous fibroids, appearing. There were no new episodes of supraventricular tachycardia, and neurological development remained normal. Echocardiographies showed progressive intramural tumors regression that almost disappeared, while the intracavitary remained with a similar size (Figure 2).

3. Discussion

Tuberous sclerosis is a neurocutaneous syndrome with autosomal dominant inheritance and has a reported incidence of 1 : 6.000. Formerly recognised by the clinical trial of epilepsy, mental retardation, and facial angiofibromatosis, it is appreciated that almost any organ of the body may be affected. The most common cardiac manifestation of the disease is the cardiac rhabdomyoma, which is thought to occur in at least 60% of children with tuberous sclerosis. A review of all papers on cardiac rhabdomyomas published up to 1990 is available [2]. At least 51% of tumours were associated with tuberous sclerosis and this rose to 86% if all patients with a possible diagnosis of tuberous sclerosis were included [2]. These benign tumours seem to originate from embryonic myocytes, representing hamartomas. The involution may be related to the inability of the tumours to divide while the heart chambers grow. Rhabdomyomas are usually highly reflective tumours, arising from the myocardium, but may be intramural, complicating the diagnosis. If a

patient with tuberous sclerosis has multiple cardiac tumours on echocardiography, they are generally considered to be cardiac rhabdomyomas [3]. Furthermore, in view of the high frequency of rhabdomyomas in infants with tuberous sclerosis, echocardiography has been proposed by some as a diagnostic tool when tuberous sclerosis is suspected in infants, even in the absence of other clinical signs, which is common at this age [1].

Cardiac rhabdomyomas have been reported to regress spontaneously in the first years of life, although the regression mechanism is not yet well understood. Recently, in a series of 154 patients with tuberous sclerosis, partial regression of the cardiac rhabdomyomas was reported in 50% of cases and complete resolution was showed in 18% of cases [4]. An earlier report found regression rates of 60% in preadolescent tuberous sclerosis patients and 18% in adult tuberous sclerosis patients [4, 5]. Our patient has the distinction of being one of the few published cases with intramural rhabdomyomas regression with persistent intracavitary rhabdomyomas, which remained in similar size in the two-year followup [6]. The explanation for the regression of only intramural rhabdomyomas is currently unknown, but it does weigh on the possible involvement of embryogenesis, which may be different in each type of rhabdomyoma.

Cardiac rhabdomyomas are typically asymptomatic and are therefore usually not operated upon unless they are obstructive, cause heart failure, or are complicated with severe intractable arrhythmias [7]. Also, they can be difficult to remove completely, because they are often located in the

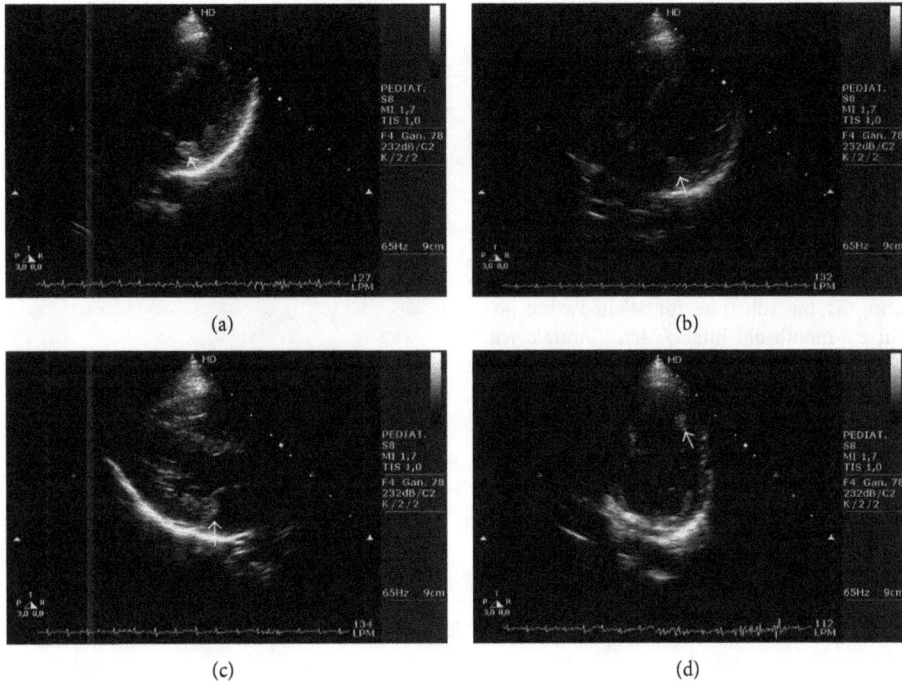

(a)

(b)

(c)

(d)

FIGURE 2: Royalty rhabdomyomas after 28-month followup. Note the disappearance of intramural rhabdomyomas and persistence of rhabdomyoma mainly located in the anterior leaflet of the mitral valve. (a) Four-chamber view with intracavitary mass in mitral valve (arrow). Disappearance of intraparietal mass in lateral wall of left atrium viewed in Figure 1(b). (b) Four-chamber doppler-colour view of intracavitary mass in tricuspid valve smaller than before, one intracavitary mass in mitral valve and disappearance of intraparietal mass in lateral wall of left atrium (arrow). (c) Longitudinal long axis of left ventricule with intracavitary mass on mitral valve (arrow). (d) Four-chamber view of intraparietal tumour in left ventricule apex smaller than before (arrow).

deep myocardium. No embolic events have been reported and there is no need for oral anticoagulation in the absence of a specific indication (e.g., atrial fibrillation). Although there are no consistent guidelines, cardiac monitoring may be proposed for all tuberous sclerosis patients with rhabdomyomas, with serial annual or biannual echocardiograms to detect haemodynamic compromise and annual Holter monitoring to detect severe arrhythmias, even if most patients are usually free from cardiac symptoms. When symptoms are present, they are generally related to the size of the tumours and their location. In our patient echocardiogram after twenty-eight months of followup showed partial regression of rhabdomyomas, as explained previously, and Holter monitoring showed sinusal rhythm with WPW syndrome with 85 beats/min.

There have also been a few isolated reports of Wolff-Parkinson-White syndrome occurring in association with tuberous sclerosis, with and without rhabdomyomas, and its prevalence is not well known. The aetiology of Wolff-Parkinson-White syndrome in tuberous sclerosis has not been explained. It has been known for some time that some of the cells in the cardiac rhabdomyomas found in patients with tuberous sclerosis are structurally identical to normal Purkinje cells, so it has been presumed that rhabdomyomatous tissue traversing the atrioventricular junction acts as the accessory pathway bypassing the atrioventricular node. This occurs more often in males and almost exclusively in association with cardiac rhabdomyomas. It presents early in life, often on day 1, and is usually associated with symptomatic supraventricular tachycardia. It responds well to medical treatment and a high proportion of cases will resolve over time, as it occurs in the present case [8] with 1 mg/8 hours of oral propranolol. To our knowledge this is the only case so far published, bringing together in one case the presence of tuberous sclerosis associated with WPW syndrome and cardiac rhabdomyomas, which present unusual regression with persistent intracardiac rhabdomyomas and disappearance of those intramurals.

Conflict of Interests

The authors report no financial relationships or conflict of interests regarding the content herein.

References

[1] G. H. Watson, "Cardiac rhabdomyomas in tuberous sclerosis," *Annals of the New York Academy of Sciences*, vol. 615, pp. 50–57, 1991.

[2] C. O. Harding and R. A. Pagon, "Incidence of tuberous sclerosis in patients with cardiac rhabdomyoma," *American Journal of Medical Genetics*, vol. 37, no. 4, pp. 443–446, 1990.

[3] C. di Liang, S. F. Ko, and S. C. Huang, "Echocardiographic evaluation of cardiac rhabdomyoma in infants and children," *Journal of Clinical Ultrasound*, vol. 28, pp. 381–386, 2000.

[4] S. Jóźwiak, K. Kotulska, J. Kasprzyk-Obara et al., "Clinical and genotype studies of cardiac tumors in 154 patients with tuberous

sclerosis complex," *Pediatrics*, vol. 118, no. 4, pp. e1146–e1151, 2006.

[5] E. G. Muhler, V. Turniski-Harder, W. Engelhardt, and G. Von Bernuth, "Cardiac involvement in tuberous sclerosis," *The British Heart Journal*, vol. 72, no. 6, pp. 584–590, 1994.

[6] H. C. Smith, G. H. Watson, R. G. Patel, and M. Super, "Cardiac rhabdomyomata in tuberous sclerosis: their course and diagnostic value," *Archives of Disease in Childhood*, vol. 64, no. 2, pp. 196–200, 1989.

[7] P. Venugopalan, J. S. Babu, and A. Al-Bulushi, "Right atrial rhabdomyoma acting as the substrate for Wolff-Parkinson-White syndrome in a 3-month-old infant," *Acta Cardiologica*, vol. 60, no. 5, pp. 543–545, 2005.

[8] F. J. K. O'Callaghan, A. C. Clarke, H. Joffe et al., "Tuberous sclerosis complex and Wolff-Parkinson-White syndrome," *Archives of Disease in Childhood*, vol. 78, no. 2, pp. 159–162, 1998.

15

Description of the First Case of Adenomyomatosis of the Gallbladder in an Infant

Yuri A. Zarate,[1,2] Katherine A. Bosanko,[1] Chaowapong Jarasvaraparn,[3] Jaime Vengoechea,[1] and Elizabeth M. McDonough[3]

[1] Section of Genetics and Metabolism, University of Arkansas for Medical Sciences College of Medicine, Little Rock, AR 72205, USA
[2] Arkansas Children's Hospital, 1 Children's Way, Slot 512-22, Little Rock, AR 72202, USA
[3] Division of Pediatric Gastroenterology, Hepatology and Nutrition, University of Arkansas for Medical Sciences College of Medicine, Little Rock, AR 72205, USA

Correspondence should be addressed to Yuri A. Zarate; yazarate@uams.edu

Academic Editor: Denis A. Cozzi

We report here the case of the youngest patient with adenomyomatosis of the gallbladder in a female infant diagnosed at 4 months of age. This diagnosis was made based on characteristic ultrasonography findings in a patient that was undergoing routine surveillance for a suspected clinical diagnosis of Beckwith-Wiedemann syndrome. The patient remains asymptomatic and currently no surgical interventions have been needed. We review the pathophysiology and ultrasonographic findings of this rare condition and present a comparison with the only other four pediatric cases of adenomyomatosis of the gallbladder.

1. Introduction

Adenomyomatosis of the gallbladder (ADMG) is an acquired condition characterized by localized or diffuse epithelial proliferation and invagination of the mucosa through a hypertrophied muscularis, forming intramural diverticula or sinus tracts. ADMG is diagnosed mainly by imaging. The pathogenesis, pathology, and indications for surgery in this condition are not well understood, especially in children. Although ADMG is benign in nature, it is possible that lithiasis and chronic inflammation secondary to ADMG may lead to dysplastic changes and cancer [1].

We report the case of a female infant diagnosed with ADMG at 4 months of age based on characteristic ultrasonography findings. This diagnosis was made incidentally on a patient that was undergoing routine surveillance for Beckwith-Wiedemann syndrome (BWS). This represents the first report of concurrent BWS and ADMG. Moreover, our case is an infant and to our knowledge is the youngest patient reported with ADMG.

2. Patient Presentation

The female proband was the first child of nonconsanguineous biracial parents (Caucasian and Brazilian). As a product of a naturally conceived full term pregnancy, she was born by cesarean section and weighed 4.932 kg (>97th centile) with no prenatal or perinatal complications. She was first evaluated at 2 months of age for possible diagnosis of BWS given her macrosomia and positive family history. Her weight was 7.2 kg (>97th centile), length was 61 cm (93rd centile), and head circumference was 42.2 cm (98th centile). There was no history of omphalocele or neonatal hypoglycemia and, on physical exam, no hemihyperplasia, ear lobe creases, or macroglossia. Dysmorphic features included narrow palpebral fissures, epicanthal folds, and tented vermilion of the upper lip.

She was subsequently evaluated at 7 months of age with persistent macrosomia. She is otherwise healthy and with normal developmental history. To complete the genetic workup, we also performed a whole genome array (Cytoscan

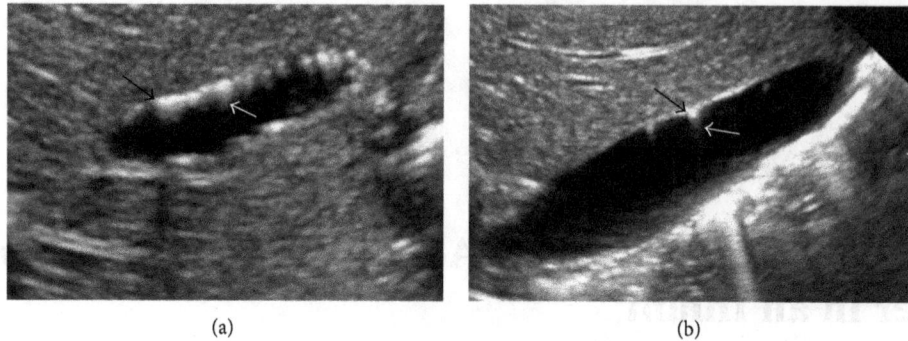

(a)   (b)

FIGURE 1: Ultrasound images at 4 months of age (a) and 7 months of age (b). Multiple nondependent echogenic foci were seen in wall of gall bladder or Rokitansky-Aschoff sinuses (black arrow) with distal sonographic shadowing or comet tail artifacts (gray arrow).

HD, Affymetrix) that was normal. The infant received the clinical diagnosis of BWS and was started on the recommended surveillance protocol. Her alpha-fetoprotein levels (AFP) were 71.2 IU/mL and 22.6 IU/mL at five and eight months of age, respectively (Normal 0–7.2 IU/mL). Liver enzymes and renal ultrasounds have been normal.

Of particular interest, however, was her initial abdominal ultrasound at 4 months of age (Figure 1(a)). The gallbladder wall was noted to have unusual echogenic foci interpreted as ADMG. A repeat ultrasound at 7 months of age showed the same finding with no change (Figure 1(b)). Since, she has been evaluated by gastroenterology and surgery. Given the lack of clinical signs of complications, the plan is to not intervene and to follow up her gallbladder on routine ultrasounds every 3 months as indicated in BWS.

Her 24-year-old mother presented to genetics clinic 34 weeks into the pregnancy. Given the history of macroglossia, hemihyperplasia, and Wilms tumor, we made a clinical diagnosis of BWS and ordered methylation analysis from peripheral blood (Methylation Specific-Multiplex Ligation Dependent Probe Amplification, MS-MLPA) which was normal. We then ordered CDKN1C sequencing which was also normal.

3. Discussion

Hyperplastic cholecystosis is a term used to differentiate from inflammatory conditions such as acute cholecystitis, since it lacks inflammatory features but exhibits features of hyperplasia. It includes two types of mucosal abnormalities of the gallbladder which are usually clinically incidental findings at the time of cholecystectomy: cholesterolosis and adenomyomatosis. Cholesterolosis is characterized by mucosal villous hyperplasia with excessive accumulation of cholesterol esters within epithelial macrophages, while ADMG describes an acquired, hyperplastic lesion of the gallbladder characterized by overgrowth of the mucosa, thickening of the muscle wall, and intramural diverticula [2].

Rokitansky-Aschoff sinuses (RAS) can appear on ultrasound as echo-poor intramural cystic structures. If they contain sludge, they become echogenic. RASs can also produce distal sonographic shadowing or ring-down (comet tail) artifacts. Such ring-down has been proposed to result from reverberation between the near and far surfaces of the sinuses themselves, closely adjacent intrasinus papillary projections, or contained cholesterol crystals. Sonographic findings of ring-down and polypoid projections of <10 mm suggest ADMG [3–5].

Although gallbladder diseases in children are reported with increasing prevalence because of the widespread use of ultrasonography as a diagnostic tool, ADMG in children was first reported in the 1990s and only in four cases to date (Table 1) [1, 6–8]. All four patients were healthy with no underlying disease except for abdominal pain. Moreover, their age range was 5–9 years (3 males and 1 female). To the best of our knowledge, we present the first case of ADMG in an infant, who was evaluated for BWS given the history of macrosomia and a positive family history (two major criteria).

ADMG is currently divided into three types: diffuse, localized, and segmental (annular type). In the localized type (fundal type), a cystic structure forms a nodule, usually in the fundus, that projects into the lumen showing a polyp on ultrasonography [4, 9]. Our patient appeared to have this type. Ultrasonography is a very sensitive and specific image modality but further imaging may be used to inform a surgical decision in cases without infection or cholelithiasis [6, 7]. Given the lack of objective evidence of complications related to ADMG, our patient has not needed further invasive imaging and continues to be monitored clinically.

Although ADMG is benign in nature, stones and chronic inflammation secondary to ADMG may lead to dysplastic changes and cancer, but the causal relationship remains questioned [1, 10]. Surgical intervention for patients with asymptomatic ADMG remains controversial [10]. All four pediatric cases previously reported had undergone cholecystectomy because they experienced abdominal pain. Our child is asymptomatic and requires regular ultrasonographic gallbladder surveillance every 3 months due to her underlying

TABLE 1: Previous cases of adenomyomatosis of the gallbladder in children.

Study	Origin	Age (years)	Sex	Symptom	Ultrasonography	Management	Type
(1) Alberti et al., 1998 [6].	Italy	5	Male	Abdominal pain	Echogenic nodule was detected next to the neck.	Laparoscopic cholecystectomy	Localized
(2) Cetinkursun et al., 2003 [7].	Turkey	6	Male	Abdominal pain, fever and bile vomiting.	A small and multiseptated gallbladder with thickened wall.	Open cholecystectomy	Diffuse
(3) Zani et al., 2005 [8].	Italy	5	Male	Abdominal pain	Multiseptated gallbladder within the lumen.	Open cholecystectomy	Segmental (annular type)
(4) Akçam et al., 2008 [1].	Turkey	9	Female	Abdominal pain	Thickening of the wall of the gallbladder with echogenic areas parallel to the wall of gallbladder.	Open cholecystectomy	Diffuse (honeycomb)
(5) Our case, 2014.	USA	4 m	Female	Incidental finding	Echoic foci within gallbladder wall.	Observation	Localized

clinical diagnosis of BWS. Therefore, we will monitor her for symptoms and for signs of gallbladder thickening and irregularity, which could be indications for cholecystectomy.

We present the case of the youngest patient with ultrasonographic findings highly suggestive of ADMG with the context of possible BWS. Ultimately, we need better knowledge to determine the long term consequences of ADMG and its potential relationship with gallbladder cancer.

Conflict of Interests

None of the authors has conflict of interests to declare.

References

[1] M. Akçam, I. Buyukyavuz, M. Çiriş, and N. Eriş, "Adenomyomatosis of the gallbladder resembling honeycomb in a child," European Journal of Pediatrics, vol. 167, no. 9, pp. 1079–1081, 2008.

[2] C. C. Owen and L. E. Bilhartz, "Gallbladder polyps, cholesterolosis, adenomyomatosis, and acute acalculous cholecystitis," Seminars in Gastrointestinal Disease, vol. 14, no. 4, pp. 178–188, 2003.

[3] P. J. Mariani and A. Hsue, "Adenomyomatosis of the gallbladder: the "good omen" comet," Journal of Emergency Medicine, vol. 40, no. 4, pp. 415–418, 2011.

[4] J.-H. Yoon, S.-S. Cha, S.-S. Han, S.-J. Lee, and M.-S. Kang, "Gallbladder adenomyomatosis: imaging findings," Abdominal Imaging, vol. 31, no. 5, pp. 555–563, 2006.

[5] V. Alessi, S. Bianco, R. Marotta, and G. Traina, "Ultrasound in the detection of focal and segmental hyperplastic cholecystoses," Radiologia Medica, vol. 75, no. 4, pp. 339–344, 1988.

[6] D. Alberti, F. Callea, G. Camoni, D. Falchetti, W. Rigamonti, and G. Caccia, "Adenomyomatosis of the gallbladder in childhood," Journal of Pediatric Surgery, vol. 33, no. 9, pp. 1411–1412, 1998.

[7] S. Cetinkursun, I. Surer, S. Deveci et al., "Adenomyomatosis of the gallbladder in a child," Digestive Diseases and Sciences, vol. 48, no. 4, pp. 733–736, 2003.

[8] A. Zani, M. Pacilli, A. Conforti, A. Casati, S. Bosco, and D. A. Cozzi, "Adenomyomatosis of the gallbladder in childhood: report of a case and review of the literature," Pediatric and Developmental Pathology, vol. 8, no. 5, pp. 577–580, 2005.

[9] M. M. Meguid, F. Aun, and M. L. Bradford, "Adenomyomatosis of the gallbladder," American Journal of Surgery, vol. 147, no. 2, pp. 260–262, 1984.

[10] T. Ootani, Y. Shirai, K. Tsukada, and T. Muto, "Relationship between gallbladder carcinoma and the segmental type of adenomyomatosis of the gallbladder," Cancer, vol. 69, no. 11, pp. 2647–2652, 1992.

16

Cutaneous Manifestation of Metastatic Infantile Choriocarcinoma

Timothy Brooks and Laura Nolting

Department of Emergency Medicine, Palmetto Health Richland, Suite 350, 14 Medical Park, Columbia, SC 29203, USA

Correspondence should be addressed to Timothy Brooks; timbrooksmd@gmail.com

Academic Editor: Piotr Czauderna

Infantile choriocarcinoma is a highly malignant rare germ cell tumor that arises from the placenta. Simultaneous intraplacental choriocarcinoma involving both mother and infant is extremely rare. Cutaneous metastasis in infantile choriocarcinoma is even rarer with only a few case reports available. Here we describe a case of a female neonate who presented to the ED with a rapidly growing and bleeding vascular lesion to her right cheek. She was eventually diagnosed by biopsy with metastatic choriocarcinoma. In addition to the cutaneous tumor, she also had metastatic disease in her lungs. Her mother was subsequently found to have choriocarcinoma with metastatic disease to the lungs as well.

1. Introduction

Choriocarcinoma is an aggressive malignant tumor of placental trophoblastic cells. Reports of the disease are presented in the literature as case reports and review articles. Metastatic spread to the fetus is rare, and diagnosis is often difficult and delayed. In this case report, we describe the clinical, laboratory, and radiographic findings of a neonate presenting to the children's emergency department who was ultimately diagnosed with metastatic choriocarcinoma.

2. Case

The infant presented to the ED the first time on the 11th day of life for evaluation of a right-sided facial mass because the mother felt it was getting bigger and darker. At the time of birth, she was noted to have a 2 cm subcutaneous mass on the right cheek (Figure 1). The lesion was dark red in color and blanched with pressure. It was firm and there was no evidence of fluctuance or surrounding cellulitis. It did not appear to be painful on palpation. It measured 2 × 2 cm in the ED. The infant had no medical history and was born at 35 weeks via spontaneous vaginal delivery, and the pregnancy was only complicated by the mother having *Trichomonas vaginalis* that was treated with metronidazole during her third trimester.

An MRI was performed and interpreted as a benign vascular lesion such as a hemangioma. It measured 17 × 18 × 19 mm with a necrotic center. There was no evidence of invasion to adjacent facial structures (Figures 2(a) and 2(b)).

Her CBC, PT, PTT, INR, and fibrinogen were all within acceptable limits.

She was subsequently admitted to the PICU for propranolol therapy to treat the hemangioma. The mother noted that the lesion had decreased in size and color intensity within 18 hours of initiation of propranolol. The child was discharged to follow-up as an outpatient.

On day 18 of life she underwent incision and drainage, without a histological sample, by ENT for what was thought at that time to be an involuted hemangioma. She had done well postoperatively until 12 days later when the lesion began to bleed prompting the mother to bring her to the ED. Vitals were stable and laboratory values were within acceptable limits. The ED physician, who examined the patient in the ED, consulted ENT who felt the infant was stable for discharge after starting her on oral prednisolone and continued the propranolol.

She returned to the ED 8 days later, on day 37 of life, with an enlarging mass and significant bleeding. The lesion had increased in size despite continuation of steroid and propranolol therapy. The mother denied any complicating

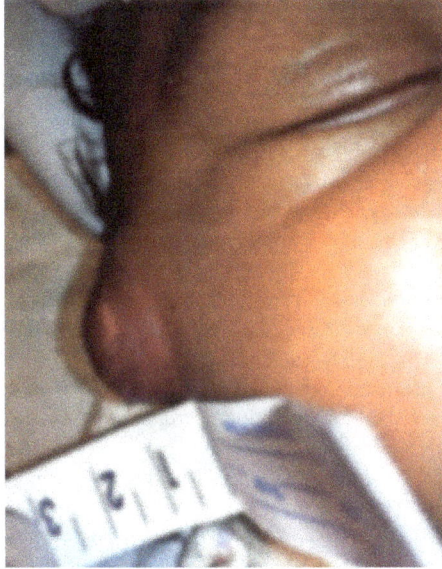

FIGURE 1: Facial lesion.

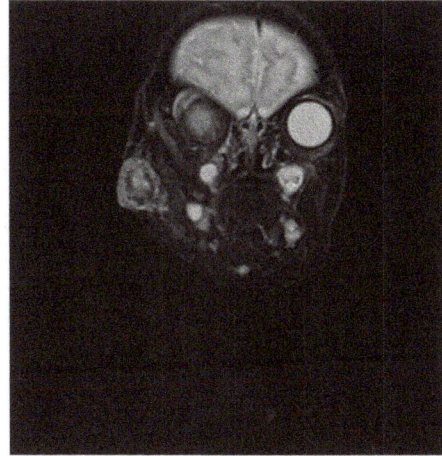

(a)

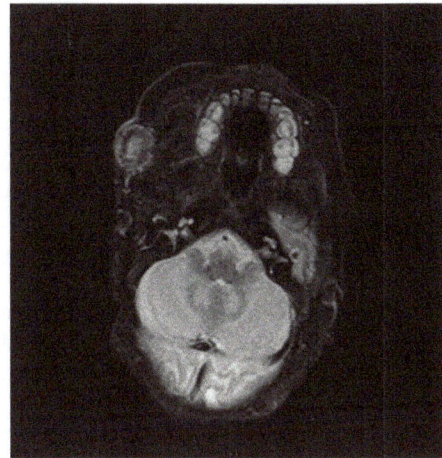

(b)

FIGURE 2: (a) Coronal MRI at 11 days. (b) Axial MRI at 11 days.

symptoms including fever, cough, congestion, increased fussiness or irritability, feeding intolerance, or change in bowel or bladder habits.

In the ED, temperature was 97.7 rectally, pulse 159, respiratory rate 44, blood pressure 67/37, and pulse ox 97%. On exam the child had a large erythematous right facial lesion with an involuting necrotic center now measuring 4 × 4 cm. There was a significant amount of clot burden stranding from the lesion. The child had appropriate behavior and neurologic findings and the remainder of the exam was normal.

There were significant normocytic anemia and leukocytosis found on CBC. Hemoglobin (MCV), RBC count, hematocrit, and platelets were 7.4 g/dL (90.3), 2.36 M/uL, 21.3%, and 297, respectively. The peripheral leukocyte count was 20,400/uL with 28% polymorphonuclear leukocytes, 59% lymphocytes, and 10% monocytes. Nineteen days prior to the hemoglobin, RBC count, hematocrit, and leukocyte count were 14.1 g/dL, 4.12 M/uL, 38.8%, and 12,300/uL, respectively.

The child was emergently transfused with packed red cells and transferred to another hospital for embolization where she was ultimately diagnosed with choriocarcinoma by biopsy. She returned to our facility and began chemotherapy, which included bleomycin, etoposide, and cisplatin. Bilateral pulmonary nodules were found on CT scan (Figure 3). There were no other areas of metastasis.

Only after the diagnosis was made histologically and chemotherapy initiated in the child was the β-hCG level checked. Subsequently, the infant's mother was evaluated and found to have metastatic disease as well and underwent chemotherapy. Both mother and child are doing well with resolving metastasis and negative β-hCG levels.

3. Discussion

Choriocarcinoma is a rare malignant disease that arises from the trophoblastic cells of the placenta. It is characterized by secretion of human chorionic gonadotropin (β-hCG). Maternal choriocarcinoma is extremely rare, occurring in an estimated 1 in 50,000 live births [1]. About 50 percent of cases of choriocarcinoma arise from complete hydatidiform mole, an additional 25 percent arise after normal pregnancies, and 25 percent follow spontaneous abortion or ectopic pregnancy [2].

Infantile choriocarcinoma is even rarer. Less than 30 cases have been described in the literature [3]. Newborn infants tend to present with a characteristic clinical picture of anemia, hepatomegaly, and precocious puberty [4]. Infantile choriocarcinoma occurs between 0 and 6 months of age. In our case, our patient was born with metastatic disease but presented with only the cutaneous manifestation making it even more difficult to diagnose. Metastasis is common and usually affects liver, lung, brain, and skin, in that order [5]. Infantile cutaneous manifestation of the disease is extremely rare. Of 208 neonates between 1955 and 2010 with malignancies and cutaneous metastases, only 4 patients (1.9%) had cutaneous metastasis due to choriocarcinoma and it was generally associated with poor prognosis [6]. Approximately

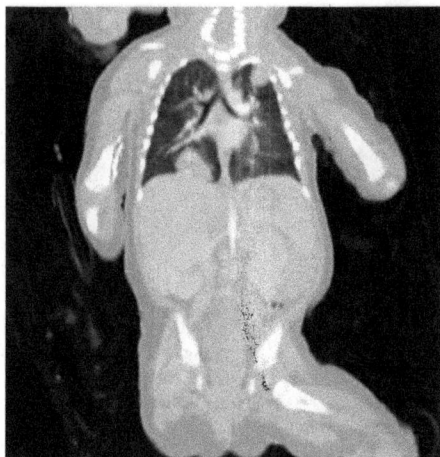

FIGURE 3: CT of the chest with metastasis.

References

[1] J. A. Tidy, G. J. S. Rustin, E. S. Newlands et al., "Presentation and management of choriocarcinoma after nonmolar pregnancy," *The British Journal of Obstetrics and Gynaecology*, vol. 102, no. 9, pp. 715–719, 1995.

[2] J. W. Chang and J. Berek, "Gestational trophoblastic disease: Epidemiology, clinical manifestations and diagnosis," Up To Date. Literature review current through: Sep 2013.

[3] M. van der Hoef, F. K. Niggli, U. V. Willi, and T. A. G. M. Huisman, "Solitary infantile choriocarcinoma of the liver: MRI findings," *Pediatric Radiology*, vol. 34, no. 10, pp. 820–823, 2004.

[4] M. E. G. Blohm, G. Calaminus, A. K. Gnekow et al., "Disseminated choriocarcinoma in infancy is curable by chemotherapy and delayed tumour resection," *European Journal of Cancer*, vol. 37, no. 1, pp. 72–78, 2001.

[5] M. E. G. Blohm and U. Göbel, "Unexplained anaemia and failure to thrive as initial symptoms of infantile choriocarcinoma: a review," *European Journal of Pediatrics*, vol. 163, no. 1, pp. 1–6, 2004.

[6] H. Isaacs, "Cutaneous metastases in neonates: a review," *Pediatric Dermatology*, vol. 28, no. 2, pp. 85–93, 2011.

[7] O. M. McNally, M. Tran, D. Fortune, and M. A. Quinn, "Successful treatment of mother and baby with metastatic choriocarcinoma," *International Journal of Gynecological Cancer*, vol. 12, no. 4, pp. 394–398, 2002.

[8] J. M. Yoon, R. C. Burns, M. H. Malogolowkin, and L. Mascarenhas, "Treatment of infantile choriocarcinoma of the liver," *Pediatric Blood and Cancer*, vol. 49, no. 1, pp. 99–102, 2007.

[9] J. Getrajdman, V. Kolev, E. Brody, and L. Chuang, "Case of maternal and infantile choriocarcinoma following normal pregnancy," *Gynecologic Oncology Case Reports*, vol. 2, no. 3, pp. 102–104, 2012.

one-quarter of infants with choriocarcinoma present with symptoms at birth and diagnosis can be easily confirmed with serum β-hCG [7]. These tumors are highly vascular and friable, so biopsy may be difficult and even dangerous [8]. Anemia may be gradual or may result from tumor rupture. Transfusion, as in our case, may be required. Failure to thrive is nonspecific and may only manifest as feeding difficulties [9]. Hemoptysis and respiratory failure may be the primary manifestations of lung involvement. Brain and skin involvement are rarely seen and usually indicated advanced disease [5].

Choriocarcinoma is a very aggressive malignancy and death may result from delays in diagnosis. Therefore, early intervention is critical for limiting the progression of disease. In infants, without appropriate treatment, death usually occurs within 3 weeks of initial presentation [8]. Fortunately, despite its aggressive nature, this cancer responds very well to chemotherapeutic agents, even in the presence of widespread metastases [9]. The chance of long-term survival, even in patients with cerebral metastases at presentation, is approximately 80% [7]. Both patients described responded very well to chemotherapy, without significant complications, and currently have shown no progression or recurrence of disease, as indicated by negative β-hCG levels, in the two years since diagnosis. Had a β-hCG level, which is universally positive in infantile choriocarcinoma and excludes the diagnosis if negative, been known early in the clinical course, chemotherapy could have been initiated sooner [4].

Because a history of maternal choriocarcinoma is associated with a risk of infantile choriocarcinoma in subsequent pregnancies, current guidelines suggest that women with such a history should be checked for β-hCG at 6 and 10 weeks following a subsequent pregnancy, regardless of the outcome [4, 7].

Conflict of Interests

The authors declare that there is no conflict of interests regarding the publication of this paper.

17

Two Cases of Progressive Familial Intrahepatic Cholestasis Type 2 Presenting with Severe Coagulopathy without Jaundice

Eric Tibesar,[1] **Christine Karwowski,**[1] **Paula Hertel,**[2]
Ann Scheimann,[1] **and Wikrom Karnsakul**[1]

[1] *Division of Pediatric Gastroenterology, Johns Hopkins University School of Medicine, 600 N. Wolfe Street, Baltimore, MD 21287, USA*
[2] *Division of Pediatric Gastroenterology, Texas Children's Hospital, 6621 Fannin Street, Houston, TX 77030, USA*

Correspondence should be addressed to Eric Tibesar; etibesa1@jhmi.edu

Academic Editor: Junji Takaya

Progressive familial intrahepatic cholestasis (PFIC) type 2 results from a mutation in the bile salt exporter pump, impeding bile acid transport. Patients usually present with jaundice, pruritus, growth failure, and fat soluble vitamin deficiencies. We present two patients diagnosed with PFIC type 2 due to severe coagulopathy and bleeding without jaundice.

Case A is a healthy 5-month-old female who presented to a local hospital with scratching to the point of bleeding and ecchymoses on her abdomen, back, and legs. She had no history of jaundice since birth and jaundice was not noted at several doctors' visits prior to this presentation. Physical examination showed neither icterus nor hepatosplenomegaly. Initial labs demonstrated AST 223 U/L, ALT 334 U/L, total bilirubin 3.4 mg/dL, direct bilirubin 2.8 mg/dL, GGT 33 U/L, partial thromboplastin time (PTT) 90.8 seconds, prothrombin time (PT) > 120.0 seconds, and INR > 13.7. She received a one-time intravenous vitamin K with repeat INR of 1.0 and then was admitted for further evaluation. Of note, she was treated with IV cefotaxime at the outside hospital due to a positive urine culture for *Escherichia coli*, and this was continued for a full seven-day course.

Cholestasis persisted with a peak direct bilirubin of 7.5 mg/dL. An abdominal ultrasound showed normal hepatic echotexture and biliary system without focal lesions. Infectious work-up included negative serologies for CMV, EBV, HIV, HSV, HCV, and HBV. As vitamin K deficiency was thought to be from cholestasis related malabsorption, fat soluble vitamin studies were performed and revealed a vitamin D (25-OH) level of <5 ng/mL, normal vitamin A, and an alpha-tocopherol level of 0.8 mg/L. Total serum bile acids were elevated at 205.3 umol/L (normal; 4.5–19.2 umol/L). Percutaneous liver biopsy revealed mild

chronic portal inflammation, periportal fibrosis, ballooning hepatocytes, significant cholestasis, and early bile duct loss with ductular proliferation (see Figures 1 and 2). No bile salt exporter pump (BSEP) staining was performed. Serum sent for genetic evaluation revealed heterozygous mutations in the ABCB11 gene (c.908(+1)G>A/c.3692 G>A (R1231Q)), confirming the diagnosis of progressive familial intrahepatic cholestasis (PFIC) type 2.

Following discharge, she suffered from intractable pruritus despite the use of ursodiol, rifampin, cholestyramine, and hydroxyzine. She underwent an internal ileal diversion at 12 months with no relief of significant pruritus and continued presence of high total bile acid level of 147.4 umol/L and subsequently an internal biliary diversion at 15 months, again without relief of pruritus and presence of even higher total bile acid level of 239.2 umol/L. Growth had been normal, but the patient had low vitamin E and D levels, despite large dose supplementation. She was listed for living related donor liver transplant at this point.

Case B is a 14-year-old male, clinically diagnosed with Alagille syndrome as an infant due to cholestasis without evidence of jaundice and a liver biopsy that showed paucity of intrahepatic bile ducts. Past medical history is significant for intracerebral hemorrhage during infancy, presumably due to vitamin K deficiency, leading to life-long seizure disorder and residual left-sided hemiparesis. He was treated with

TABLE 1: Initial presenting clinical and laboratory data.

Case	Age at diagnosis	ALT (U/L)	Total bilirubin (mg/dL)	Direct bilirubin (mg/dL)	Serum bile acids (umol/L)	GGT (U/L)	Prothrombin time (seconds)	INR	Vitamin D (25-OH) (ng/mL)
A	5 months	334	3.4	2.8	205.3	33	>120.0	>13.7	<5
B	14 years	57	0.6	0.1	n/a	35	40	4.2	n/a

Values marked n/a mean that no data was available for that patient. Normal reference values: ALT, 0–31 U/L; total bilirubin, 0.1–1.2 mg/dL; direct bilirubin, 0.0–0.4 mg/dL; serum bile acids, 4.5–19.2 umol/L; GGT, 8–51 U/L; prothrombin time, 9.4–11.6 seconds; INR, 0.9–1.1; vitamin D (25-OH), 32–100 ng/mL.

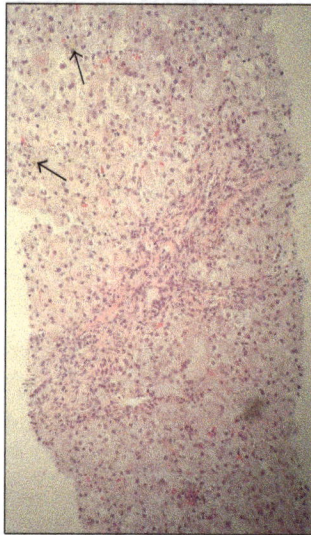

FIGURE 1: Liver biopsy at 100x magnification showing bile duct plugs (arrows) along with multinuclear giant/hydropic cells.

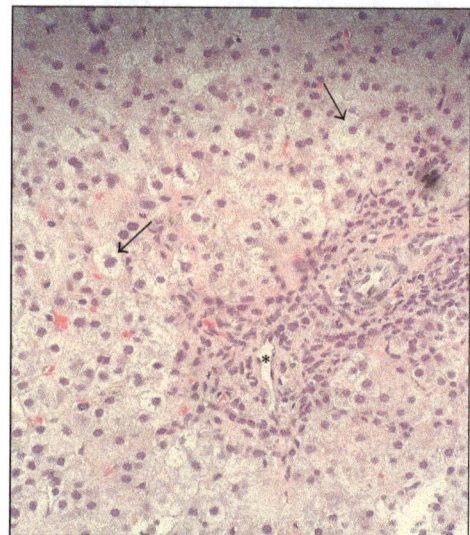

FIGURE 2: Liver biopsy at 200x magnification showing ballooning hepatocytes (arrows) with inflammation around the portal vein (*).

phenytoin for seizure control and followed up closely by the pediatric liver service due to concerns about fat soluble vitamin deficiencies, cholestasis, and poor growth.

At the age of 14, he presented to an outside emergency room with leg pain and increased bruising. Jaundice was not noted. Labs showed PT of 40 seconds and PTT of 120 seconds. He received a one-time intramuscular dose of 30 mg vitamin K, and repeat labs showed PT of 16.7 seconds and PTT of 35.0 seconds. Total bilirubin was 0.6 mg/dL and GGT was normal (see Table 1 for comparison to Case A). No antibiotics were given and he was discharged home the next day, with close follow-up arranged in the pediatric GI clinic.

Over the following 15–18 months, he developed jaundice with worsening cholestasis and increased pruritus. At the age of 16, due to increased jaundice, he underwent endoscopic retrograde cholangiopancreatography (ERCP) and percutaneous liver biopsy. The ERCP was normal. Liver biopsy showed marked canalicular and hepatocellular cholestasis, with mild to moderate portal and lobular fibrosis including BSEP staining (see Figures 3 and 4). There was no paucity of intrahepatic bile ducts, with findings inconsistent with Alagille syndrome. Because of continued jaundice and cholestasis, genetic testing was done, showing mutations in the ABCB11 gene (c.890A>G; p.Q297G/c.2343+1 G>T), confirming the diagnosis of PFIC type 2 [1]. Case B reached adult age without transplantation.

Discussion. These two cases demonstrate an unusual presentation of PFIC type 2 in that both had severe coagulopathy without the presence or the history of jaundice in their clinical manifestations. Although both patients eventually developed a more obvious feature of jaundice, their initial presentations of cholestasis and coagulopathy in the absence of jaundice were concerning enough to warrant further investigations in order to provide proper management. In a recent analysis of presenting signs and symptoms of patients with BSEP mutations, the most common finding was jaundice (73% of patients), with 9% of patients presenting with manifestations of vitamin deficiency [2]. Of those 9% of patients, 58% presented without clinical signs of jaundice, although the exact vitamin deficiency and presence of clinical bleeding were not mentioned [2]. There was no mention of any patient specifically presenting with coagulopathy or clinical bleeding, corrected with vitamin K, in the absence of jaundice.

Patients with PFIC type 2 can be diagnosed based on mutations in the ABCB11 gene, which encodes the BSEP protein. To date, there are more than 100 mutations that have been discovered in the ABCB11 gene, leading to a 70% reduction or complete absence of bile salts removed from the liver [3]. Two of the more common mutations that have been found include the missense mutations E297G and D482G, found in up to 30% of European patients with PFIC type 2 [4]. A retrospective analysis of 84 patients with

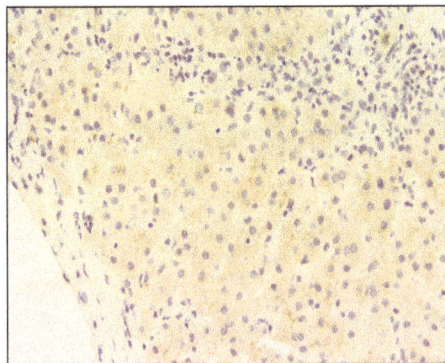

FIGURE 3: Liver biopsy of Case B, at 20x magnification showing staining for BSEP protein.

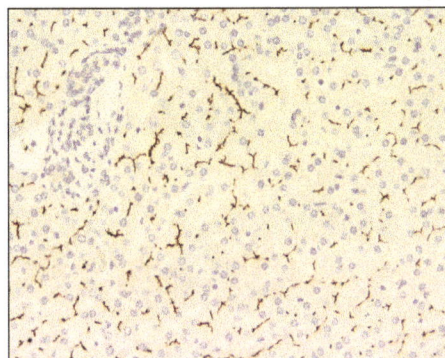

FIGURE 4: Liver biopsy at 20x magnification, used as a positive control for biopsy in Figure 3. BSEP protein stains are brown.

ABCB11 gene mutations found that 61% of them had one or two alleles with these more common missense mutations [2]. Ten were noted to have coagulopathy from vitamin deficiency upon presentation, with three being noted to have the D482G mutation [2]. Both patients in this report had genetic analysis, without evidence of either of the two more common mutations.

In Case A the first mutation is c.3692 G>A in exon 27 [5]. The predicted protein effect is R1231Q, which does not lead to an abnormal splice site but causes a missense mutation. This results in an immature protein or delayed maturation of BSEP, presumably lowering its function [6]. This mutation was also reported in 2 patients who had homozygous and compound heterozygous mutations [5, 7]. The patient with homozygous mutations developed severe fibrosis and underwent liver transplantation at the age of 2.9 years. The other mutation at the splice site, c.908+1G>A in intron 9 of *ABCB11*, has also been reported by Strautnieks et al. [5]. In that study, this mutation was found in a compound heterozygote for c.908+1G>A with another common missense mutation c.1445A>G. The c.1445A>G is predicted to cause p.Asp482Gly; however, its true effect is aberrant splicing which leads to translation of a truncated protein [6]. The progression of liver disease in this patient was actually slow.

In Case B, his first mutation is 890 A>G in exon 9 [5]. The predicted protein effect is E297G or p.Glu297Gly. The other mutation is c.2343+1 G>T which is a mutation at splice site, 5′ intron 19, a novel splice site change. This compound heterozygous mutation was reported in Case B's sister who developed persistent cholestasis and bridging fibrosis at the age of 2 years, biliary cirrhosis at the age of 3 years, and cholangiocarcinoma and died at the age of 4 [1].

There are technical challenges to the exploration of the mRNA consequences of the splice site mutations by sequencing the corresponding cDNA. Since expression of BSEP protein in extrahepatic tissues is low, the only way to get sufficient mRNA is sampling the explanted liver and conserving the RNAse inhibitors immediately at the time of surgery, which was not feasible in both cases. We can assume that Case B must have similar mutations as his sister whose mRNA sequencing was performed and published by Scheimann et al. [1]. On the other hand, from a clinical perspective, one would assume that homozygotes of c.3692 G>A would manifest a more severe presentation compared to a compound heterozygote of c.908(+1)G>A/c.3692 G>A, similar to Case A. In theory, the expected result of c.908+1G>A could be exon 9 skipping with deletion, frameshift mutation resulting in a premature stop codon and protein truncation. However, less likely events include skipping of more than one exon or cryptic splice site activation. More importantly, the absence of the wild type transcript, which originates from the allele carrying the splice site mutation, is rather complicated in a compound heterozygote, especially with a normally transcribed allele carrying a 2.3 kb downstream missense mutation. In one report, biallelic BSEP mutations were described in PFIC type 2 children with a tendency to have lower bile acid concentration and lower age at liver transplantation than those with one truncating and one missense mutation; an expected correlation with a severe mutation with vitamin malabsorption and deficiencies was not reported [8]. Perhaps there is yet more to learn about genotype and phenotype association to understand the molecular function of the BSEP protein.

In this report we conclude that patients who present with cholestasis and significant coagulopathy that respond to vitamin K should have congenital liver diseases such as PFIC included in their differential diagnosis though cholestasis may not be pronounced as a common clue in the diagnosis. Genetic analysis for mutations in the ABCB11 gene can aid in diagnosis after ruling out common causes of cholestasis. Further study in larger cohorts of PFIC type 2 populations may reveal more specific genotype-phenotype correlations.

Abbreviations

PTT: Partial thromboplastin time
PT: Prothrombin time
BSEP: Bile salt exporter pump
PFIC: Progressive familial intrahepatic cholestasis.

Conflict of Interests

The authors declare that there is no potential conflict of interests to disclose.

Acknowledgments

The authors would like to acknowledge the help of Dr. Milton Finegold and Dr. Robert Anders with assistance in interpretation of the pathology slides and Dr. Milan Jirsa for interpretation of PFIC2 mutations in Case A in preparing this paper.

References

[1] A. O. Scheimann, S. S. Strautnieks, A. S. Knisely, J. A. Byrne, R. J. Thompson, and M. J. Finegold, "Mutations in bile salt export pump (ABCB11) in two children with progressive familial intrahepatic cholestasis and cholangiocarcinoma," *The Journal of Pediatrics*, vol. 150, no. 5, pp. 556–559, 2007.

[2] L. Pawlikowska, S. Strautnieks, I. Jankowska et al., "Differences in presentation and progression between severe FIC1 and BSEP deficiencies," *Journal of Hepatology*, vol. 53, no. 1, pp. 170–178, 2010.

[3] Genetics Home Reference, ABCB11 gene, 2013, http://ghr.nlm.nih.gov/gene/ABCB11.

[4] H. Hayashi, T. Takada, H. Suzuki, H. Akita, and Y. Sugiyama, "Two common PFIC2 mutations are associated with the impaired membrane trafficking of BSEP/ABCB11," *Hepatology*, vol. 41, no. 4, pp. 916–924, 2005.

[5] S. S. Strautnieks, J. A. Byrne, L. Pawlikowska et al., "Severe bile salt export pump deficiency: 82 different ABCB11 mutations in 109 families," *Gastroenterology*, vol. 134, no. 4, pp. 1203–1214, 2008.

[6] J. A. Byrne, S. S. Strautnieks, G. Ihrke et al., "Missense mutations and single nucleotide polymorphisms in ABCB11 impair bile salt export pump processing and function or disrupt pre-messenger RNA splicing," *Hepatology*, vol. 49, no. 2, pp. 553–567, 2009.

[7] L. Alvarez, P. Jara, E. Sánchez-Sabaté et al., "Reduced hepatic expression of farnesoid X receptor in hereditary cholestasis associated to mutation in ATP8B1," *Human Molecular Genetics*, vol. 13, no. 20, pp. 2451–2460, 2004.

[8] A. Davit-Spraul, M. Fabre, S. Branchereau et al., "ATP8B1 and ABCB11 Analysis in 62 children with normal gamma-glutamyl transferase Progressive Familial Intrahepatic Cholestasis (PFIC): phenotypic differences between PFIC1 and PFIC2 and natural history," *Hepatology*, vol. 51, no. 5, pp. 1645–1655, 2010.

18

A Case of Diprosopus: Perinatal Counseling and Management

Kimberly M. Thornton,[1,2] **Timothy Bennett,**[2,3] **Vivekanand Singh,**[2,4] **Neil Mardis,**[2,5]
Jennifer Linebarger,[2,6] **Howard Kilbride,**[1,2] **and Kristin Voos**[1,2]

[1] Division of Neonatology, Children's Mercy Hospital, 2401 Gillham Road, Kansas City, MO 64108, USA
[2] University of Missouri-Kansas City School of Medicine, 2411 Holmes Road, Kansas City, MO 64108, USA
[3] Department of Obstetrics and Gynecology, Elizabeth J. Ferrell Fetal Health Center, Children's Mercy Hospital,
   2401 Gillham Road, Kansas City, MO 64108, USA
[4] Department of Pathology, Children's Mercy Hospital, 2401 Gillham Road, Kansas City, MO 64108, USA
[5] Department of Radiology, Children's Mercy Hospital, 2401 Gillham Road, Kansas City, MO 64108, USA
[6] Department of Pediatrics, Palliative Care Center, Children's Mercy Hospital, 2401 Gillham Road, Kansas City, MO 64108, USA

Correspondence should be addressed to Kimberly M. Thornton; kimmcdonaldthornton@gmail.com

Academic Editor: Nan-Chang Chiu

Diprosopus is a rare congenital malformation associated with high mortality. Here, we describe a patient with diprosopus, multiple life-threatening anomalies, and genetic mutations. Prenatal diagnosis and counseling made a beneficial impact on the family and medical providers in the care of this case.

1. Introduction

Advances in perinatal imaging and diagnostic tools often allow for recognition of complex, rare, and even life-threatening congenital malformations prior to birth. Prenatal diagnosis of these conditions provides time for earlier counseling and planning for perinatal management options. Guiding a family through this process can be difficult for the medical team, but is an attempt to improve the overall outcome and experience for everyone involved. We present a case of diprosopus associated with multiple congenital malformations which were prenatally diagnosed. The parents received extensive multidisciplinary, prenatal counseling allowing both the family and the medical providers to be well prepared for the birth and postnatal management.

2. Case

A 29-year-old gravida 2 para 1 Caucasian female was referred for maternal-fetal-medicine consultation at 26-week gestation due to suspected fetal anomalies. Obstetrical ultrasound examination, confirmed by fetal magnetic resonance imaging (MRI), demonstrated craniofacial duplication, several abnormalities of the brain and skull, thoracolumbosacral dysraphism with neural tube defect and likely Chiari II malformation, large congenital diaphragmatic hernia (CDH) with liver and bowel noted in the left chest, hypoplastic left lung, and possible horseshoe kidney (Figure 1). Fetal echocardiogram findings were consistent with Tetralogy of Fallot (TOF). The parents had a multidisciplinary consultation with maternal-fetal medicine, neonatology, genetics, cardiology, radiology, and palliative care. Given the multiple, severe congenital anomalies, the medical team and family planned for limited resuscitative efforts and anticipated comfort care after birth.

A 2440 g male infant was delivered via repeat cesarean section at 36-week gestation secondary to preterm labor. At birth, the infant was pale and cyanotic with no spontaneous cry and poor tone. He had shallow spontaneous respirations with poor aeration on auscultation. The left mouth was small and fixed. No glottis was visualized when the laryngoscope was inserted into the right mouth. The infant was then

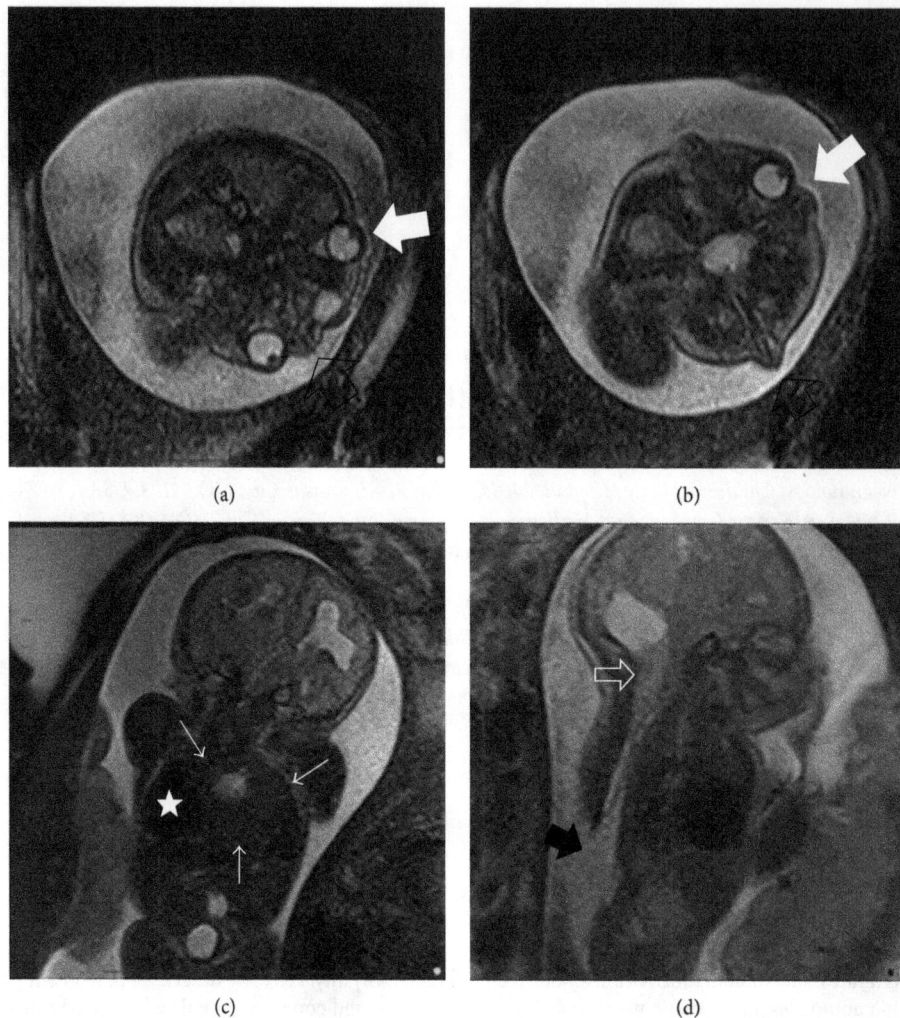

(a)

(b)

(c)

(d)

FIGURE 1: Axial images from fetal MRI (a and b) showing the left-sided (open black arrows) and right-sided (solid white arrows) fetal faces. Coronal image from fetal MRI (c) reveals a left-sided diaphragmatic hernia (thin white arrows) containing liver and bowel with displacement of the fetal heart (white star) to the right. Chiari II malformation with tonsillar herniation through the posterior foramen magnum (open white arrow) and associated lumbosacral spinal dysraphism (solid black arrow) is noted on a sagittal image (d).

wrapped in a warm blanket and given to the family to hold. He died in his parents' arms a few minutes after birth.

The parents consented to a complete postmortem evaluation. Physical exam demonstrated complete facial duplication with tetrophthalmos (four eyes), two noses, two mouths, two chins, and one fully formed ear on each side of the head with a hypoplastic pinna in the midline. Two anterior and two posterior fontanels were palpable. There was also a ruptured myelomeningocele measuring 6.3 cm × 3.9 cm in the thoracolumbar region and a scaphoid abdomen. The first and second toes of each foot overlapped and the nails were hypoplastic.

Dissection of the cranial cavity revealed brain duplication with fusion of the parietal and occipital lobes of each brain. The right and left brains fused at the mesencephalon and brainstem. Each brain had an optic chiasm, a pituitary gland, and a single large ventricle with loss of the ependymal lining

and no third ventricle identified. There was a single midbrain, rudimentary cerebellar tissue and fourth ventricle, atresia of the cerebral aqueduct with rudimentary and hypoplastic cerebral peduncles, bilateral absence of the corpus callosum, bilateral polymicrogyria, and dysplasia of the right and left cortices. Dissection of the thorax and abdomen revealed left CDH with intestine, stomach, spleen, and the left lobe of the liver herniated into the left pleural cavity with concomitant pulmonary hypoplasia. Cardiac findings included TOF (pulmonary atresia, ventricular septal defect, overriding aorta, and pulmonary arteries), atrial septal defect, patent ductus arteriosus, superior pulmonary veins draining to the left atrium (no inferior pulmonary veins), dilated right atrium, and hypoplastic left atrium. A common oropharynx connected two separate nasopharynxes and two separate oral cavities. There was a single larynx and esophagus. The intestines were malrotated with the appendix located in the

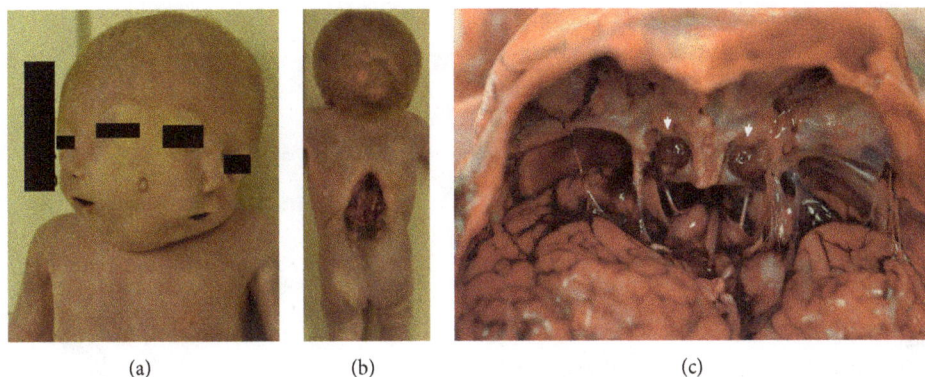

FIGURE 2: (a) Facial duplication with a hypoplastic pinna in the midline. (b) Open thoracolumbar myelomeningocele measuring 6.3 cm × 3.9 cm. (c) Anterior cranial fossa with two pituitary glands (white arrows).

left upper abdominal quadrant. Ectopic right and left kidneys were located in the lower abdomen and an accessory spleen was present. Testes were undescended bilaterally and the right testis was atrophic. The placental pathology revealed normal fetal membranes and chorionic villi consistent with third trimester gestation with a two-vessel umbilical cord (Figure 2).

Whole-genome microarray-based comparative genomic hybridization (aCGH) using Oxford Gene Technology revealed a male karyotype (46 X,Y), a 983 kb deletion on chromosome 4q34.3, a 562 kb gain on chromosome Xp22.31p22.2, and a 32 kb gain on chromosome 13q12.11. Quantitative polymerase chain reaction of maternal blood indicated the duplications on chromosomes Xp22.31p22.2 and 13q12.11 were maternally inherited. The 4q34.3 deletion was not maternally inherited, however. Unfortunately, due to the family's financial burden, genetic testing was not completed on the father.

3. Discussion

Diprosopus or craniofacial duplication is the rarest form of conjoined twinning, with an incidence of approximately 0.4% of all types of conjoined twins [1]. Historically, two main theoretical embryologic explanations have been considered: either a "fusion" of two parallel notochords in close proximity occurs or a "fission" of a single notochord occurs during the first few weeks after conception [2]. More recent theories include duplication of neural crest cell derivatives and mutations of the *Dlx* homeobox gene [3, 4]. A spectrum of diprosopus exists from a duplication of only the nose to complete facial duplication similar to that of our patient [5]. Many other congenital anomalies have been reported to occur in conjunction with diprosopus, including various neurologic, cardiac, pulmonary, skeletal, and gastrointestinal system defects [5–8]. Conjoined twins have a high mortality, especially if they have other major congenital anomalies [8, 9].

There have been no previous reports of genetic mutations associated with diprosopus. The clinical significance of the maternally inherited duplications at Xp22.31p22.2 and 13q12.11 is unknown. There is a theoretical possibility

of an X-linked recessive inheritance pattern since the X chromosome duplication has caused no disease or malformation in the mother, but this is unlikely as no reports of familial recurrence have previously been reported in the literature. The 4q34.3 deletion has been associated with cardiovascular abnormalities such as TOF [10, 11], but none of these genes are located in the deletion region in our case. Given the rare incidence of this disease and our inability to complete genetic testing of both parents, we are unable to conclude that any of the genetic findings are associated with our patient's congenital malformations and the family was counseled accordingly. However, a lack of genetic association for diprosopus continues to support an embryologic theory of abnormal twinning.

It should be noted that the prenatal diagnosis at 26 weeks somewhat limited perinatal management options. However, the combination of detailed ultrasound and MRI imaging provided accurate prenatal diagnoses so that the family and medical providers were able to develop a comprehensive plan of care in advance of the delivery. Almost three months before the birth, medical providers compassionately informed the family that a successful resuscitation was unlikely. The parents asked that providers to make an attempt to resuscitate, but if unsuccessful, they wanted to hold and baptize their son. During follow-up counseling, the family stated that the birth and death experiences were more peaceful than anticipated. They felt that the medical, emotional, and spiritual support provided by the multidisciplinary team significantly reduced their anxiety, facilitated their decision-making, and, ultimately, aided them in coping with their loss.

Conflict of Interests

The authors declare no conflict of interest.

References

[1] L. D. Edmonds and P. M. Layde, "Conjoined twins in the United States, 1970–1977," *Teratology*, vol. 25, no. 3, pp. 301–308, 1982.

[2] R. Spencer, "Conjoined twins: theoretical embryologic basis," *Teratology*, vol. 45, no. 6, pp. 591–602, 1992.

[3] D. Carles, W. Weichhold, E. M. Alberti, F. Leger, F. Pigeau, and J. Horovitz, "Diprosopia revisited in light of the recognized role of neural crest cells in facial development," *Journal of Craniofacial Genetics and Developmental Biology*, vol. 15, no. 2, pp. 90–97, 1995.

[4] M. J. Depew, T. Lufkin, and J. L. R. Rubenstein, "Specification of jaw subdivisions by *Dlx* genes," *Science*, vol. 298, no. 5592, pp. 381–385, 2002.

[5] S. Hähnel, P. Schramm, S. Hassfeld, H. H. Steiner, and A. Seitz, "Craniofacial duplication (diprosopus): CT, MR imaging, and MR angiography findings—case report," *Radiology*, vol. 226, no. 1, pp. 210–213, 2003.

[6] M. D'Armiento, J. Falleti, G. Maria Maruotti, and P. Martinelli, "Diprosopus conjoined twins: radiologic, autoptic, and histologic study of a case," *Fetal and Pediatric Pathology*, vol. 29, no. 6, pp. 431–438, 2010.

[7] T. Laor, J. Stanek, and J. L. Leach, "Diprosopus tetraophthalmus: CT as a complement to autopsy," *The British Journal of Radiology*, vol. 85, no. 1009, pp. e10–e13, 2012.

[8] G. L. Fernandes, F. K. Matsubara, F. K. Marques et al., "Three-dimensional prenatal diagnosis of monocephalus diprosopus tetraophthalmos," *Journal of Ultrasound in Medicine*, vol. 29, no. 3, pp. 501–503, 2010.

[9] L. Spitz and E. M. Kiely, "Conjoined Twins," *Journal of the American Medical Association*, vol. 289, no. 10, pp. 1307–1310, 2003.

[10] W. Xu, A. Ahmad, S. Dagenais, R. K. Iyer, and J. W. Innis, "Chromosome 4q deletion syndrome: Narrowing the cardiovascular critical region to 4q32.2-q34.3," *The American Journal of Medical Genetics A*, vol. 158, no. 3, pp. 635–640, 2012.

[11] T. Huang, A. E. Lin, G. F. Cox et al., "Cardiac phenotypes in chromosome 4q- syndrome with and without a deletion of the dHAND gene," *Genetics in Medicine*, vol. 4, no. 6, pp. 464–467, 2002.

19

Update Review and Clinical Presentation in Congenital Insensitivity to Pain and Anhidrosis

L. M. Pérez-López,[1] M. Cabrera-González,[1] D. Gutiérrez-de la Iglesia,[1] S. Ricart,[2] and G. Knörr-Giménez[1]

[1]Pediatric Orthopaedic Surgery Department, Sant Joan de Déu Children's Hospital, University of Barcelona, Barcelona, Spain
[2]Pediatric Rheumatology Department, Sant Joan de Déu Children's Hospital, University of Barcelona, Barcelona, Spain

Correspondence should be addressed to L. M. Pérez-López; lperezl@hsjdbcn.org

Academic Editor: Piero Pavone

Introduction. Congenital insensitivity to pain and anhidrosis (CIPA) or hereditary sensory and autonomic neuropathy type IV is an extremely rare syndrome. Three clinical findings define the syndrome: insensitivity to pain, impossibility to sweat, and mental retardation. This pathology is caused by a genetic mutation in the NTRK1 gene, which encodes a tyrosine receptor (TrkA) for nerve growth factor (NGF). *Methods.* The consultation of a child female in our center with CIPA and a tibia fracture in pseudoarthrosis encouraged us to carefully review literature and examine the therapeutic possibilities. A thorough review of literature published in Pubmed was done about CIPA and other connected medical issues mentioned in the paper. *Conclusions.* The therapeutic approach of CIPA remains unclear. The preventive approach remains the only possible treatment of CIPA. We propose two new important concepts in the therapeutic approach for these patients: (1) early surgical treatment for long bone fractures to prevent pseudoarthrosis and to allow early weight bearing, decreasing the risk of further osteopenia, and (2) bisphosphonates to avoid the progression of osteopenia and to reduce the number of consecutive fractures.

1. Introduction

Congenital insensitivity to pain and anhidrosis (CIPA), also known as hereditary sensory and autonomic neuropathy type IV, is an extremely rare syndrome. The first reference to a similar pathology was mentioned by Dearborn in the early 1900s [1], and it was published in 1963 by Swanson [2]. Three clinical findings define the syndrome: insensitivity to pain, inability to sweat, and mental retardation [3, 4]. Only a few hundreds of cases of CIPA have been recently published worldwide [5, 6]. This condition occurs with an incidence of 1 in 125 million newborns [7].

The pathogenesis of CIPA is characterized by a genetic loss-of-function mutation of the NTKR1 gene (locus 1q 21-22) [8, 9]. Multiple new mutations have been progressively described [10–16]. NTRK1 mutations imply an alteration in TrkA, a NGF receptor. NGF is involved in surveillance of nociceptive sensory neurons and sympathetic autonomic neurons and collaborates in the activation and homeostasis of other cellular types so that a NTRK1 mutation will cause deficient development of [17–20]

(1) the afferent somatic sensory system for pain and temperature, located in the dorsal root ganglion sensory neurons,

(2) the autonomic sympathetic neuronal system, which implies loss of the innervation of eccrine sweat glands by sympathetic neurons,

(3) the central nervous system,

(4) the bidirectional communication between the immune system and the nervous system (NGF has a relevant role in the signal pathway of B lymphocytes through three processes: Trk A phosphorylation, cytoskeleton assemblage, and MAP kinase activation).

The molecular alteration in the function of NGF in turn also alters the normal process of fracture consolidation [21].

Normal osteoblast/osteoprogenitor differentiation and proliferation are hindered, tending to result in fibroblast differentiation of multipotent stromal mesenchymal cells and periosteal cells.

Bone metabolism is also affected by the lack of nociceptive fibers, present not only in the skin but also in the skeletal system [22]. Due to the trophic role that nociceptive fibers may play in the skeletal system, bone fractures are very common [23].

2. Case Presentation

Medical record and radiographic data of the present case were reviewed and reported in a study approved by the department of documentation of our hospital. The patient's parents also gave their consent. A thorough review of the PubMed literature on CIPA and associated medical conditions mentioned in this paper was performed (Table 1). This case report is an illustrative example of a patient affected by CIPA.

We present a case involving a seven-year-old, female child of Spanish nationality. She had been evaluated in another center for episodes of recurrent fever. After a long diagnostic process including a pertinent genetic study which detected two mutations in the NTRK1 gene responsible for CIPA, she was diagnosed with the syndrome [8]. Her parents were healthy, and no consanguinity was present.

Clinical exploration revealed absence of a pain response, recurrent episodes of fever, sweating deregulation, mental retardation, cutaneous autolesions, fracture without consolidation, avascular necrosis (Figure 1), demineralized bones, generalized osseous destruction (Figure 2), warm and dry skin with thickening of the soles and palms, and lower limb edema (Figures 3(a), 3(b), and 3(c)) [5, 24–26].

The patient was referred to our center four months after fracture of the middle shaft of the right tibia. Radiologic signs of hypertrophic pseudoarthrosis were present (Figure 4). An elastic intramedullary nailing was carried out [27]. Complete radiological consolidation of the fracture was achieved five months after the surgery (Figure 5).

In the following months, several fractures occurred, including a fifth metatarsal fracture in the right foot (Figure 1) and a fourth metatarsal fracture in the left foot, a right femoral middle shaft fracture that was surgically treated with good results (Figures 6(a), 6(b), and 6(c)), and an epiphysiolysis at the distal shaft of the right tibia. In CIPA, due to the alteration of the bone fracture metabolism, hypertrophic bone callus (Figures 1, 4, and 6(c)) and pseudoarthrosis (Figure 4) are very common. In the present patient, bone consolidation was only achieved when a surgical technique was applied.

During this period of time with recurrent fractures, treatment with bisphosphonates was started. A dose of 1 mg/Kg/day during 3 consecutive days of intravenous pamidronate was administered every four months, for one year. We obtained good results in preventing new fractures at upper and lower limbs, skull, and spine bones at 5 years of follow-up. No adverse effects were seen regarding pamidronate infusion or during the follow-up.

At 5 years of follow-up, patient has progressed.

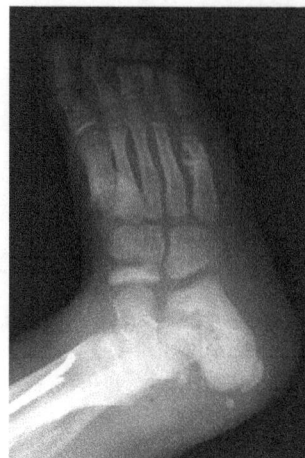

FIGURE 1: Navicular avascular necrosis and fifth metatarsal fracture in the right foot with hypertrophic bone callus.

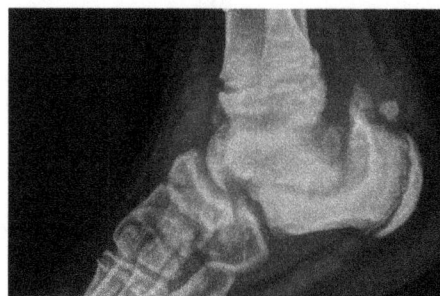

FIGURE 2: Demineralized bones and generalized osseous destruction.

3. Discussion

CIPA is an autosomal recessive disorder [8]. Some cases of consanguinity have been described among affected patients [7, 28]. Apart from the already well-defined genetic transmission of CIPA, there is an infrequent non-Mendelian inheritance characterized by uniparental disomy of chromosome 1 [10]. It is described by the transmission of an autosomal recessive pathology from only one affected parent. The molecular genetic analysis of the presented patient detected two heterozygous mutations in the NTRK1 gene (c.2205+1G>T in intron 16 and c.360-45C>A in intron 3), found also in her mother, suggesting then uniparental disomy.

The therapeutic approach to CIPA is still evolving and remains controversial [7]. There is no definitive agreement regarding its management, and therapeutic options are restricted to treatment of symptoms and protection from self-mutilation, fractures, and wound infections, which may lead to amputation. Such limited treatment options imply potentially catastrophic consequences of the natural pathologic evolution of the disease. Fractures associated with CIPA may be devastating and deeply affect the patient's functionality. Surgical treatment provides stability to the focal point of the fracture, helping to provide definitive consolidation. Moreover, immobilization contributes to accelerated bone

TABLE 1: Thorough review of the PubMed literature on CIPA and associated medical conditions mentioned in this paper was performed.

References	Year of publication	Particularity of the observation and remarks for each reading
Dearborn [1]	1932	First reference, in literature, to a similar disease
Swanson [2]	1963	First reference, in literature, to CIPA
Nishida [3]	1951	Three clinical representative findings: insensitivity to pain, inability to sweat, and mental retardation
Tunçbilek et al. [4]	2005	
Rosemberg et al. [5] review	1994	Only 32 cases have been published worldwide
Gao et al. [6]	2013	Only some hundreds of cases have been published worldwide
Daneshjou et al. [7]	2012	Incidence 1 in 125 million newborns
Indo et al. [8]	1996	CIPA pathogenesis: genetic loss-of-function mutation of the NTKR1 gene (locus 1q 21-22). NTKR1 mutations imply an alteration in TrKA, A NGF receptor
Indo et al. [9]	1997	
Indo et al. [8]	1996	Autosomal recessive disorder
Indo [10]	2001	Not only autosomal recessive inheritance, but also uniparental disomy (non-Mendelian inheritance of autosomal recessive disease from a single carrier parent, as the exposed case)
Indo [10] review	2001	
Indo et al. [15]	2001	
Bonkowsky et al. [11]	2003	
Lin et al. [12]	2010	Novel mutation and polymorphism in the NTRK1 gene causing CIPA
Mardy et al. [16]	2001	
Miura et al. [13]	2000	
Weier et al. [14]	1995	
Bonkowsky et al. [11]	2003	
Indo [25] review	2002	A very profuse resume of clinical and genetic characteristics of CIPA
Indo [18]	2010	NGF receptor failure causes a deficient development of dorsal root neurons (pain and temperature sensory system) autonomic sympathetic neural system (eccrine sweat glands innervation) Central nervous system The signal pathway of B lymphocytes
Indo [19]	2012	
Tanaka et al. [20]	1990	
Schwarzkopf et al. [17] review	2005	
Indo [25]	2002	
Melamed et al. [21]	2004	
Grills and Schuijers [24]	1998	NGF function disruption also causes an altered process of fracture consolidation
Fruchtman et al.[26]	2013	Descriptive clinical presentation including morbidity conditions (some of these clinical facts are also present in the case reported)
Yang et al. [27]	2013	
Jarade et al. [35] review	2002	Ocular manifestations
Brandes and Stuth [39]	2006	Anaesthetic considerations
Oliveira et al. [40]	2009	
Abdulla et al. [33]	2014	Heterotopic ossification and callus formation following fractures, eventually Charcot's joint
Schreiber et al. [41]	2005	Insulin-related difficulties

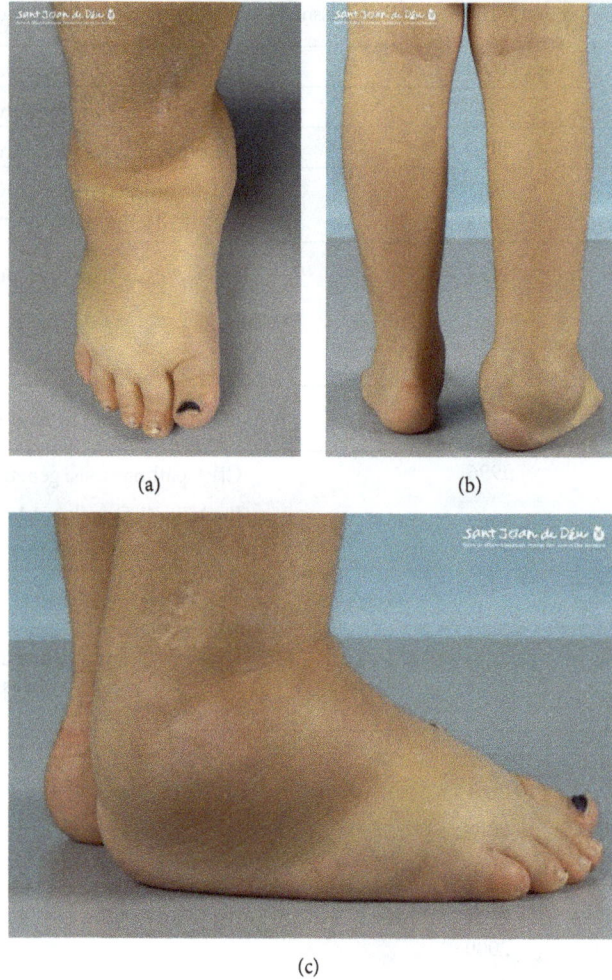

(a)

(b)

(c)

FIGURE 3: Lower limb edema.

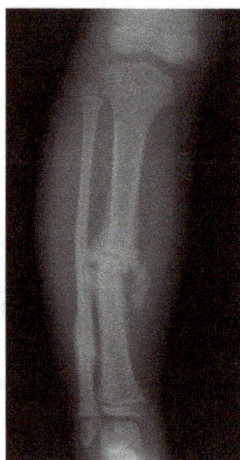

FIGURE 4: Hypertrophic bone callus.

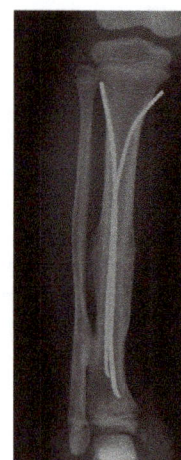

FIGURE 5: Complete radiological consolidation of the tibia fracture was achieved five months after the surgery.

demineralization. Surgical fracture repair allows for early weight bearing, diminishing the risk of further osteopenia, which is also usually present in these patients as a part of their associated neurogenic arthropathy (Figure 3) [21].

For all of these reasons, we recommend early surgical treatment of fractures. It allows for more rapid functional recovery, reducing the risk of accelerated osteopenia due to immobilization.

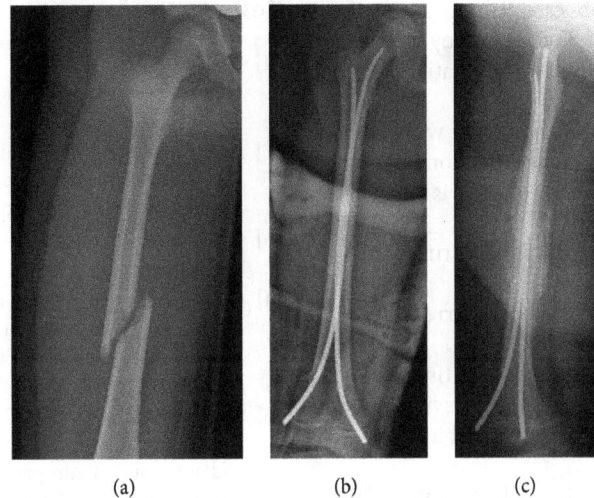

FIGURE 6: Right femoral middle shaft fracture that was surgically treated with good results. Hypertrophic bone callus associated.

The use of bisphosphonates in patients affected by CIPA had never been mentioned before in literature. Due to our previous good experience with pamidronate in treating osteoporotic fractures for disuse in children with different medical conditions [29, 30], we made a therapeutic approach with pamidronate as a compassionate use in this child. We obtained good results in preventing new fractures.

These two therapeutic observations might be relevant in the absence of specific treatment for CIPA. However, we may not forget that further studies addressing CIPA management are needed to provide more rigorous and scientific conclusions.

CIPA may present various signs and symptoms that can be misleading. The differential diagnoses of this pathology include radicular hereditary sensory neuropathy (HSN I); hereditary sensory and autonomic neuropathy (HSN II); familial dysautonomia or Riley-Day syndrome (HSN III) [31]; congenital indifference to pain (HSN V) [32]; and Lesch-Nyhan syndrome. Corneal ulcers are also relatively frequent in patients with CIPA. A differential diagnosis of neurotrophic keratitis may be taken into consideration [33, 34]. Among all these diagnostic possibilities and according to Raspall-Chaure [29],

CIPA must be the first diagnostic hypothesis when assessing a patient with insensitivity to pain, anhidrosis, and self-mutilation.

According to literature, the first step in the diagnosis of CIPA syndrome is consideration of the clinical presentation based on the combination of three basic signs: insensitivity to pain, anhidrosis, and mental retardation [3, 4]. Other possible signs may be associated: impaired temperature sensation [5], facial alterations [6], mandibular osteolysis [7], dental caries [6], and premature tooth loss [6]; repetitive soft tissue and osseous infections of hematogenous origin [33], mainly caused by *S. aureus* [25]; self-mutilating behavior [7]; occasional microcephaly [5, 24]; urine and fecal incontinence [11]; growth disturbances; and heterotopic ossification [7, 35, 36].

Neurological laboratory tests may provide additional information. Short-latency somatosensory evoked potentials show marked prolongation of the central conduction time [19] and microneurography reveals abnormal activity of somatic A-delta and C fibers in the nerves of the skin [6, 37, 38]. A negative sympathetic skin response may also be helpful in the diagnosis due to the lack of sudomotor nerves in skin biopsy [38].

Pharmacologic tests that evaluate autonomic function are also useful. The Mecholyl test produces prompt pupillary miosis [24], pain test results abnormal [6, 13, 24], there is an absence of a flare reaction to the histamine test [24] (although we may find some normal responses to subdermal histamine injection) [11], and the sweat test using pilocarpine reveals a disruption of sweat gland function. Histopathologic evaluation shows a hyperplastic epidermis with acanthosis and hyperkeratosis and a decreased amount of sweat and sebaceous glands [6].

Finally, molecular evaluation that reveals mutations of the NTKR1 gene provides a definitive diagnosis [19, 24].

About the anesthetic considerations [39, 40], although pain stimuli are absent, anxiety associated with surgical procedures may generate stress and consequent hemodynamic instability. It is necessary to minimize preoperative apprehension and anxiety with the use of sedatives. Also the autonomic response to surgery is inconsistent and erratic, which results in difficulty determining the necessary anesthetic doses in advance. Finally, temperature control is crucial. Malignant hyperthermia or hypothermia may be lethal.

NGF-TrkA pathway has a role in the morphogenesis of the endocrine pancreas, in insulin secretion *in vitro*, and in insulin secretion in response to glucose. Patients with CIPA present with alterations of the first phase of insulin secretion [41].

The similarities between CIPA and reflex sympathetic dystrophy are very interesting. Both are characterized by neurogenic inflammation, skin alterations with vasomotor disruption, and osteopenia.

Some authors have focused on establishing a specific treatment for complex regional pain syndrome by studying the role of receptor tyrosine kinase for NGF in patients with CIPA [29].

The high incidence of infections in patients with CIPA is also problematic. Skin and deep bone infections are the most common types, and *Staphylococcus aureus* is the most commonly involved pathogen.

Resistance to antibiotics is a frequently occurring limitation in the treatment of these patients [25].

Temperature deregulation may cause recurrent fever, which may lead to death if not recognized early.

Other complications such as trauma or soft tissue/bone infection may decrease condition of the survival rate, although all are treatable conditions if diagnosed in a timely manner [7].

The best therapeutic approach to patients with CIPA appears to be based on prophylactic measures such as braces for early weight bearing in nonsurgical fractures and accurate follow-up to avoid missing complications. We propose an unusual treatment challenge, with an early surgical treatment for long bone fractures and early use of bisphosphonates as follows.

Therapeutic proposals are as follows:

(1) Surgical fracture repair to achieve an early functional recovery that avoids a final destructive situation.

(2) Bisphosphonates use to manage osteoporosis.

Addressing the cause of CIPA as opposed to solely symptomatic treatment seems to be the optimal therapeutic approach. If CIPA results from loss-of-function mutations in the NTRK1 gene encoding TrkA, then molecular treatment involving a receptor tyrosine kinase for NGF would be the most effective therapeutic technique.

Disclosure

There were not any financial relationships that could be broadly relevant to the work. Our institution has not received any sort of support state. We have not received any financial support. None of the authors has received or may receive any personal payment or in-kind benefit or other professional benefits from a commercial entity. We have also followed the rules of good scientific practice, according to ethical responsibilities of all authors.

Conflict of Interests

None of the authors has directly received research funding and/or has potential conflict of interests.

Acknowledgments

The authors thank the patient and her parents for their kind collaboration. Also, they would like to express their gratitude for Carlos Aláez (Department of Photography, Sant Joan de Déu University Children's Hospital, Barcelona) for his help with preparation of the images.

References

[1] G. Dearborn, "A case of congenital general pure analgesia," *Journal of Nervous & Mental Disease*, vol. 75, no. 6, pp. 612–615, 1932.

[2] A. G. Swanson, "Congenital insensitivity to pain with anhydrosis. A unique syndrome in two male siblings," *Archives of Neurology*, vol. 8, no. 3, pp. 299–306, 1963.

[3] G. Nishida, "Congenital anhidrosis," *Saishin Igaku*, vol. 6, pp. 1100–1104, 1951.

[4] G. Tunçbilek, C. Öztekin, and A. Kayikçioğlu, "Calcaneal ulcer in a child with congenital insensitivity to pain syndrome," *Scandinavian Journal of Plastic and Reconstructive Surgery and Hand Surgery*, vol. 39, no. 3, pp. 180–183, 2005.

[5] S. Rosemberg, S. K. Nagahashi Marie, and S. Kliemann, "Congenital insensitivity to pain with anhidrosis (hereditary sensory and autonomic neuropathy type IV)," *Pediatric Neurology*, vol. 11, no. 1, pp. 50–56, 1994.

[6] L. Gao, H. Guo, N. Ye et al., "Oral and craniofacial manifestations and two novel missense mutations of the NTRK1 gene identified in the patient with congenital insensitivity to pain with anhidrosis," *PLoS ONE*, vol. 8, no. 6, Article ID e66863, 2013.

[7] K. Daneshjou, H. Jafarieh, and S.-R. Raaeskarami, "Congenital insensitivity to pain and anhydrosis (CIPA) syndrome; a report of 4 cases," *Iranian Journal of Pediatrics*, vol. 22, no. 3, pp. 412–416, 2012.

[8] Y. Indo, M. Tsuruta, Y. Hayashida et al., "Mutations in the TRKA/NGF receptor gene in patients with congenital insensitivity to pain with anhidrosis," *Nature Genetics*, vol. 13, no. 4, pp. 485–488, 1996.

[9] Y. Indo, S. Mardy, M. Tsuruta, M. A. Karim, and I. Matsuda, "Structure and organization of the human TRK A gene encoding a high affinity receptor for nerve growth factor," *Japanese Journal of Human Genetics*, vol. 42, no. 2, pp. 343–351, 1997.

[10] Y. Indo, "Molecular basis of congenital insensitivity to pain with anhidrosis (CIPA): mutations and polymorphisms in TRKA (NTRK1) gene encoding the receptor tyrosine kinase for nerve growth factor," *Human Mutation*, vol. 18, no. 6, pp. 462–471, 2001.

[11] J. L. Bonkowsky, J. Johnson, J. C. Carey, A. G. Smith, and K. J. Swoboda, "An infant with primary tooth loss and palmar hyperkeratosis: a novel mutation in the *NTRK1* gene causing congenital insensitivity to pain with anhidrosis," *Pediatrics*, vol. 112, part 1, no. 3, pp. e237–e241, 2003.

[12] Y.-P. Lin, Y.-N. Su, W.-C. Weng, and W.-T. Lee, "Novel neurotrophic tyrosine kinase receptor type 1 gene mutation associated with congenital insensitivity to pain with anhidrosis," *Journal of Child Neurology*, vol. 25, no. 12, pp. 1548–1551, 2010.

[13] Y. Miura, S. Mardy, Y. Awaya et al., "Mutation and polymorphism analysis of the TRKA (NTRK1) gene encoding a high-affinity receptor for nerve growth factor in congenital insensitivity to pain with anhidrosis (CIPA) families," *Human Genetics*, vol. 106, no. 1, pp. 116–124, 2000.

[14] H.-U. G. Weier, A. P. Rhein, F. Shadravan, C. Collins, and D. Polikoff, "Rapid physical mapping of the human trk protooncogene (NTRK1) to human chromosome 1q21-q22 by P1 clone selection, fluorescence in situ hybridization (FISH), and computer-assisted microscopy," *Genomics*, vol. 26, no. 2, pp. 390–393, 1995.

[15] Y. Indo, S. Mardy, Y. Miura et al., "Congenital insensitivity to pain with anhidrosis (CIPA): novel mutations of the TRKA

(NTRK1) gene, a putative uniparental disomy, and a linkage of the mutant TRKA and PKLR genes in a family with CIPA and pyruvate kinase deficiency," *Human Mutation*, vol. 18, no. 4, pp. 308–318, 2001.

[16] S. Mardy, Y. Miura, F. Endo, I. Matsuda, and Y. Indo, "Congenital insensitivity to pain with anhidrosis (CIPA): effect of TRKA (NTRK1) missense mutations on autophosphorylation of the receptor tyrosine kinase for nerve growth factor," *Human Molecular Genetics*, vol. 10, no. 3, pp. 179–188, 2001.

[17] R. Schwarzkopf, V. Pinsk, Y. Weisel, D. Atar, and Y. Gorzak, "Clinical and genetic aspects of congenital insensitivity to pain with anhidrosis," *Harefuah*, vol. 144, no. 6, pp. 433–437, 2005.

[18] Y. Indo, "Nerve growth factor, pain, itch and inflammation: lessons from congenital insensitivity to pain with anhidrosis," *Expert Review of Neurotherapeutics*, vol. 10, no. 11, pp. 1707–1724, 2010.

[19] Y. Indo, "Nerve growth factor and the physiology of pain: lessons from congenital insensitivity to pain with anhidrosis," *Clinical Genetics*, vol. 82, no. 4, pp. 341–350, 2012.

[20] M. Tanaka, A. Sotomatsu, H. Kanai, and S. Hirai, "Iron-dependent cytotoxic effects of dopa on cultured neurons of the dorsal root ganglia," *Clinical Neurology*, vol. 30, no. 4, pp. 379–383, 1990.

[21] I. Melamed, J. Levy, R. Parvari, and E. W. Gelfand, "A novel lymphocyte singnaling defect: trk A mutation in the syndrome of congenital insensitivity to pain and anhidrosis (CIPA)," *Journal of Clinical Immunology*, vol. 24, no. 4, pp. 441–448, 2004.

[22] K. A. Derwin, R. A. Glover, and E. M. Wojtys, "Nociceptive role of substance-P in the knee joint of a patient with congenital insensitivity to pain," *Journal of Pediatric Orthopaedics*, vol. 14, no. 2, pp. 258–262, 1994.

[23] E. L. Hill and R. Elde, "Distribution of CGRP-, VIP-, DβH-, SP-, and NPY-immunoreactive nerves in the periosteum of the rat," *Cell and Tissue Research*, vol. 264, no. 3, pp. 469–480, 1991.

[24] B. L. Grills and J. A. Schuijers, "Immunohistochemical localization of nerve growth factor in fractured and unfractured rat bone," *Acta Orthopaedica Scandinavica*, vol. 69, no. 4, pp. 415–419, 1998.

[25] Y. Indo, "Genetics of congenital insensitivity to pain with anhidrosis (CIPA) or hereditary sensory and autonomic neuropathy type IV. Clinical, biological and molecular aspects of mutations in TRKA(NTRK1) gene encoding the receptor tyrosine kinase for nerve growth factor," *Clinical Autonomic Research*, vol. 12, supplement 1, pp. I20–I32, 2002.

[26] Y. Fruchtman, Z. H. Perry, and J. Levy, "Morbidity characteristics of patients with congenital insensitivity to pain with anhidrosis (CIPA)," *Journal of Pediatric Endocrinology and Metabolism*, vol. 26, no. 3-4, pp. 325–332, 2013.

[27] L. Yang, S. F. Ji, R. J. Yue, J. L. Cheng, and J. J. Niu, "Old fractures in two patients with congenital insensitivity to pain with anhidrosis: radiological findings," *Clinical Imaging*, vol. 37, no. 4, pp. 788–790, 2013.

[28] J. P. Metaizeau and J. N. Ligier, "Surgical treatment of fractures of the long bones in children. Interference between osteosynthesis and the physiological processes of consolidation. Therapeutic indications," *Journal de Chirurgie*, vol. 121, no. 8-9, pp. 527–537, 1984.

[29] M. Raspall-Chaure, M. Del Toro-Riera, M. Gratacós et al., "Congenital insensitivity to pain with anhidrosis associated with congenital myasthenic syndrome," *Revista de Neurologia*, vol. 41, no. 4, pp. 218–222, 2005.

[30] J. F. Sebestyen, T. Srivastava, and U. S. Alon, "Bisphosphonates use in children," *Clinical Pediatrics*, vol. 51, no. 11, pp. 1011–1024, 2012.

[31] N. J. Shaw, "Management of osteoporosis in children," *European Journal of Endocrinology*, vol. 159, supplement 1, pp. S33–S39, 2008.

[32] R. A. Boraz, "Familial dysautonomia (Riley-Day Syndrome): report of case," *ASDC Journal of Dentistry for Children*, vol. 51, no. 1, pp. 64–65, 1984.

[33] M. Abdulla, S. S. Khaled, Y. S. Khaled, and H. Kapoor, "Congenital insensitivity to pain in a child attending a paediatric fracture clinic," *Journal of Pediatric Orthopaedics B*, vol. 23, no. 5, pp. 406–410, 2014.

[34] M. Karthikeyan, T. Sreenivas, J. Menon, and D. K. Patro, "Congenital insensitivity to pain and anhydrosis: a report of two cases," *Journal of Orthopaedic Surgery*, vol. 21, no. 1, pp. 125–128, 2013.

[35] E. F. Jarade, H. F. El-Sheikh, and K. F. Tabbara, "Indolent corneal ulcers in a patient with congenital insensitivity to pain with anhidrosis: a case report and literature review," *European Journal of Ophthalmology*, vol. 12, no. 1, pp. 60–65, 2002.

[36] G. Szöke, A. Rényi-Vámos, and M. A. Bider, "Osteoarticular manifestations of congenital insensitivity to pain with anhidrosis," *International Orthopaedics*, vol. 20, no. 2, pp. 107–110, 1996.

[37] M. Nolano, C. Crisci, L. Santoro et al., "Absent innervation of skin and sweat glands in congenital insensitivity to pain with anhidrosis," *Clinical Neurophysiology*, vol. 111, no. 9, pp. 1596–1601, 2000.

[38] Z. Shorer, S. W. Moses, E. Hershkovitz, V. Pinsk, and J. Levy, "Neurophysiologic studies in congenital insensitivity to pain with anhidrosis," *Pediatric Neurology*, vol. 25, no. 5, pp. 397–400, 2001.

[39] I. F. Brandes and E. A. E. Stuth, "Use of BIS monitor in a child with congenital insensitivity to pain with anhidrosis," *Paediatric Anaesthesia*, vol. 16, no. 4, pp. 466–470, 2006.

[40] C. R. D. Oliveira, V. C. Paris, R. A. Pereira, and F. S. T. de Lara, "Anesthesia in a patient with congenital insensitivity to pain and anhidrosis," *Revista Brasileira de Anestesiologia*, vol. 59, no. 5, pp. 602–609, 2009.

[41] R. Schreiber, J. Levy, N. Loewenthal, V. Pinsk, and E. Hershkovitz, "Decreased first phase insulin response in children with congenital insensitivity to pain with anhidrosis," *Journal of Pediatric Endocrinology and Metabolism*, vol. 18, no. 9, pp. 873–877, 2005.

20

A Case of Acute Myeloid Leukemia (FAB M2) with Inversion 16 Who Presented with Pelvic Myeloid Sarcoma

Mustafa Çakan,[1] Ahmet Koç,[1] Kıvılcım Cerit,[2] Süheyla Bozkurt,[3] Rabia Ergelen,[4] and Irmak Vural[5]

[1]Department of Pediatric Hematology and Oncology, Faculty of Medicine, Marmara University, Mimar Sinan Caddesi No. 41, Pendik, 34899 Istanbul, Turkey
[2]Department of Pediatric Surgery, Faculty of Medicine, Marmara University, Mimar Sinan Caddesi No. 41, Pendik, 34899 Istanbul, Turkey
[3]Department of Pathology, Faculty of Medicine, Marmara University, Mimar Sinan Caddesi No. 41, Pendik, 34899 Istanbul, Turkey
[4]Department of Radiology, Faculty of Medicine, Marmara University, Mimar Sinan Caddesi No. 41, Pendik, 34899 Istanbul, Turkey
[5]Department of Pediatrics, Faculty of Medicine, Marmara University, Mimar Sinan Caddesi No. 41, Pendik, 34899 Istanbul, Turkey

Correspondence should be addressed to Mustafa Çakan; mustafacakan@hotmail.com

Academic Editor: Ozgur Cogulu

Acute leukemias are the most common childhood cancer in all age groups. Acute myeloid leukemias (AML) constitute about 15–20% of acute leukemias. Fatigability, pallor, fever, and bleeding are the most common presenting symptoms of AML. Hepatosplenomegaly and lymphadenopathy are commonly encountered during physical examination. In rare instances eruptions due to skin involvement and localized tumor masses (myeloid sarcoma) may be found. Myeloid sarcoma is especially seen in AML-M2 subtype. By cytogenetic analysis, in AML-M2 subtype t(8;21) is often seen and it is more probable to find inversion 16 in AML-M4Eos subtype. Herein, we present a 15-year-old girl whose initial symptom was abdominal pain for three days and her pathological sign was a large abdominal mass which was verified by imaging studies and diagnosed as myeloid sarcoma by biopsy. On bone marrow examination, she had diagnosis of AML-M2 and by cytogenetic analysis inversion 16 was positive. She was treated with AML-BFM 2004 protocol and she is being followed up in remission on her ninth month of the maintenance therapy.

1. Introduction

Acute myeloid leukemia (AML) comprises 15–20% of all childhood acute leukemias. In most of the patients, fever, pallor, weight loss, and mucosal bleeding are seen. In more than half of the cases, liver, spleen, and lymph nodes are palpable [1, 2].

Myeloid sarcoma (chloroma and granulocytic sarcoma) is defined as a tumoral mass which is formed by immature myeloid cells in the extramedullary area. It is seen in less than 5% of all AML cases. The most common locations are head and neck region, skin, gingival region, and intracranial and paravertebral areas [3–6].

In FAB classification, AML is classified according to myeloblasts' morphology into 10 subtypes [7]. In 2008,

WHO classification was developed and AML was reclassified according to accompanying cytogenetic abnormalities [8]. AML-M2 comprises 10–15% of all AML cases. Myeloid sarcoma may accompany AML-M2 more commonly than other subgroups. By cytogenetic analysis t(8; 21) is often found in this subgroup. It is more probable to see inversion 16 [inv(16)] in AML-M4Eos [1, 2, 9].

2. Case Report

A 15-year-old girl was admitted to the emergency room with the complaint of abdominal pain for 3 days. On physical examination a solid mass was palpable on the left lower quadrant of the abdomen. She had neither organomegaly nor lymphadenopathy. On ultrasound examination, a uniform,

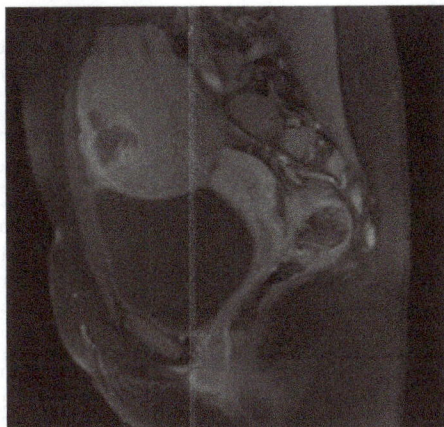

FIGURE 1: Sagittal T2-contrast-enhanced, fat saturated MR image of the mass.

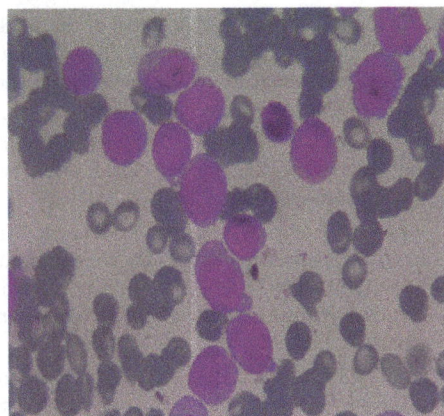

FIGURE 2: The view of myeloblasts on bone marrow aspiration material (×1000, Giemsa stain).

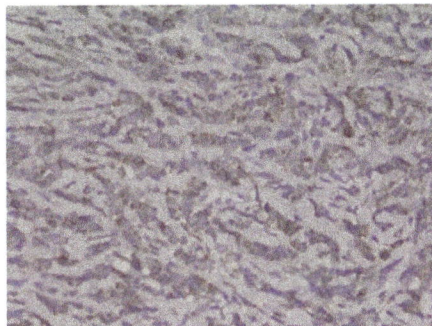

FIGURE 3: Immunohistochemistry showing MPO immunoreactivity in the cytoplasm of the neoplastic cells (×400, myeloperoxidase stain).

well-demarcated mass with 70×58 mm size was seen on the left superolateral part of the uterus. On MRI examination, $92 \times 70 \times 80$ mm sized, encapsulated, well-demarcated mass was observed at the same location (Figure 1). The right ovary was seen in both of the imagining techniques but the left one was not seen. Complete blood count revealed hyperleukocytosis with a leukocyte count of $100.6 \times 10^9/L$, anemia (hemoglobin: 107 g/L), and mild thrombocytopenia (platelets: $125 \times 10^9/L$). Lactate dehydrogenase level was 1144 U/L and other biochemical tests were at normal ranges. On peripheral blood smear examination 20% of cells were blasts. On bone marrow aspiration, 85% of cells were large myeloid blasts with fine chromatin and striking nucleoli (Figure 2). Eosinophilia or Auer rods were not observed. Since the rate of myeloid maturation was over 10%, findings of bone marrow aspiration were correlated with AML-M2 with maturation type. By flow cytometric analysis, 77% of mononuclear cells were positive for CD33, CD34, CD13, HLA-DR, CD117, and cytoplasmic MPO. CD14 was positive in 8% of the cells. Tru-cut biopsy was performed from the pelvic mass and there were atypical, large neoplastic cells with round, fine hyperchromatic nuclei spreading as single

cell lines and in some areas they were showing cohesive aggregates. There was an extensive fibrotic stroma causing widespread squeezing artefact in neoplastic cells. CD34, CD117, MPO, and lysozyme were diffusely positive in neoplastic cells (Figure 3). These findings were consistent with myeloid sarcoma. By cytogenetic analysis inv(16) was positive and t(8; 21), t(15; 17), t(4; 11), and t(9; 22) were negative.

The induction chemotherapy of AML-BFM 2004 protocol was started. An MRI was performed just before the beginning of the third block and 60% of shrinkage was achieved. Apart from the third block of chemotherapy, high-dose methylprednisolone was given for 7 days [10]. Two weeks after this therapy, on ultrasound examination, the mass still persisted. Laparoscopy was performed and the mass was extracted, preserving the left ovarian tissue. It was verified that the mass was originating from the left ovary. Total necrosis was seen on pathological examination of the material. Our patient completed 5 blocks of AML-BFM 2004 protocol without any problem. On control bone marrow examinations there were no blasts and control inv(16) became negative. She is being followed up on her ninth month of the maintenance therapy.

3. Discussion

AML is a hematological malignancy characterized by proliferation of myeloid cell precursors with or without maturation. The initial symptoms of AML are related to anemia, neutropenia, and thrombocytopenia which develop due to bone marrow infiltration of leukemic blasts [1, 2]. Myeloid sarcoma is defined as the accumulation of immature myeloid cells or myeloblasts in the extramedullary area. It is seen in 1–5% of all AML cases. It is more probable to encounter myeloid sarcoma in childhood AML than adults [11]. In the report of Ohanian et al. myeloid sarcoma was seen in 9% of all age groups of AML cases and in 40% of childhood AML cases [12]. The signs and symptoms of myeloid sarcoma are related to pressure effect on the adjacent structures [4–6]. Our patient's initial symptom was related to myeloid sarcoma mass. Myeloid sarcomas are commonly located at bone, periost, soft tissues of head and neck region, skin, and orbita. Rarely they can be located at intestine, mediastinum, pleura, peritoneum, biliary tract, breast, uterus, and ovaries [4–6, 13]. There are reports of case series about orbitally located myeloid sarcomas in Turkish children [3]. If there are associated cytogenetic abnormalities like inv(16) or t(8; 21), myeloid sarcoma is more commonly encountered [4, 5, 14]. Our case had inv(16) and supports this information. At the time of diagnosis since the pelvic mass was very big, we could not figure out the origin of the mass. During laparoscopy it was clearly seen that the mass was originating from the left ovary.

AML with maturation (FAB AML-M2) comprises 10–15% of all AML cases. To fulfill morphological diagnostic criteria, in the bone marrow, blast percentage must be over 20%, mature myeloid cell percentage must be over 10%, and monocytic component must be less than 20%. Immunophenotypically expression of CD13, CD33, CD65, CD11b, CD15, CD34, CD38, and HLA-DR is present [15, 16].

By cytogenetic analysis in cases of AML-M2, generally t(8; 21) is present. Inv(16) and t(16; 16) which are abnormalities of the 16th chromosome are seen in 7-8% of AML cases [17–19]. Inv(16) generally accompanies AML-M4Eos, but as in our case there are reports of AML-M2 cases with inv(16) positivity. He et al. reported in their paper that, in 15 of inv(16) positive AML patients, 12 of them had AML-M4Eos and one of them had AML-M2 [20]. In the research of Chan et al. 5 of the 43 AML patients had inv(16) and 3 of them had AML-M2 [21].

The prognosis of AML patients with inv(16) is generally better than other AML subtypes. Because the response to chemotherapy is satisfactory, it is recommended that bone marrow transplantation should be reserved for relapsed cases [1, 2, 9]. In our case, after the third block of chemotherapy total remission was achieved and inv(16) became negative.

In conclusion, in children who present with a solid mass, the possibility of myeloid sarcoma should be kept in mind. Our case also supported the opinion that inv(16) is not restricted to AML-M4Eos subtype.

Disclosure

This case report was presented as a poster at the 1st Marmara Pediatric Congress, 17–19 January 2014, İstanbul.

Conflict of Interests

The authors declare that there is no conflict of interests regarding the publication of this paper.

References

[1] R. J. Arceci and T. R. Golub, "Acute myelogenous leukemia," in *Principles and Practice of Pediatric Oncology*, P. Pizzo and D. G. Poplack, Eds., pp. 591–644, Lippincott Williams & Wilkins, Philadelphia, Pa, USA, 5th edition, 2006.

[2] J. E. Rubnitz, B. I. Razzouk, and R. C. Riberio, "Acute myeloid leukemia," in *Childhood Leukemias*, C.-H. Pui, Ed., pp. 499–539, Cambridge University Press, Memphis, Tenn, USA, 2nd edition, 2006.

[3] A. O. Cavdar, E. Babacan, S. Gozdasoglu et al., "High risk subgroup of acute myelomonocytic leukemia (AMML) with orbito-ocular granulocytic sarcoma (OOGS) in Turkish children," *Acta Haematologica*, vol. 81, no. 2, pp. 80–85, 1989.

[4] D. Reinhardt and U. Creutzig, "Isolated myelosarcoma in children—update and review," *Leukemia and Lymphoma*, vol. 43, no. 3, pp. 565–574, 2002.

[5] R. Schwyer, G. G. Sherman, R. J. Cohn, J. E. Poole, and P. Willem, "Granulocytic sarcoma in children with acute myeloblastic leukemia and t(8;21)," *Medical and Pediatric Oncology*, vol. 31, no. 3, pp. 144–149, 1998.

[6] J. C. Byrd, W. J. Edenfield, D. J. Shields, and N. A. Dawson, "Extramedullary myeloid cell tumors in acute nonlymphocytic leukemia: a clinical review," *Journal of Clinical Oncology*, vol. 13, no. 7, pp. 1800–1816, 1995.

[7] J. M. Bennett, D. Catovsky, M. T. Daniel et al., "Proposed revised criteria for the classification of acute myeloid leukemia. A report of the French-American-British Cooperative Group," *Annals of Internal Medicine*, vol. 103, no. 4, pp. 620–625, 1985.

[8] J. W. Vardiman, J. Thiele, D. A. Arber et al., "The 2008 revision of the World Health Organization (WHO) classification of myeloid neoplasms and acute leukemia: rationale and important changes," *Blood*, vol. 114, no. 5, pp. 937–951, 2009.

[9] A. Redler, "Leukemias," in *Manual of Pediatric Hematology and Oncology*, P. Lanzkowsky, Ed., pp. 550–563, Elsevier, San Diego, Calif, USA, 5th edition, 2011.

[10] G. Hiçsönmez, M. Cetin, D. Aslan, and E. Ozyürek, "The role of short course of high-dose methylprednisolone in children with acute myeloblastic leukemia (FAB M2) presented with myeloid tumor," *Pediatric Hematology and Oncology*, vol. 20, no. 5, pp. 373–379, 2003.

[11] G. M. Dores, S. S. Devesa, R. E. Curtis, M. S. Linet, and L. M. Morton, "Acute leukemia incidence and patient survival among children and adults in the United States, 2001-2007," *Blood*, vol. 119, no. 1, pp. 34–43, 2012.

[12] M. Ohanian, S. Faderl, F. Ravandi et al., "Is acute myeloid leukemia a liquid tumor?" *International Journal of Cancer*, vol. 133, no. 3, pp. 534–543, 2013.

[13] J. S. Nigam, V. Misra, V. Kumar, and K. Varma, "Aleukemic granulocytic sarcoma presenting at multiple sites: ovary, breast and soft tissue," *Rare Tumors*, vol. 4, no. 3, pp. 115–117, 2012.

[14] S. Paydas, S. Zorludemir, and M. Ergin, "Granulocytic sarcoma: 32 cases and review of the literature," *Leukemia and Lymphoma*, vol. 47, no. 12, pp. 2527–2541, 2006.

[15] R. B. Walter, M. Othus, A. K. Burnett et al., "Significance of FAB subclassification of "acute myeloid leukemia, NOS" in the 2008 WHO classification: analysis of 5848 newly diagnosed patients," *Blood*, vol. 121, no. 13, pp. 2424–2431, 2013.

[16] E. Campo, S. H. Swerdlow, N. L. Harris, S. Pileri, H. Stein, and E. S. Jaffe, "The 2008 WHO classification of lymphoid neoplasms and beyond: evolving concepts and practical applications," *Blood*, vol. 117, no. 19, pp. 5019–5032, 2011.

[17] D. Grimwade, R. K. Hills, A. V. Moorman et al., "Refinement of cytogenetic classification in acute myeloid leukemia: determination of prognostic significance of rare recurring chromosomal abnormalities among 5876 younger ad ult patients treated in the United Kingdom Medical Research Council trials," *Blood*, vol. 116, no. 3, pp. 354–365, 2010.

[18] E. Forestier, S. Heim, E. Blennow et al., "Cytogenetic abnormalities in childhood acute myeloid leukaemia: a Nordic series comprising all children enrolled in the NOPHO-93-AML trial

between 1993 and 2001," *British Journal of Haematology*, vol. 121, no. 4, pp. 566–577, 2003.

[19] K. N. Manola, "Cytogenetics of pediatric acute myeloid leukemia," *European Journal of Haematology*, vol. 83, no. 5, pp. 391–405, 2009.

[20] Y.-X. He, Y.-Q. Xue, H.-Y. Wang et al., "Clinical and laboratory features of pediatric acute myeloid leukemia with inversion of chromosome 16," *Zhonghua Er Ke Za Zhi*, vol. 50, no. 8, pp. 593–597, 2012.

[21] N. P. H. Chan, W. S. Wong, M. H. L. Ng et al., "Childhood acute myeloid leukemia with *CBFβ-MYH11* rearrangement: study of incidence, morphology, cytogenetics, and clinical outcomes of Chinese in Hong Kong," *American Journal of Hematology*, vol. 76, no. 3, pp. 300–303, 2004.

21

Aspiration Pneumonitis Caused by Polyethylene Glycol-Electrolyte Solution Treated with Conservative Management

Ricardo A. Mosquera, Mark McDonald, and Cheryl Samuels

High Risk Children Comprehensive Care Clinic, University of Texas Health Science of Houston, 6410 Fannin Street, Suite 500, Houston, TX 77030, USA

Correspondence should be addressed to Ricardo A. Mosquera; ricardo.a.mosquera@uth.tmc.edu

Academic Editor: Doris Fischer

Polyethylene glycol (PEG) electrolyte solution, Golytely, is an osmotic laxative commonly used in preoperative bowel cleansing. In this case report, a 9-year-old boy developed aspiration pneumonitis following accidental infusion of PEG solution into his right lung following migration of his nasogastric tube (NGT). Hypoxemia and tachypnea without respiratory failure were observed after infusion. Because PEG is a nonabsorbable toxic material, previous case reports have advocated for the performance of bronchoalveolar lavage (BAL) in the treatment of PEG pneumonitis. With close monitoring, our patient was able to be successfully treated without the need for invasive interventions including BAL or intubation. Generalizations about PEG absorption in the lung based on its permeability in the gastrointestinal tract should not deter the use of more conservative treatment in the appropriate patient.

1. Introduction

Polyethylene glycol (PEG) is a complex organic polymer that can be combined with sodium sulfate to form a highly efficacious osmotic laxative with a variety of medical applications [1]. This PEG-electrolyte solution is commonly used in preoperative bowel cleansing as it has been demonstrated that PEG is both effective and well tolerated in pediatric and adult populations [1, 2]. A major disadvantage of using PEG in bowel preparation is the unpleasant taste and the relatively large volume that must be ingested [1, 3]. This limitation can be overcome by administering the solution via nasogastric tube [1]. Common adverse effects of PEG include nausea, vomiting, and bloating though more serious gastrointestinal (GI) complications like pancreatitis can occur in addition to anaphylaxis, angioedema, and ventricular arrhythmia [4]. Additionally, the introduction of PEG solution into the lungs causes significant inflammation and an intraluminary fluid shift resulting in pulmonary edema [3]. These complications can be life-threatening and even fatal [3, 5–10]. Current treatment recommendations from previous case reports

include the use of prophylactic antibiotics, IV corticosteroids, and early bronchoscopy with bronchoalveolar lavage (BAL) and intubation with ventilation [6, 8, 9, 11]. In this report, we describe a pediatric patient who developed aspiration pneumonitis secondary to accidental PEG aspiration and was successfully treated with careful monitoring, IV antibiotics, and IV steroids without BAL. His symptoms disappeared after four days. Chest radiograph revealed complete resolution of right lower lobe opacities 7 days later.

2. Case Presentation

A 9-year-old Hispanic boy with spina bifida, hydrocephalus status post-VP shunt with normal neurological cognitive function, and neurogenic bladder with ileovesicostomy was scheduled for bladder augmentation and revision of his urinary diversion. He was admitted to the hospital for preoperative bowel preparation consisting of polyethylene lavage (1400cc over 4 hours) via nasogastric feeding tube (NGT) with a kangaroo feeding pump. The NGT placement

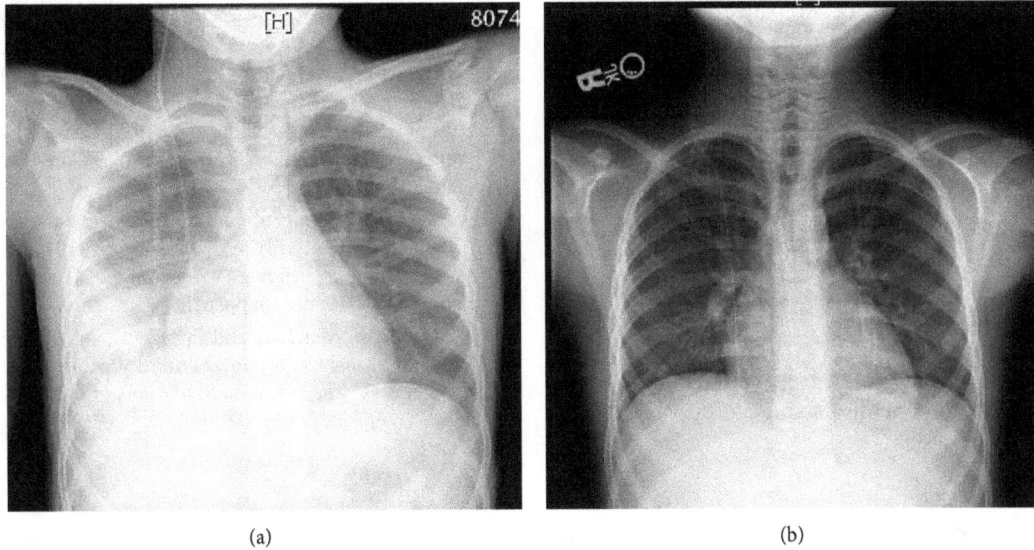

FIGURE 1: (a) CXR obtained immediately after nasogastric infusion of 283 mL of PEG in the right lung revealed right lower lobe opacities. (b) CXR 7 days after infusion showed significant clearance of right lower lobe opacities.

was confirmed with auscultation. Shortly after the infusion was begun, the patient developed significant coughing and gagging with small amount of emesis of clear fluid. The infusion was immediately stopped and a radiograph showed placement of the NG tube in the right lung. A review of the feeding pump revealed the patient had received a total of 283 mL of solution. The primary care provider and the pediatric and pulmonary services were notified and consulted.

Prior to the incident the patient's vitals were stable with a heart rate of 80 beats/minute, blood pressure 90/64 mm Hg, respiratory rate 18 breaths/minute, and oxygen saturation 100% in room air. When the infusion was stopped, the patient's vitals were mildly elevated with a heart rate of 126 beats/min, blood pressure 111/55 mm Hg, a respiratory rate 28 breaths/min, and oxygen saturation 93% in room air. On exam the patient had decreased breath sounds over the right lung field with no crackles or wheezing and did not appear to be in significant distress. A chest X-ray showed a right lower lobe aspiration pneumonitis (Figure 1). IV clindamycin was begun and the patient was transferred to the Pediatric IMU (intermediate medical unit) for continuous cardiopulmonary monitoring with recommendations to start supplemental oxygen and intravenous steroids if his condition deteriorated. Overnight, the patient had an increase in tachypnea and his oxygen desaturated to 87–89% on room air. He subsequently received 2 liters of oxygen via nasal cannula to maintain oxygen saturations above 92% and IV Solu-Medrol was begun at a dose of 2 mg/kg/day. A subsequent X-ray was performed the following day that showed worsening of his pneumonitis though his PCO2 and pH remained within normal limits and he appeared clinically stable. Two days after the ingestion, the patient was transitioned to room air and his condition began to steadily improve. The patient was discharged 4 days after the infusion and a final chest X-ray obtained demonstrated complete resolution of pneumonitis (Figure 1).

3. Discussion

In the present case, the patient had respiratory compromise secondary to the accidental infusion. However, his respiratory compromise did not deteriorate to respiratory failure. With careful, continuous cardiopulmonary monitoring, the decision was made not to perform bronchoscopy with BAL. This decision was made with the family after all options were discussed in detail. They expressed concern for him to be taken to the bronchoscopy procedure room and to be sedated/anesthetized. Authors in previous case studies have recommended BAL as the treatment of choice for aspiration pneumonitis from PEG infusion [6, 11]. One assumption that supports this recommendation is that PEG is nonabsorbable [6]. However, this may be a generalization based on the permeability of PEG in the gastrointestinal tract which significantly differs from the permeability in the pulmonary epithelium [2]. Given that in the current case the aspiration pneumonitis resolved without invasive intervention to remove the offending agent, we speculate, based on this experience, that aspirated PEG can be absorbed or neutralized. This interpretation is consistent with the finding that in the rodent lung only half of a solution of 3.4 kDa PEG (similar size to PEG) remained in the alveoli after 9-10 hours [12, 13]. While bronchoscopy is a relatively safe procedure with a risk of approximately 5% for minor complications and <2% for major complications, it is still an invasive procedure that requires sedation and may not be necessary in an otherwise clinically stable patient [14]. Our finding is supported by another case study in which an adult patient was only given antibiotics, corticosteroids, and diuretics following PEG aspiration and the clinical and radiographic manifestations of his pneumonitis resolved after 3 days [4]. In most of the case reports the use of BAL and/or intubation with ventilation for treatment of PEG aspiration are recommended. These interventions may have been very appropriate as the conditions of the patients in these cases were more severe [3, 7–11]. Given the absence of designed studies assessing the costs and benefits of using bronchoscopy with BAL or intubation with ventilation for treatment of PEG aspiration, we recommend that the stability of the patient be an important determinant when deciding on treatment modalities. Additionally, we believe that treatment decisions should not be rooted in generalizations about the absorption of PEG based solely on its permeability in the GI tract.

Conflict of Interests

The authors declare that there is no conflict of interests regarding the publication of this paper.

References

[1] A. Dahshan, C. H. Lin, J. Peters, R. Thomas, and V. Tolia, "A randomized, prospective study to evaluate the efficacy and acceptance of three bowel preparations for colonoscopy in children," *The American Journal of Gastroenterology*, vol. 94, no. 12, pp. 3497–3501, 1999.

[2] R. W. Pelham, L. C. Nix, R. E. Chavira, M. V. Cleveland, and P. Stetson, "Clinical trial: single- and multiple-dose pharmacokinetics of polyethylene glycol (PEG-3350) in healthy young and elderly subjects," *Alimentary Pharmacology and Therapeutics*, vol. 28, no. 2, pp. 256–265, 2008.

[3] P. de Graaf, C. Slagt, J. L. C. A. de Graaf, and R. J. L. F. Loffeld, "Fatal aspiration of polyethylene glycol solution," *The Netherlands Journal of Medicine*, vol. 64, no. 6, pp. 196–198, 2006.

[4] J. Belsey, O. Epstein, and D. Heresbach, "Systematic review: adverse event reports for oral sodium phosphate and polyethylene glycol," *Alimentary Pharmacology and Therapeutics*, vol. 29, no. 1, pp. 15–28, 2009.

[5] A. Argent, M. Hatherill, L. Reynolds, and L. Purves, "Fulminant pulmonary oedema after administration of a balanced electrolyte polyethylene glycol solution," *Archives of Disease in Childhood*, vol. 86, no. 3, article 209, 2002.

[6] G. Y. Hur, S. Y. Lee, J. J. Shim, K. H. In, K. H. Kang, and S. H. Yoo, "Aspiration pneumonia due to polyethylene glycol-electrolyte solution (Golytely) treated by bronchoalveolar lavage," *Respirology*, vol. 13, no. 1, pp. 152–154, 2008.

[7] H. U. Marschall and F. Bartels, "Life-threatening complications of nasogastric administration of polyethylene glycol-electrolyte solutions (Golytely) for bowel cleansing," *Gastrointestinal Endoscopy*, vol. 47, no. 5, pp. 408–410, 1998.

[8] U. Narsinghani, M. Chadha, H. C. Farrar, and K. S. Anand, "Life-threatening respiratory failure following accidental infusion of polyethylene glycol electrolyte solution into the lung," *Journal of Toxicology—Clinical Toxicology*, vol. 39, no. 1, pp. 105–107, 2001.

[9] C. M. Paap and R. Ehrlich, "Acute pulmonary edema after polyethylene glycol intestinal lavage in a child," *The Annals of Pharmacotherapy*, vol. 27, no. 9, pp. 1044–1047, 1993.

[10] A. Wong and G. L. Briars, "Acute pulmonary oedema complicating polyethylene glycol intestinal lavage," *Archives of Disease in Childhood*, vol. 87, no. 6, article 537, 2002.

[11] P. Liangthanasarn, D. Nemet, R. Sufi, and E. Nussbaum, "Therapy for pulmonary aspiration of a polyethylene glycol solution," *Journal of Pediatric Gastroenterology and Nutrition*, vol. 37, no. 2, pp. 192–194, 2003.

[12] H. Gursahani, J. Riggs-Sauthier, J. Pfeiffer, D. Lechuga-Ballesteros, and C. S. Fishburn, "Absorption of polyethylene glycol (PEG) polymers: the effect of PEG size on permeability," *Journal of Pharmaceutical Sciences*, vol. 98, no. 8, pp. 2847–2856, 2009.

[13] K. Knop, R. Hoogenboom, D. Fischer, and U. S. Schubert, "Poly(ethylene glycol) in drug delivery: pros and cons as well as potential alternatives," *Angewandte Chemie International Edition*, vol. 49, no. 36, pp. 6288–6308, 2010.

[14] J. de Blic, V. Marchac, and P. Scheinmann, "Complications of flexible bronchoscopy in children: prospective study of 1,328 procedures," *The European Respiratory Journal*, vol. 20, no. 5, pp. 1271–1276, 2002.

22

Cooccurrence of Darier's Disease and Epilepsy: A Pediatric Case Report and Review of the Literature

Tamer Celik,[1] Umit Celik,[2] Cigdem Donmezer,[2] Mustafa Komur,[1] Orkun Tolunay,[2] and Pelin Demirtürk[3]

[1] Pediatric Neurology, Adana Numune Research and Training Hospital, Adana, Turkey
[2] Pediatrics, Adana Numune Research and Training Hospital, Adana, Turkey
[3] Pathology Department, Adana Numune Research and Training Hospital, Adana, Turkey

Correspondence should be addressed to Umit Celik; ucelik32@gmail.com

Academic Editor: Piero Pavone

Darier's disease is a skin disorder characterized by multiple eruptions of hyperkeratosis or crusted papules at seborrheic areas with histologic acantholysis and dyskeratosis. It is caused by mutations in a single gene, being *ATP2A2* and that is expressed in the skin and brain. The cooccurrence of various neurologic and psychiatric diseases with Darier's disease has been reported frequently in literature. They include mood disorders, epilepsy, encephalopathy, and schizophrenia. In this study, we report a pediatric case with the cooccurrence of Darier's disease and epilepsy. We also revised current English literature on this topic.

1. Introduction

Darier's disease (DD, Lutz-Darier-White disease, keratosis follicularis; MIM 124200) is a skin disorder characterized by multiple eruptions of hyperkeratotic or crusted papules and plaques at seborrheic areas, palmoplantar pits, and nail abnormalities [1]. The prevalence of the disease is estimated to be 1 in 50000 people [2]. DD is autosomal, dominantly inherited with high penetrance, although phenotypic expression is variable [2]. The linear form of DD is not inherited; it rather occurs as a result of somatic mutations. No family history is common and it represented a third of cases reported in a study [3].

DD is caused by mutations in the *ATP2A2* gene, which maps to chromosome 12q23-q24.1 and encodes the sarcoplasmic/endoplasmic reticulum calcium ATPase isoform 2 (SERCA2), a calcium pump located in the endoplasmic reticulum membrane [4, 5]. Darier's disease is caused by reduction in the SERCA2b function leading to abnormal intracellular Ca+2 signalling and abnormal organization or maturation of complexes responsible for cell adhesion [6].

DD is presenting in adolescence or adulthood with the onset of multiple focal keratotic skin lesions [4, 5]. Skin lesions may be severe, with widespread itchy malodorous crusted plaques, painful erosions, blistering, and mucosal lesions. Sun, heat, and sweating exacerbate the disease. Males and females are affected equally by the disease. Several variants of cutaneous lesions have been reported in literature [4]. Bullous, erosive, vegetative form, familial haemorrhagic variant, and hypopigmented macules were seen in DD patients. Seborrheic dermatitis, Hailey-Hailey disease, and transient acantholyticdermatosis should be assessed in differential diagnosis [7]. The cooccurrence of various neurologic and psychiatric diseases including mood disorders, mental retardation, and schizophrenia has been reported with DD [8, 9]. However, there are only a few reports that indicate the cooccurrence of epilepsy and DD.

In this study, we report a pediatric case with cooccurrence of DD and epilepsy. We also revised the current English literature existing on this topic.

2. Case Report

A sixteen-year-old female patient was referred to the Pediatric Neurology Department because of seizures. The history

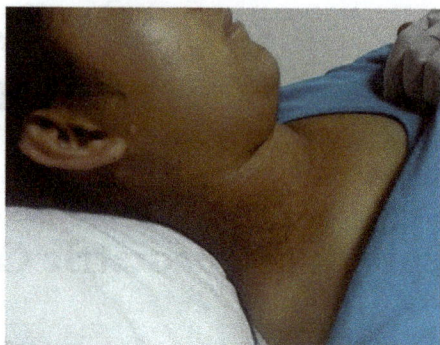

FIGURE 1: Hyperkeratotic dark papules on the neck.

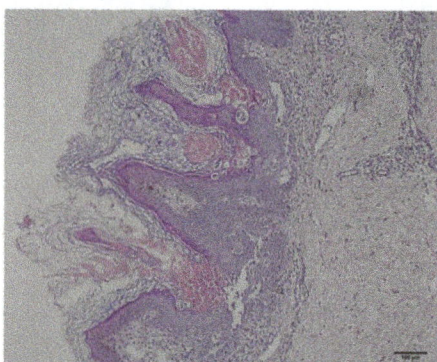

FIGURE 2: Skin biopsy showing hyperkeratosis, dyskeratosis, papillomatosis, suprabasal acantholysis, and dermal chronic inflammatory infiltrate (H&E ×100).

of the patient revealed ordinary vaginal birth of 3 kg and no problems in neonatal and early childhood but some learning difficulties and low success in the school at the time the patient started primary school. There is no similar disease history in the family. Within the last year, she also had a history of 3 generalized tonic-clonic seizures that lasted for 3-4 minutes. However, it was learned that she has never applied to a physician. According to the medical history, she had rash in the neck and behind the ears that had begun two years ago. Although the skin lesions were sometimes itchy, heat or sweating did not worsen them. In her examination, hyperkeratotic papules in 0.3 × 0.5 cm dimensions were detected, being hard with palpation, presented on a postauricular area, and ranging in length from neck and covering the scalp and ears (Figure 1). Neurologic and other system examinations, biochemical tests and complete blood cell count, electrocardiogram, cerebral magnetic resonance imaging, and finally awake and sleep electroencephalogram were normal. The patient consulted a dermatologist and punch biopsy of the skin was taken. On histopathological examination; hyperkeratosis, dyskeratosis, papillomatosis, suprabasal acantholysis, and dermal chronic inflammatory infiltrate were seen and Darier's disease was confirmed (Figure 2).

3. Discussion

DD appears in association with an increased prevalence of neuropsychiatric disorders including mental retardation, epilepsy, schizophrenia, bipolar disorder, and sociopathic behaviour [4, 10, 11]. The majority of DD patients have no neuropsychiatric problems. The reported prevalence rates and types of neuropsychiatric features in studies vary greatly. It is not known if neuropsychiatric symptoms are a psychological reaction to having a skin disease or a direct consequence of mutations in the ATP2A2 gene [12]. DD gene has pleiotropic effects in skin and brain [5]. These tissues share a common ectodermal origin and intracellular calcium signalling in neurons is involved in neuronal excitability and neurotransmission [13]. SERCA2 is a calcium pump of the endoplasmic reticulum transporting calcium from the cytosol to the lumen of endoplasmic reticulum [12]. ATP2A2 mutations lead to loss of calcium transport by SERCA2 resulting in decreased endoplasmic reticulum calcium concentration in Darier's keratinocytes [12]. The role of SERCA2 in neurological development or function remains highly plausible since the gene is widely expressed in the brain [14]. One study suggests that a susceptibility locus for bipolar disorder cosegregates with the keratosis follicularis region, but it is distinct from the keratosis follicularis-causing mutation [15]. Missense, nonsense, frameshift, and splicing mutations in the ATPA2 gene of families with DD have been described [1]. Up to date, more than 120 familial and sporadic mutations in ATP2A2 have been identified in DD patients but attempts at identifying genotype-phenotype correlation have not been successful [7]. Ruiz-Perez et al. reported that variant cutaneous phenotypes associated with missense mutations. Contrarily, they also reported that neuropsychiatric features are not associated with a spesific type of mutation but rather depend on concomitant genetic and environmental factors [16]. On the other hand, Jacobsen et al. reported that missense mutations in ATP2A2 correlate with the presence of neuropsychiatric phenotypes and more specifically that the ATP binding domain may have relevance in mood disorders [5]. Comparison of molecular data and association with neuropsychiatric disorders do not reveal an obvious genotype-phenotype correlation in Ringpfeil et al.'s study [17]. In a study in North African population, no obvious phenotype-genotype correlation was established [18].

Our patient was referred to the Pediatric Neurology Department for evaluation of her seizures. There, we detected skin lesions (Figure 1). Seborrheic dermatitis and transient acantholysis dermatosis in differential diagnosis were excluded. By evaluation of the clinical characteristics and following biopsy, DD was diagnosed. Here, genetic analysis was not performed. The patient had epileptic and also learning problems. While the reported lifetime prevalence rates of epilepsy in the general population are variable, with the percentage 1.3%, the overall prevalence of epilepsy is 30–42.9 in 1000 DD patients [4, 19, 20]. A higher prevalence of epilepsy in individuals with DD was seen compared with that in general population [4, 20]. In the study of Gordon-Smith et al., mood disorders (50%), specifically major depression (30%), bipolar disorder (4%), suicide attempts (13%), suicidal thoughts (31%), and epilepsy (3%), in 100 DD patients were reported [20]. The association does not appear as a specific subtype of epilepsy. In some DD cases with epilepsy, cerebral atrophy was reported in computed tomography of the brain [21] but our patient's MRI findings were normal.

DD patients may show moderate learning and behavioral problems [1]. Learning difficulties are related not only to the IQ level but also to many factors such as social isolation, and low social condition may contribute to this situation. In the study of Gordon-Smith et al., the IQ level of DD patients was found to be indifferent to the general population [20]. However, in a study limited to just a few cases, the IQ of 2 of the 5 patients was detected to be below the average [10]. Mental retardation has been reported in some families. In a British report, 5% of 163 patients were mentally retarded and the same proportion was epileptic [4]. A study conducted in Denmark provides us with the information that seven of the 37 patients were mentally subnormal and nine others were destitute [22].

In conclusion, both pediatric neurologists and dermatologists should be aware of a possible cooccurrence of Darier's disease and epilepsy. The recognition and treatment of epilepsy will prevent complications that may develop and can also improve the patient's life quality.

Conflict of Interests

The authors declare that there is no conflict of interests regarding the publication of this paper.

References

[1] A. Sakuntabhai, S. Burge, S. Monk, and A. Hovnanian, "Spectrum of novel ATP2A2 mutations in patients with Darier's disease," Human Molecular Genetics, vol. 8, no. 9, pp. 1611–1619, 1999.

[2] C. S. Munro, "The phenotype of Darier's disease: penetrance and expressivity in adults and children," British Journal of Dermatology, vol. 127, no. 2, pp. 126–130, 1992.

[3] J. D. Wilkinson, R. A. Marsden, and R. P. R. Dawber, "Review of Darier's disease in the Oxford region," British Journal of Dermatology, vol. 97, no. 15, pp. 15–16, 1977.

[4] S. M. Burge and J. D. Wilkinson, "Darier-White disease: a review of the clinical features in 163 patients," Journal of the American Academy of Dermatology, vol. 27, no. 1, pp. 40–50, 1992.

[5] N. J. Jacobsen, I. Lyons, B. Hoogendoorn et al., "ATP2A2 mutations in Darier's disease and their relationship to neuropsychiatric phenotypes," Human Molecular Genetics, vol. 8, no. 9, pp. 1631–1636, 1999.

[6] J. Dhitavat, R. J. Fairclough, A. Hovnanian, and S. M. Burge, "Calcium pumps and keratinocytes: lessons from Darier's disease and Hailey-Hailey disease," British Journal of Dermatology, vol. 150, no. 5, pp. 821–828, 2004.

[7] P.-Y. Kwok and T. Hsu, "Keratosis Follicularis (Darier Disease)," 2014, http://www.emedicine.com/.

[8] A. S. Pendlebury, "Darier's disease and epilepsy," Nursing Times, vol. 60, pp. 449–450, 1964.

[9] S.-L. Wang, S.-F. Yang, C.-C. Chen, P.-T. Tsai, and C.-Y. Chai, "Darier's disease associated with bipolar affective disorder: a case report," Kaohsiung Journal of Medical Sciences, vol. 18, no. 12, pp. 622–626, 2002.

[10] R. S. Medansky and A. A. Woloshin, "Darier's disease. An evaluation of its neuropsychiatric component," Archives of Dermatology, vol. 84, pp. 482–484, 1961.

[11] N. A. Getzler and A. Flint, "Keratosis follicularis: a study of one family," Archives of Dermatology, vol. 93, no. 5, pp. 545–549, 1966.

[12] M. Savignac, A. Edir, M. Simon, and A. Hovnanian, "Darier disease: a disease model of impaired calcium homeostasis in the skin," Biochimica et Biophysica Acta, vol. 1813, no. 5, pp. 1111–1117, 2011.

[13] M. J. Berridge, M. D. Bootman, and P. Lipp, "Calcium—a life and death signal," Nature, vol. 395, no. 6703, pp. 645–648, 1998.

[14] F. Baba-Aissa, L. Raeymaekers, F. Wuytack, L. Dode, and R. Casteels, "Distribution and isoform diversity of the organellar Ca^{2+} pumps in the brain," Molecular and Chemical Neuropathology, vol. 33, no. 3, pp. 199–208, 1998.

[15] I. Jones, N. Jacobsen, E. K. Green, G. P. Elvidge, M. J. Owen, and N. Craddock, "Evidence for familial cosegregation of major affective disorder and genetic markers flanking the gene for Darier's disease," Molecular Psychiatry, vol. 7, no. 4, pp. 424–427, 2002.

[16] V. L. Ruiz-Perez, S. A. Carter, E. Healy et al., "ATP2A2 mutations in Darier's disease: variant cutaneous phenotypes are associated with missense mutations, but neuropsychiatric features are independent of mutation class," Human Molecular Genetics, vol. 8, no. 9, pp. 1621–1630, 1999.

[17] F. Ringpfeil, A. Raus, J. J. DiGiovanna et al., "Darier disease—novel mutations in ATP2A2 and genotype–phenotype correlation," Experimental Dermatology, vol. 10, no. 1, pp. 19–27, 2001.

[18] M. Bchetnia, C. Charfeddine, S. Kassar et al., "Clinical and mutational heterogeneity of Darier disease in Tunisian families," Archives of Dermatology, vol. 145, no. 6, pp. 654–656, 2009.

[19] J. W. A. S. Sander and S. D. Shorvon, "Epidemiology of the epilepsies," Journal of Neurology Neurosurgery and Psychiatry, vol. 61, no. 5, pp. 433–443, 1996.

[20] K. Gordon-Smith, L. A. Jones, S. M. Burge, C. S. Munro, S. Tavadia, and N. Craddock, "The neuropsychiatric phenotype in Darier disease," British Journal of Dermatology, vol. 163, no. 3, pp. 515–522, 2010.

[21] A. López-Hernández, L. Tamayo de Malo, and R. Cuéllar Alvarenga, "Mental retardation convulsions and cerebral atrophy; main neurological changes in Darier's disease," Boletín Médico del Hospital Infantil de México, vol. 37, pp. 531–537, 1980.

[22] I. B. Svensen and B. Albrechtsen, "The prevalence of dyskeratosisfollicularis in Denmark," Acta Dermato-Venereologica, vol. 30, pp. 256–269, 1961.

23

Smith-Lemli-Opitz Syndrome: A Case with Annular Pancreas

Mehmet Demirdöven,[1,2] **Hamza Yazgan,**[1] **Mevlit Korkmaz,**[3]
Arzu Gebeşçe,[1] **and Alparslan Tonbul**[1]

[1] Department Of Pediatrics, School Of Medicine, Fatih University, Turkey
[2] Fatih Üniversitesi Tıp Fakültesi, Sahil Yolu Sokak No. 16 Dragos Maltepe, 34844 Istanbul, Turkey
[3] Department Of Pediatrics Surgery, School Of Medicine, Fatih University, Turkey

Correspondence should be addressed to Mehmet Demirdöven; mdemirdoven@fatih.edu.tr

Academic Editor: William B. Moskowitz

Smith-Lemli-Opitz syndrome is an autosomal recessive disease of cholesterol metabolism. It is a multiple malformation syndrome with typical dysmorphic features such as bitemporal narrowing, ptosis, epicanthus, microcephaly, micrognathia, and cardiovascular, skeletal, urogenital, and gastrointestinal anomalies. This report presents a typical case of Smith-Lemli-Opitz syndrome with annular pancreas which is an unreported gastrointestinal abnormality.

1. Introduction

Smith-Lemli-Opitz syndrome (SLOS) is an autosomal recessive disease caused by an inborn error of cholesterol metabolism due to the deficiency of the enzyme 7-dehydrocholesterol reductase. It is by far the most common disorder of the postsqualene cholesterol biosynthesis. The incidence is reported to be approximately 1/20 000-1/70 000 and is more common in people of European descent [1]. The clinical phenotype ranges from mild to severe with classic SLOS patients having characteristic faces that include microcephaly, ptosis, anteverted nares, and micrognathia; growth and mental retardation; hypogenitalism in males; and skeletal abnormalities, the most common being 2,3 toe syndactyly and postaxial polydactyly. Many gastrointestinal abnormalities were also reported in SLOS patients including colonic aganglionosis, cholestatic liver disease, and pyloric stenosis [2].

Herein we report a case of SLOS with annular pancreas resulting in duodenal obstruction that is not reported so far.

2. Case

The patient was a male baby born at 34 gw from 24-year-old primigravid mother by spontaneous vaginal delivery. There was a first degree consanguinity between parents.

The physical examination revealed a 3200 gr (>90 p), 48 (75–90 p) cm hypotonic, cyanotic baby with hydrops fetalis. Head circumference was 35 cm (>90 p). Bitemporal narrowing, ptosis, cataracts, short nasal root, anteverted nares, micrognathia, low-set ears, overriding fingers, and scrotal hypoplasia with cryptorchidism were noted (Figures 1 and 2). There was a 2/6 grade systolic mesocardiac murmur. Abdominal distention was also remarkable with 4 cm hepatic and 2 cm splenic enlargement. Ultrasonographic evaluation of abdomen demonstrated right ptotic kidney and grade 2 pelvicaliceal ectasia in left kidney. Echocardiography revealed VSD, ASD, PDA, and pericardial effusion. Cranial ultrasound was normal. Because of the typical dysmorphic features, SLOS was the clinical diagnosis. Serum cholesterol and dehydrocholesterol levels were 74 mg/dL and 4.2 μg/mL, respectively. 7-Dehydrocholesterol (DHC7)/cholesterol ratio was 0.56 (normal: 0.16 ± 0.09 μg/mL). Basal serum cortisol level was 32 μg/dL. During followup in NICU the patient had feeding intolerance with bile stained vomitus. Radiologic evaluation of gastrointestinal system delineated delayed passage from pylorus, a filling defect at the base of the duodenal bulb and also a filling defect at the antral region that is consistent with a web. At the surgical exploration, stomach and the first part of the duodenum were dilated and there was an obstruction at the second part of the duodenum caused by

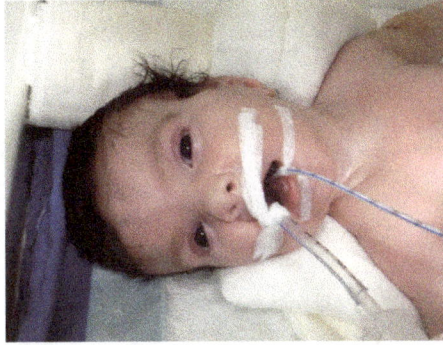

FIGURE 1: Typical dysmorphic face of the patient.

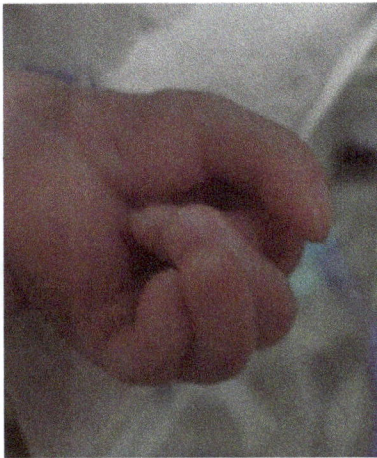

FIGURE 2: Overriding fingers.

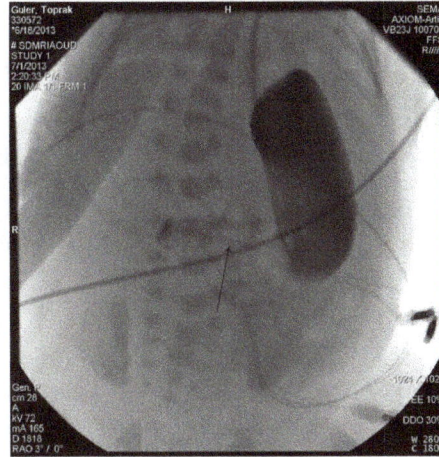

FIGURE 3: Upper GI series showing difficulty in gastric emptying and insufficient distention at the pylorus and duodenum (arrow) due to the encircled pancreatic tissue.

annular pancreas (Figure 3). After operation, his condition was deteriorated and he died of respiratory failure 37 days after birth.

3. Discussion

Cholesterol is an important lipid molecule that is essential for cellular membrane for proper membrane permeability and fluidity. It is also a precursor for the synthesis of steroid hormones, bile acids, and vitamin D. Cholesterol also functions in intracellular transport, cell signaling, and nerve conduction.

Abnormalities in cholesterol biosynthesis result in some of the several dysmorphology syndromes, namely, desmosterolosis, lathosterolosis, CHILD syndrome (a form of chondrodysplasia punctata), Greenberg dysplasia, and the more common SLOS [3]. The pathogenesis of these multisystem malformations has not been clear yet. Some of them have been attributed to impaired sonic hedgehog (SHH) functioning which plays a key regulatory role in vertebrate organogenesis, such as in the growth of digits and organization of the brain [4, 5].

SLOS is a multiple congenital malformation syndrome caused by deficiency of the enzyme 7-dehydrocholesterol reductase encoded by DHCR7 gene located on chromosome 11q13.4. The diagnosis requires measurement of serum cholesterol and 7-dehydrocholesterol levels. Although most affected individuals have hypocholesterolemia, there may be an overlap in cholesterol levels of normal and affected individuals especially when the affected individuals are older or have a milder phenotype. Age-appropriate values must be considered for diagnosis (85–165 mg/dL in neonates) [6]. Serum cholesterol was low (74 mg/dL) in our patient. Normal range for 7DHC is $0.16 \pm 0.09\,\mu g/mL$ [7]. In our patient, the level of 7DHC was high ($4.2\,\mu g/mL$) and the ratio was 0.56 confirming the diagnosis of SLOS.

Clinical characteristics include mental retardation, developmental delay, failure to thrive, autism, photosensitivity, microcephaly, bitemporal narrowing, broad nose with anteverted nares, micrognathia, ptosis, epichantal folds, cataracts, optic nerve hypoplasia, ASD, VSD, PDA, pyloric stenosis, Hirschsprung disease, hypospadias, cryptorchidism, renal anomalies, and skeletal abnormalities like rhizomelia, 2-3 toe syndactyly, and polydactyly [8].

Infants with SLOS frequently have feeding problems secondary to a combination of hypotonia, oral-motor incoordination, cleft palate, dysmotility, hypomotility, gastrointestinal reflux, constipation, and formula intolerance [9]. Hirschsprung disease and hypertrophic pyloric stenosis have been described [10, 11]. The frequency of hepatic manifestation is reported to be 2.5–16% [12]. Cholestatic liver disease and isolated hypertransaminasemia are among them. In addition to typical dysmorphic features of SLOS, our patient had duodenal obstruction caused by annular pancreas that has not been described so far.

Conflict of Interests

The authors declare that there is no conflict of interests regarding the publication of this paper.

References

[1] F. D. Porter, "Smith-Lemli-Opitz syndrome: pathogenesis, diagnosis and management," *European Journal of Human Genetics*, vol. 16, no. 5, pp. 535–541, 2008.

[2] G. E. Herman, "Disorders of cholesterol biosynthesis: Prototypic metabolic malformation syndromes," *Human Molecular Genetics*, vol. 12, no. 1, pp. R75–R88, 2003.

[3] H. Yu and S. B. Patel, "Recent insights into the Smith-Lemli-Opitz syndrome," *Clinical Genetics*, vol. 68, no. 5, pp. 383–391, 2005.

[4] J. A. Porter, K. E. Young, and P. A. Beachy, "Cholesterol modification of hedgehog signaling proteins in animal development," *Science*, vol. 274, no. 5285, pp. 255–259, 1996.

[5] R. L. Kelley, E. Roessler, R. C. Hennekam et al., "Holoprosencephaly in RSH/Smith-Lemli-Opitz syndrome: does abnormal cholesterol metabolism affect function of Sonic Hedgehog?" *American Journal of Medical Genetics*, vol. 66, no. 4, pp. 478–484, 1996.

[6] P. M. Yip, M. K. Chan, J. Nelken, N. Lepage, G. Brotea, and K. Adeli, "Pediatric reference intervals for lipids and apolipoproteins on the VITROS 5,1 FS Chemistry System," *Clinical Biochemistry*, vol. 39, no. 10, pp. 978–983, 2006.

[7] G. Koo, S. K. Conley, C. A. Wassif, and F. D. Porter, "Discordant phenotype and sterol biochemistry in Smith-Lemli-Opitz syndrome," *American Journal of Medical Genetics A*, vol. 152, no. 8, pp. 2094–2098, 2010.

[8] A. E. DeBarber, Y. Eroglu, L. S. Merkens, A. S. Pappu, and R. D. Steiner, "Smith-Lemli-Opitz syndrome," *Expert Reviews in Molecular Medicine*, vol. 13, p. e24, 2011.

[9] M. J. M. Nowaczyk, "Smith-Lemli-Opitz Syndrome.," in *GeneReviews*, R. A. Pagon, M. P. Adam, T. D. Bird, C. R. Dolan, C. T. Fong, and K. Stephens, Eds., University of Washington, Seattle, Wash, USA, 1993.

[10] K. Patterson, K. E. Toomey, and R. S. Chandra, "Hirschsprung disease in a 46,XY phenotypic infant girl with Smith-Lemli-Opitz syndrome," *Journal of Pediatrics*, vol. 103, no. 3, pp. 425–427, 1983.

[11] C. Mueller, S. Patel, M. Irons et al., "Normal cognition and behavior in a Smith- Lemli—opitz syndrome patient who presented with Hirschsprung disease," *The American Journal of Medical Genetics*, vol. 123, no. 1, pp. 100–106, 2003.

[12] J. S. Ko, B. S. Choi, J. K. Seo et al., "A novel *DHCR7* mutation in a Smith-Lemli-Opitz syndrome infant presenting with neonatal cholestasis," *Journal of Korean Medical Science*, vol. 25, no. 1, pp. 159–162, 2010.

24

Serious Delayed Hair Toe Tourniquet Syndrome with Bone Erosion and Flexor Tendon Lesion

Nicola Bizzotto, Andrea Sandri, Dario Regis, Guillherme Carpeggiani, Franco Lavini, and Bruno Magnan

Department of Orthopaedic and Trauma Surgery, Integrated University Hospital, Piazzale A. Stefani 2, 37126 Verona, Italy

Correspondence should be addressed to Nicola Bizzotto; info@nicolabizzotto.eu

Academic Editor: Anselm Chi-wai Lee

Hair toe tourniquet syndrome (HTTS) is an uncommon pediatric condition occurring when the toe is circumferentially strangulated by human hair or fibers. An 8-week-old little girl was admitted to the Emergency Department because of the worsening swelling in the right second and third toes, which had been been previously treated with a local antibiotic thinking of an infection. An unrecognized HTTS was leading the third toe to necrosis. An urgent release of the constricting band on the two toes was performed and bone erosion and partial flexor tendon lesion on the third toe were detected. We would like to raise awareness in the community and in colleagues about HTTS in children, because early recognition and urgent treatment are mandatory to provide an adequate management and prevent severe complications.

1. Introduction

Hair toe tourniquet syndrome (HTTS) is an unusual condition that occurs when toe is circumferentially strangulated by a strand of hair, thread, or fiber [1]. HTTS infrequently occurs in adolescents or cognitively impaired adults and the incidence is higher in infants under the age of 2 years. In most cases etiology is accidental, although bad hygiene habits are considered risk factors [2]. Clinical presentations are edema, redness up to tissue necrosis, depending on duration and entity of constriction [1, 2]. Mat Saad et al. [3] reported a unique case of HTTS in a 3-month-old baby with erosion of the middle phalanx of the third toe. We present a rare case of a HTTS with bone erosion and partial flexor tendon lesion. To the best our knowledge, these combined injuries have not previously described.

2. Case Report

An 8-week-old girl was admitted to the Emergency Department with a worsening swelling and redness of the right second and third toes. Four days earlier, the mother had noticed the swelling and had taken her baby to the pediatrician.

Local antibiotic and bandaging were started thinking of an infection, but swelling and redness rapidly increased.

At admission to the Orthopedic Department, the patient was quiet and afebrile, with no signs of systemic involvement. No congenital deformity or trauma was reported. Inflammatory blood markers were normal. The third toe revealed significant swelling, congestion, and violet color; the second toe appeared to be edematous, with normal color (Figure 1). Capillary refilling appeared to be good in both toes. With magnifying loupes, a three-millimeter black hair was found protruding dorsally from the base of the swollen third toe. The hair was rolled around the base of the toe, but the deep constriction was invisible because of severe skin swelling. The second toe appeared less edematous with normal color; another black hair was noticed rolled at the base. Diffuse skin and deep-tissue maceration was recognized at the base of the third toe on plantar region. Surgical inspection of the wound revealed partial flexor tendon lesion and bone erosion. The hair was taken and circumferentially unwound from the third toe using a surgical forceps. It was rolled around the metatarsophalangeal joint and the interphalangeal joint. Diffuse deep-tissue maceration and ulceration prevented repairing the tendon. A second hair was noticed and unrolled

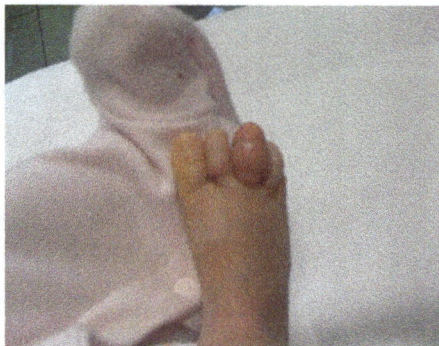

FIGURE 1: Right foot on admission. Note swelling and redness of the second and third toes.

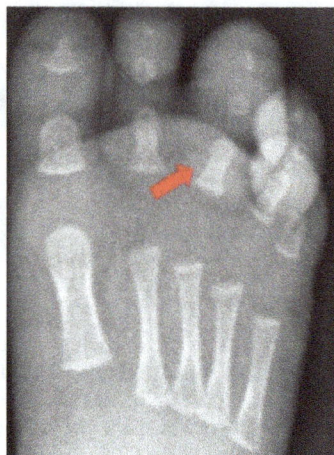

FIGURE 2: Plan X-ray showing bone erosion (arrow).

from the base of the second toe. Bandaging without sutures was performed. Postoperative X-rays confirmed bone erosion crossing the proximal phalanx of the third toe (Figure 2).

Systemic antibiotic therapy (ceftriaxone 250 mg and teicoplanin 40 mg infusion) was administered for 7 days. Swelling decreased and the wound healed satisfactorily in 5 weeks with no signs of tissue necrosis, infection, or neurovascular problems, but a decreased flexion of the third toe was evident (Figure 3).

3. Discussion

Hair toe tourniquet syndrome (HTTS) indicates a pediatric emergency where toe is constricted by hair or fibers causing ischemic strangulation [1, 2]. Although the first case of HTTS was seen in 1612, in modern society it is still rarely recognized [4]. The third toe is most frequently involved in 31.5% of cases, and two toes are involved in 23.5% of cases. Incidence is higher in infants under the age of 2 years, with a median age of 4 months [5].

HTTS has been recognized to be mostly an accidental injury, although the hypothesis of child abuse must be considered [2]. Many causes may be taken into account, such as the telogen effluvium in the mother's hair-loss period

after pregnancy or loss of fibers using old clothes or socks [6]. Some authors have postulated that it occurs by chance, with the baby's digital movements within the loose fabric of clothing such as mittens or socks [7]. Moreover, cases have been described in babies living in extreme poverty and where bad behavior by the parents is also found [2].

The only sign of HTTS in neonates could be excessive prolonged crying, because the hair cuts the skin and can be buried under it; older infants can complain of pain and difficulty in ambulation [3]. The constriction blocks lymphatic drainage, creates local tissue edema, and reduces the venous outflow; an ischemic condition develops hour by hour. If not promptly diagnosed and treated, the constriction can lead to tissue necrosis [3].

Diagnosis of HTTS is essentially clinical. Radiographs should be taken to identify bone erosions in cases of serious and prolonged constriction [3]. Differential diagnosis of HTTS includes infections, ainhum (dactylosis spontanea), and congenital constriction band syndrome [2]. In the literature, HTTS is usually described only with swelling and circulatory suffering of toes; only one case has been reported of a bone lesion due to prolonged constriction and local tissue ulceration [3]. In our unique case, a progressive deepening of the hair into the soft tissue of the third toe produced a partial lesion of flexor tendon and bone erosion as confirmed on X-ray.

The goal of treatment for HTTS is to remove constriction. Many different techniques have been described. Some authors suggest that techniques using scalpels or needles to get under the hair tourniquet are difficult because of the swelling; the risk of damaging healthy tissues is high [8]. O'Gorman and Ratnapalan [9] used a depilatory cream to destroy such hair, concluding that this is safe and can be performed with minimal discomfort to the patient. However, this technique cannot be used if the hair fibers are deeply embedded in the edematous skin and not clearly visible; we do not suggest the use of creams if there are wounds or deep-tissue exposure. A surgical technique with dorsal peritendinous incisions of a strangulated finger has been described. Serour and Gorenstein [10] suggest a short, deep, longitudinal incision over the area of strangulation on the dorsal aspect of the toe as far as the phalanx bone, using a surgical blade. Complete trans-section and release of the constricting fibers are effected in this way. The technique is simple and allows the complete release of strangulation without risks of iatrogenic soft tissue damage. Fortunately, in our case we unwound and removed hair constriction because a small part of the hairs coming out dorsally from the toes was seen.

4. Conclusion

HTTS has to be considered as a cause of toe swelling and discoloration in children. An accurate search of the hair must be performed using magnifying loupes because the hair tourniquet may not be detectable to the naked eye. Early recognition and urgent treatment are mandatory to avoid potential complications.

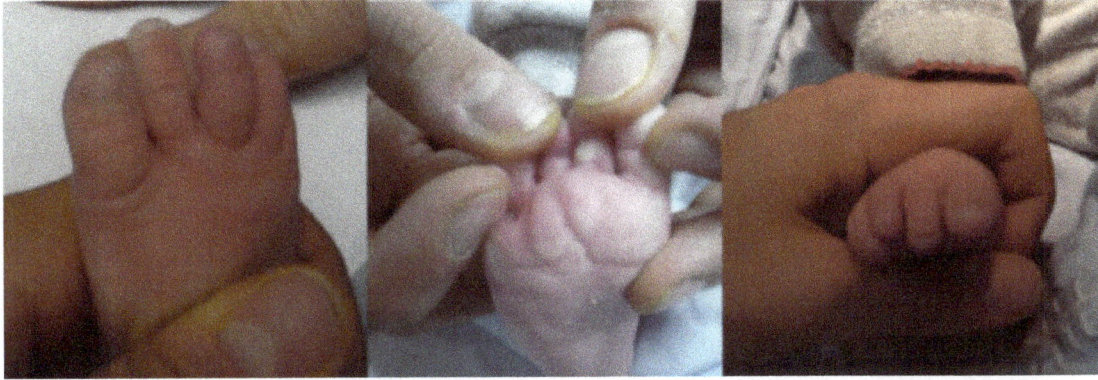

FIGURE 3: Right foot 5 weeks after treatment, demonstrating reduction of swelling and limited flexion of the third toe.

Consent

Written informed consent was obtained from the parents for publication of this case report and any accompanying images.

Conflict of Interests

The authors declare that there is no conflict of interests regarding the publication of this paper.

References

[1] J. L. Bacon and J. T. Burgis, "Hair thread tourniquet syndrome in adolescents: a presentation and review of the literature," *Journal of Pediatric and Adolescent Gynecology*, vol. 18, no. 3, pp. 155–156, 2005.

[2] A. Klusmann and H.-G. Lenard, "Tourniquet syndrome—accident or abuse?" *European Journal of Pediatrics*, vol. 163, no. 8, pp. 495–498, 2004.

[3] A. Z. Mat Saad, E. M. Purcell, and J. J. McCann, "Hair-thread tourniquet syndrome in an infant with bony erosion: a case report, literature review, and meta-analysis," *Annals of Plastic Surgery*, vol. 57, no. 4, pp. 447–452, 2006.

[4] M. Corazza, E. Carlà, E. Altieri, and A. Virgili, "What syndrome is this?" *Pediatric Dermatology*, vol. 19, no. 6, pp. 555–556, 2002.

[5] P. Lohana, G. N. Vashishta, and N. Price, "Toe-tourniquet syndrome: a diagnostic dilemma!," *Annals of the Royal College of Surgeons of England*, vol. 88, no. 4, pp. W6–W8, 2006.

[6] R. S. Strahlman, "Toe tourniquet syndrome in association with maternal hair loss," *Pediatrics*, vol. 111, no. 3, pp. 685–687, 2003.

[7] N. J. Quinn Jr., "Toe tourniquet syndrome," *Pediatrics*, vol. 48, no. 1, pp. 145–146, 1971.

[8] H. V. Kurup, M. Gnanapavan, and L. McSweeney, "Hair-tourniquet syndrome: unwind or incise?" *Emergency Medicine Australasia*, vol. 18, no. 4, article 415, 2006.

[9] A. O'Gorman and S. Ratnapalan, "Hair tourniquet management," *Pediatric Emergency Care*, vol. 27, no. 3, pp. 203–204, 2011.

[10] F. Serour and A. Gorenstein, "Treatment of the toe tourniquet syndrome in infants," *Pediatric Surgery International*, vol. 19, no. 8, pp. 598–600, 2003.

25

Pulmonary Hemosiderosis in Children with Bronchopulmonary Dysplasia

**David Kurahara, Marina Morie, Maya Yamane, Sarah Lam,
Wallace Matthews, Keolamau Yee, and Kara Yamamoto**

Department of Pediatrics, John A. Burns School of Medicine, University of Hawaii, Honolulu, HI, USA

Correspondence should be addressed to David Kurahara; davidk@kapiolani.org

Academic Editor: Pietro Strisciuglio

We describe a possible association between pulmonary hemosiderosis (PH) and a history of bronchopulmonary dysplasia (BPD). Both patients were born at 28-week gestation and presented with PH at ages 22 months and 6 years, respectively. Both initially presented with cough and tachypnea, and bronchoalveolar lavage showed evidence of hemosiderin-laden macrophages. Initial hemoglobin levels were < 4 g/dL and chest radiographs showed diffuse infiltrates that cleared dramatically within days after initiation of intravenous corticosteroids. In the first case, frank pulmonary blood was observed upon initial intubation, prompting the need for high frequency ventilation, immediate corticosteroids, and antibiotics. The mechanical ventilation wean was made possible by the addition of mycophenolate mofetil (MMF) and hydroxychloroquine. Slow tapering off of medications was accomplished over 6 years. These cases represent a possible correlation between prematurity-associated BPD and PH. We present a review of the literature regarding this possible association. In addition, MMF proved to be life-saving in one of the PH cases, as it has been in pulmonary hemorrhage related to systemic lupus erythematosus. Further studies are warranted to investigate the possible association between PH and prematurity-related BPD, as well as the use of MMF in the treatment of PH.

1. Introduction

Pulmonary hemosiderosis (PH) can present with a catastrophic lung hemorrhage in previously healthy young children. It has rarely been described to occur in children with previous lung disease like bronchopulmonary dysplasia (BPD). In idiopathic pulmonary hemosiderosis (IPH) no underlying cause can be found and it can present with iron-deficiency anemia, recurrent hemoptysis, and diffuse parenchymal infiltrates on chest radiograph (CXR) [1]. Iron-deficiency anemia results due to hemosiderin iron deposition in the alveoli [2]. Recurrent episodes of alveolar hemorrhage may occur and the clinical course of IPH is variable. The finding of hemosiderin-laden macrophages (HLM) by bronchoalveolar lavage (BAL) is helpful to confirm the diagnosis [3]. IPH most commonly affects children, although adult cases have been reported [1]. IPH has been treated with corticosteroids and/or immunosuppressive drugs with variable success [1, 2]. Here we investigate a possible association between PH and history of prematurity-associated

bronchopulmonary dysplasia (BPD), as well as the utility of mycophenolate mofetil (MMF) as a treatment option for PH.

2. Case History

2.1. Case 1. The patient was a 22-month-old Filipino female born at 28-week gestation at a weight of 1,073 g. Neonatal course was complicated by BPD, grade I intraventricular hemorrhage (IVH), retinopathy of prematurity (ROP), and necrotizing enterocolitis requiring a sigmoid resection. She was discharged home at 3 months of life at a weight of 3000 g and required one year of oxygen therapy without further complications.

At 22 months of age, she presented to the Emergency Department with hemoglobin of 3.5 g/dL and fluffy infiltrates on CXR. Upon immediate transfer to the pediatric intensive care unit, intubation was attempted, but gross red blood was noted to be coming out of the endotracheal tube (ET). Intubation was reattempted and ET placement was confirmed visually, but gross red blood continued to flow from the ET.

CXR showed diffuse pulmonary infiltrates and bronchoscopy revealed abundant HLM which was helpful in the diagnosis of PH. She was put on high frequency ventilation and started on intravenous (IV) methylprednisolone (2 mg/kg/d) and broad spectrum antibiotics. At this point she was critically ill and it was felt that a lung biopsy was not possible. She improved dramatically and was successfully weaned to a conventional ventilator in 2 days, then continuous positive airway pressure (CPAP) 7 days later. She was not able to be tapered off of CPAP until the addition of MMF upon pediatric rheumatology consult. PH work-up including antinuclear (ANA), antineutrophil cytoplasmic (ANCA), antiglomerular basement, cardiolipin, cow's milk preciptins, gliadin, and reticulin antibodies was all negative. Urinalysis and complement studies were also normal. After successful CPAP wean, she was discharged home after 1 month of hospitalization.

Over the next 2 years, she had recurrent episodes of respiratory distress requiring hospitalization. Each episode showed diffuse pulmonary infiltrates on CXR and rapid improvement upon IV corticosteroid administration. When hydroxychloroquine (HC) was added to her medication regimen, she stabilized significantly and has not required further hospitalizations.

Her medications were slowly tapered off over the next 6 years: corticosteroids first, then MMF, and finally the HC. Follow-up CXRs, hemoglobin, pulmonary function tests, and growth velocity have all normalized.

2.2. Case 2. The patient was a 6-year-old Filipino female born at 28-week gestation, with neonatal course complicated by BPD requiring oxygen therapy for 15 months, congenital tracheal stenosis and tracheal ring s/p reconstructive surgery, grade II IVH, developmental delay, ROP, and neurosensory hearing loss s/p cochlear implant. After an initial prolonged hospitalization in the neonatal ICU, she did well until she presented with intermittent cough and rapid breathing for 2 weeks. She had tactile fever and tachycardia but no history of hemoptysis, hematemesis, or hematochezia.

In the emergency room she was tired and pale with mild hypoxia and conjunctival pallor. Complete blood count showed likely iron-deficiency anemia (hemoglobin = 3.3 g/dL, hematocrit = 11.9, MCV = 77.2, iron = 21, TIBC = 531, and reticulocyte count = 14.8). CXR showed bilateral pulmonary infiltrates. In addition, CRP = 0.1 and ESR = 24.

With suspicion of PH, she was given a packed red blood cell transfusion, diuretics, and IV corticosteroids (2 mg/kg/d). BAL showed abundant HLM which was useful in the diagnosis of PH. Due to prior tracheal ring surgery and the history of BPD it was felt that lung biopsy would have put her at high risk for complications so this was not performed. Further work-up revealed elevated ANA of 320 (nl < 40), positive SSA/Ro titer of 99.6 (nl < 20), and positive antimyeloperoxidase ANCA (anti-MPO) of 11.5 (nl < 9). The rest of her ANA studies, anti-GBM, cow's milk precipitins, gliadin, and reticulin antibodies were negative. Her Hb stabilized with IV corticosteroids, no further bleeding occurred, and she was discharged home after one week. Parents were counseled on the use of other immunosuppressant drugs in PH but decided against these unless she had

another episode. Her corticosteroids were slowly tapered off over 4 years with no further episodes of bleeding and normal CXRs and pulmonary function tests. Her anti-MPO antibody disappeared after the initial positive finding. ANA and SSA/Ro antibodies remain positive and continue to be followed by pediatric rheumatology, but she has not fulfilled criteria for SLE.

3. Discussion

Very few cases in the literature describe a history of prematurity in children who develop PH. However, there may be an unrecognized association between prematurity-related BPD and later development of PH. One case in the German literature describes IPH in a 3-year-old child with history of ductus ligation at 32 weeks and birth weight of 1405 g [4]. Another article describes a male, born at 32-week gestation, diagnosed with IPH at 2 years of age [2]. There is no mention of BPD during the neonatal course, but BPD was less likely to develop given a 32-week gestational infant.

Could earlier lung damage have predisposed these children to develop PH later in life? BPD is defined as the need for supplemental oxygen for ≥ 28 days of life [5]. Both of our cases fulfill the criteria for BPD. BPD is characterized by diffuse airway damage and alternating areas of overinflation with atelectasis, fibrosis, smooth muscle hypertrophy, and prominent vascular hypertensive lesions with airway wall thickening [5]. As children with BPD get older, they have higher rates of wheezing, pneumonia, long-term medication use, and respiratory symptoms and higher hospitalization rates than controls without BPD [6–8]. Therefore, prior history of BPD and its associated lung damage may predispose to increased risk of recurrent pulmonary hemorrhage and lower respiratory tract infections. Similarly, a 9-year-old male developed postinfectious bronchiolitis obliterans with PH, confirmed by lung biopsy and CT scan, following a viral infection at 7 months of age with years of persistent respiratory symptoms [9]. Further studies are needed to delineate a link between prematurity-related BPD and IPH. A history for any child suspected to have IPH should include a detailed birth history.

The treatment for IPH has been well described to include corticosteroids and immunosuppressive agents [2] as this illness includes both inflammatory and immune components. Hydroxychloroquine has been used successfully [10] and in our first case proved to be helpful in reducing bleeding episodes, which prevented further hospitalizations. In a series of 26 children with IPH by Kabra et al., symptoms did not recur in 17 individuals initially started on both prednisolone and HC [10]. A retrospective study looking at prognosis of IPH showed improved outcome with long-term immunosuppression via corticosteroids, HC, and/or azathioprine [11].

MMF is used increasingly in severe SLE and other autoimmune diseases [12]. It has been lifesaving in retractable pulmonary hemorrhage refractory to corticosteroids, cyclophosphamide, and even plasmapheresis, which usually carries a very high mortality rate of 70–95% [13–15]. MMF is a potent immunosuppressive agent that inhibits proliferation of T and B lymphocytes and suppresses antibody formation by B lymphocytes, without hepatotoxicity, nephrotoxicity, or mutagenicity [16]. It is an immunosuppressive agent used in transplantation, with evidence of superior protection against acute transplant rejection compared to azathioprine-containing regimens [12]. This medication proved effective in our first case. It allowed for successful wean from the ventilator after a very severe pulmonary hemorrhage. It was felt that monthly pulse cyclophosphamide would not be effective rapidly enough to avoid a fatality, and the side effects of daily cyclophosphamide would surpass those of daily MMF. No published reports of MMF used in IPH were found, but we feel that it was instrumental in our patient's improvement. Further studies are needed, but MMF may provide added immunosuppression during life-threatening pulmonary hemorrhage in IPH and other autoimmune disorders.

Our cases illustrate the often-difficult decision of obtaining a lung biopsy on an actively hemorrhaging lung. Both cases were started on corticosteroids prior to pulmonary and rheumatology involvement, so it was felt that biopsy risk would outweigh the benefit, especially on two children with a previous history of BPD and possible lung scarring. Earlier literature describes the importance of getting a lung biopsy to rule out other vasculitic illnesses [2, 3]. However, more recent literature supports making the diagnosis using BAL [1, 10, 17]. Calculating the percent of HLM may improve the sensitivity to 100% and the specificity to 96% when an index of 35% or more is used [17]. Biopsy may be helpful in some cases of protracted pulmonary disease as in the case with bronchiolitis obliterans described by Pinto et al. [9]. The logistics and risk of lung biopsy in a child with an active pulmonary hemorrhage should be considered carefully.

Previous chronic lung disease may be a risk factor for the development of PH. We report two cases of PH in children with history of prematurity-related BPD. Since they had previous lung damage related to prematurity they were classified as PH as the idiopathic description is a diagnosis made from exclusion of other possible coexistent lung diseases. Further studies are needed to investigate this association, and detailed birth histories should be elicited for all cases of suspected IPH. In one case, the use of MMF and hydroxychloroquine was helpful in improving the disease outcome. MMF may be a useful agent in PH management as seen in SLE-related pulmonary hemorrhage.

Conflict of Interests

The authors declare that there is no conflict of interests regarding the publication of this paper.

References

[1] V. Poggi, A. Lo Vecchio, F. Menna, and G. Menna, "Idiopathic pulmonary hemosiderosis: a rare cause of iron-deficiency anemia in childhood," *Journal of Pediatric Hematology/Oncology*, vol. 33, no. 4, pp. e160–e162, 2011.

[2] O. C. Ioachimescu, S. Sieber, and A. Kotch, "Idiopathic pulmonary haemosiderosis revisited," *European Respiratory Journal*, vol. 24, no. 1, pp. 162–170, 2004.

[3] N. Milman and F. M. Pedersen, "Idiopathic pulmonary haemosiderosis. Epidemiology, pathogenic aspects and diagnosis," *Respiratory Medicine*, vol. 92, no. 7, pp. 902–907, 1998.

[4] I. Mutz, R. Hirschmann, and W. D. Muller, "Idiopathic pulmonary hemosiderosis in a 3 year old child following ductus surgery in the neonatal period," *Klinische Padiatrie*, vol. 197, no. 2, pp. 130–134, 1985.

[5] I. Narang, "Long-term follow-up of infants with lung disease of prematurity," *Chronic Respiratory Disease*, vol. 7, no. 4, pp. 259–269, 2010.

[6] W. H. Northway Jr., R. B. Moss, K. B. Carlisle et al., "Late pulmonary sequelae of bronchopulmonary dysplasia," *The New England Journal of Medicine*, vol. 323, no. 26, pp. 1793–1799, 1990.

[7] I. Narang, M. Rosenthal, D. Cremonesini, M. Silverman, and A. Bush, "Longitudinal evaluation of airway function 21 years after preterm birth," *The American Journal of Respiratory and Critical Care Medicine*, vol. 178, no. 1, pp. 74–80, 2008.

[8] E. C. Walter, W. J. Ehlenbach, D. L. Hotchkin, J. W. Chien, and T. D. Koepsell, "Low birth weight and respiratory disease in adulthood: a population-based case-control study," *The American Journal of Respiratory and Critical Care Medicine*, vol. 180, no. 2, pp. 176–180, 2009.

[9] L. A. Pinto, A. Oliveira, S. Collaziol et al., "Postinfectious bronchiolitis obliterans accompanied by pulmonary hemosiderosis in childhood," *Jornal Brasileiro de Pneumologia*, vol. 32, no. 6, pp. 587–591, 2006.

[10] S. K. Kabra, S. Bhargava, R. Lodha, A. Satyavani, and M. Walia, "Idiopathic pulmonary hemosiderosis: clinical profile and follow up of 26 children," *Indian Pediatrics*, vol. 44, no. 5, pp. 333–338, 2007.

[11] M. M. Saeed, M. S. Woo, E. F. MacLaughlin, M. F. Margetis, and T. G. Keens, "Prognosis in pediatric idiopathic pulmonary hemosiderosis," *Chest*, vol. 116, no. 3, pp. 721–725, 1999.

[12] C. N. Pisoni, Y. Karim, and M. J. Cuadrado, "Mycophenolate mofetil and systemic lupus erythematosus: an overview," *Lupus*, vol. 14, no. 1, pp. s9–s11, 2005.

[13] A. S. Samad and C. B. Lindsley, "Treatment of pulmonary hemorrhage in childhood systemic lupus erythematosus with mycophenolate Mofetil," *Southern Medical Journal*, vol. 96, no. 7, pp. 705–707, 2003.

[14] M. H. Moradinejad, "Treatment of intractable pulmonary hemorrhage in two patients with childhood systemic lupus erythematosus," *Rheumatology International*, vol. 29, no. 9, pp. 1113–1115, 2009.

[15] R. A. Dweik, A. C. Arroliga, and J. M. Cash, "Alveolar hemorrhage in patients with rheumatic disease," *Rheumatic Disease Clinics of North America*, vol. 23, no. 2, pp. 395–410, 1997.

[16] R. L. Hoffmann and S. J. Reeder, "Mycophenolate mofetil (CellCept): the newest immunosuppressant," *Critical care nurse*, vol. 18, no. 3, pp. 50–57, 1998.

[17] Z. N. Salih, A. Akhter, and J. Akhter, "Specificity and sensitivity of hemosiderin-laden macrophages in routine bronchoalveolar lavage in children," *Archives of Pathology and Laboratory Medicine*, vol. 130, no. 11, pp. 1684–1686, 2006.

26

Hodgkin's Lymphoma Revealed by Hemophagocytic Lymphohistiocytosis in a Child

Sarra Benmiloud,[1,2] Mohamed Hbibi,[1] Sana Chaouki,[1]
Sana Abourazzak,[1] and Moustapha Hida[1]

[1] Unit of Pediatric Hematology-Oncology, Department of Pediatrics, University Hospital Hassan II, Faculty of Medicine and Pharmacy,
University of Sidi Mohamed Ben Abdellah, 30000 Fez, Morocco
[2] Unit of Pediatric Hematology-Oncology, Department of Pediatrics, Mother-Child Hospital, University Hospital Hassan II,
Faculty of Medicine and Pharmacy, University of Sidi Mohamed Ben Abdellah, BP 1893, Km 2.200, Sidi Hrazem Road,
30000 Fez, Morocco

Correspondence should be addressed to Sarra Benmiloud; benmiloudsarra@yahoo.fr

Academic Editor: Yusuke Shiozawa

Hemophagocytic lymphohistiocytosis (HLH) is a severe life-threatening disorder, responsible for extensive phagocytosis of hematopoietic cells and causing a multisystem organ failure. If lymphomas are common causes of HLH, the association with Hodgkin's lymphoma is rarely described in children. We report a case of a 9-year-old boy presenting with HLH as an initial manifestation of Hodgkin's lymphoma. He has been suffering from persistent high fever, asthenia, weight loss, and hepatosplenomegaly with no lymphadenopathy. The diagnosis of HLH secondary to infectious disease was initially worn. The patient received high-dose intravenous immunoglobulin with broad-spectrum antibiotics. However, his state got worse with the onset of dry cough and pleural effusion. Histopathologic examination of pleural fluid showed the presence of Reed-Sternberg cells. The outcome was favorable after treatment by corticosteroid and chemotherapy. Hodgkin's lymphoma revealed by HLH is a source of delayed diagnosis and should be borne in mind in children.

1. Introduction

Hemophagocytic lymphohistiocytosis (HLH) is a severe life-threatening disorder causing a multisystem organ failure. It is characterized by an excessive and uncontrolled immune response, due to cytokine dysregulation and lymphohistiocytic proliferation [1, 2]. The HLH is usually a secondary reaction to infection, medication, autoimmune, or neoplastic diseases. Hematologic malignancies are a well-known HLH etiology, but the combination of Hodgkin's lymphoma (HL) and HLH in the pediatric population is rarely reported at the time of diagnosis.

We report a novel pediatric case of HL revealed by HLH as an initial manifestation, illustrating the diagnostic difficulties and the interest of rapid treatment.

2. Case Report

A 9-year-old boy, with no past medical history, was admitted for a persistent high fever that reached 40°C, evolving for one month, associated with anorexia, asthenia, vomiting, and significant weight loss. Clinical examination found the child in poor physical condition, febrile to 39.5°C, and pale. Abdominal palpation found a hepatosplenomegaly. The rest of the physical examination demonstrated lenticular cervical and inguinal lymph nodes.

Laboratory tests revealed leukopenia (white blood count = 1080/mm^3, normal: 4000–10000/mm^3), neutropenia (neutrophil = 750/mm^3, normal: 3000–5600/mm^3), lymphopenia (lymphocytes = 120/mm^3, normal: 3000–5500/mm^3), anemia (hemoglobin = 6.6 g/dL, normal: 11.5–14.5 g/dL),

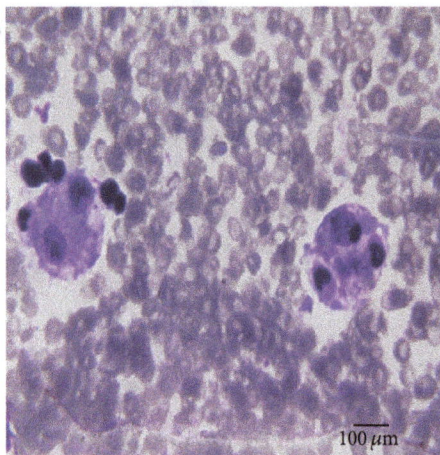

FIGURE 1: Image showing two macrophages with hemophagocytosis in bone marrow aspiration smear (magnification ×1000).

thrombocytopenia (platelet count = 79000/mm^3, normal: 150000–450000/mm^3), elevated C-reactive protein (171 mg/L, normal: 0–6 mg/L), abnormal liver function (serum glutamate oxaloacetic transaminase = 258 IU/L, normal: 5–34 IU/L; serum glutamate pyruvate transaminase = 168 IU/L, normal: 0–55 IU/L), elevated lactate dehydrogenase (973 IU/L, normal: 0–248 IU/L), hyperferritinemia (703 μg/L, normal: 20–250 μg/L), hypertriglyceridemia (3.7 g/L, normal: 0–1.50 g/L), normal fibrinogenemia (3.9 g/L, normal: 2–4 g/L), and hypoalbuminemia (19.2 g/L, normal: 33–50 g/L). The bone marrow aspiration showed the presence of numerous macrophages with hemophagocytosis without evidence of malignancy (Figure 1).

The diagnosis of HLH was worn based on six of eight diagnostic criteria: fever, hepatosplenomegaly, pancytopenia, hyperferritinemia, hypertriglyceridemia, and bone marrow hemophagocytosis [1]. The bacteriological (blood, urine and stool cultures, tuberculosis tests, and mycoplasma serology), viral (serology of Epstein-Barr virus (EBV), cytomegalovirus, parvovirus B19, human immunodeficiency virus, and hepatitis A, B, and C), and parasite (toxoplasmosis, leishmaniasis) evaluations were negative. Immune tests (antinuclear antibodies and anti-DNA and rheumatoid factor) were normal. The search for EBV by polymerase chain reaction (PCR) could not be performed due to the lack of financial patient's resources.

The diagnosis of HLH secondary to infectious disease was initially suspected. The patient received broad-spectrum antibiotics and high-dose intravenous immunoglobulin. However, his condition had worsened with the onset of dry cough and dyspnea. The chest X-ray demonstrated an alveolar syndrome in the lower lobe of the right lung and a bilateral minimal pleural effusion. The thoracoabdominopelvic computed tomography revealed the presence of scattered nodules at different parenchymal lung segments, measuring 15 mm for the largest diameter, a right parenchymal lung condensation, multiple mediastinal enlarged lymph

nodes measuring 14 mm for the largest, minimal pleural and pericardial effusions, hepatosplenomegaly containing multiple millimetric nodular hypodense lesions, and hilar and para-aortic infracentimetric lymph nodes (Figure 2). Echocardiography objectified minimal pericardial effusion with normal cardiac function. Bacteriological examination of pleural fluid was negative. Histopathological examination of pleural fluid revealed the presence of Reed-Sternberg cells that was positive for the anti-CD15 and anti-CD30 antibodies (Figure 3); some of these cells were positive for the anti-CD20 antibody. The anti-CD3 antibody was positive in the reactive lymphocytes. EBV-encoded RNA (EBER) in situ hybridization for detecting and localizing latent EBV in patient's HL cells was not done, because this technique is not available in our country's laboratory. Bone marrow biopsy showed no bone marrow infiltration by tumor cells. Due to a drop of patient's performance status, a biopsy of mediastinal lymph nodes or pulmonary lesions could not be made.

The diagnosis of a HL associated with a HLH was worn based on the pathological study of pleural fluid and imaging data. However, no genetic mutation could be studied due to the lack of financial patient's resources. The patient received initially three bolus of methylprednisolone, followed by chemotherapy combining two monthly courses of OPPA (vincristine, doxorubicin, procarbazine, and prednisone) and four monthly cycles of COPP (cyclophosphamide, vincristine, procarbazine, and prednisone). The evolution was slowly favorable. After 6 weeks, the pleural effusion and the hepatosplenomegaly disappeared; the laboratory tests were normal. Currently we are at 20-month follow-up; the child is asymptomatic with no residual disease or relapse.

3. Discussion

HLH is an excessive and uncontrolled immune response producing large quantities of inflammatory cytokines. It can be primary, related to several molecular defects (mutations in perforin 1, UNC 13D, syntaxin 11, syntaxin-binding protein-2, SH2D1A, RAB27A, and XIAP or a defect on chromosome 9q21.3-22), or secondary to infections, autoimmune diseases, chronic inflammatory disorders, acquired immunodeficiencies, and various malignancies, mainly hematological malignancies [1, 2]. Clinically, there is a persistent high fever associated with hepatosplenomegaly. Biologically, the diagnosis is suggested by the association of bicytopenia with hyperferritinemia, altered liver function, hypertriglyceridemia or hypofibrinogenemia, increased soluble CD25 levels, and low or absence of natural killer (NK) cells activity. Histologically, there is a significant hemophagocytosis in bone marrow, spleen, or lymph nodes [1]. The identification of the causal disease in the secondary forms is mandatory because only its treatment will stop HLH.

HLH occurring during malignancies has been reported previously in the literature, most commonly in the case of leukemia and lymphomas (more often T or NK phenotype) especially in adult patients [3–5]. It is probably the secretion

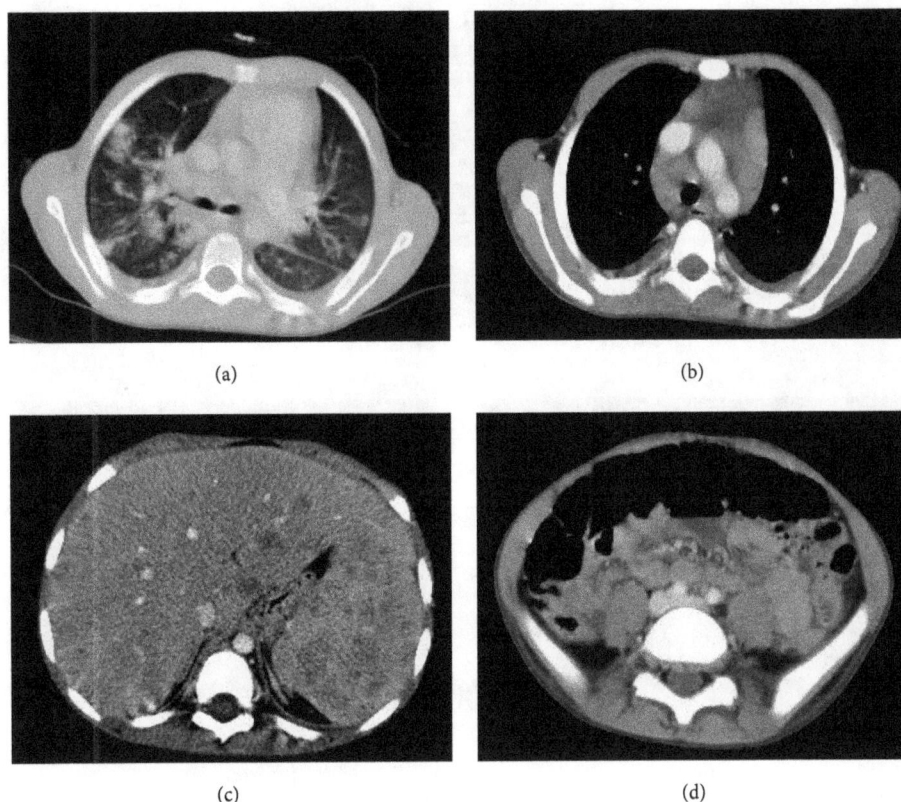

(a)

(b)

(c)

(d)

FIGURE 2: Thoracoabdominopelvic computed tomography in axial sections demonstrating scattered nodules at different parenchymal lung segments, a right parenchymal lung condensation, and minimal pleural effusion (a), multiple mediastinal enlarged lymph nodes (b), hepatosplenomegaly containing multiple nodular hypodense lesions (c), and hilar and para-aortic infracentimetric lymph nodes (d).

of proinflammatory cytokines (interferon-γ, tumor necrosis factor α, interleukin-2 (IL-2), IL6, IL-8, IL-10, IL-12, IL-18, and IL-4), by malignant cells, which contribute to this immune dysregulation. In T or NK lymphomas, it seems that the uncontrolled production of cytokines is caused by EBV [3]. Studies in children, who developed HLH in the sitting of acute lymphoblastic leukemia, suggested that the chemotherapy combined with malignancy predisposes to defects in T-cell and NK-cell function and also to infections which triggered HLH [6]. Sometimes, HLH was reported as the first presentation of malignancies, as in our case, probably due to the release of cytokines induced by activated macrophages and T cells [4, 6, 7].

Among HLH secondary to lymphoma, HL is often described in children [6–9]. Even though EBV is significantly associated with HL, the association of HLH and HL is uncommon at the time of diagnosis [7–9]. It seems that HLH could have a role in determining the clinical manifestations of the primary disease, from silent clinical forms to fulminant evolutions, which often lead to delay in diagnosis as in our case [3]. The largest study of patients with HL and HLH shows that the main features of this association are male predominance, disseminated disease, a high proportion of lymphocyte depletion and mixed cellularity histological subtypes, and a strong association with EBV which was

detected in the tumor cells of 94% of cases that suggest a major pathogenic role of EBV in this association [8, 10].

When HLH is diagnosed, the search for a trigger is imperative for the prognosis. In our observation, diagnostic difficulties were due to the rarity of the association of HL and HLH in children at the time of diagnosis and the major alteration of physical condition which made delicate explorations. The diagnosis is easy when the HL manifests as diffuse adenomegalies accessible for biopsy. However, in case of atypical manifestations, histological studies with biopsies are required. Studies in patients with malignancy reported that the presence of HLH is a negative prognosis factor with a high mortality rate, imposing an early and appropriate therapy [3, 6]. According to the literatures, the prognosis of patients in the case of association of HL and HLH is extremely poor [8, 10]. Despite therapy, survival is short. But if the treatment is successful, the survival rate comes back as expected [3].

4. Conclusion

HLH as an initial presentation of HL is rare in children. This association is a source of delayed diagnosis and should be borne in mind, especially as the prognosis depends on

(a)

(b)

(c)

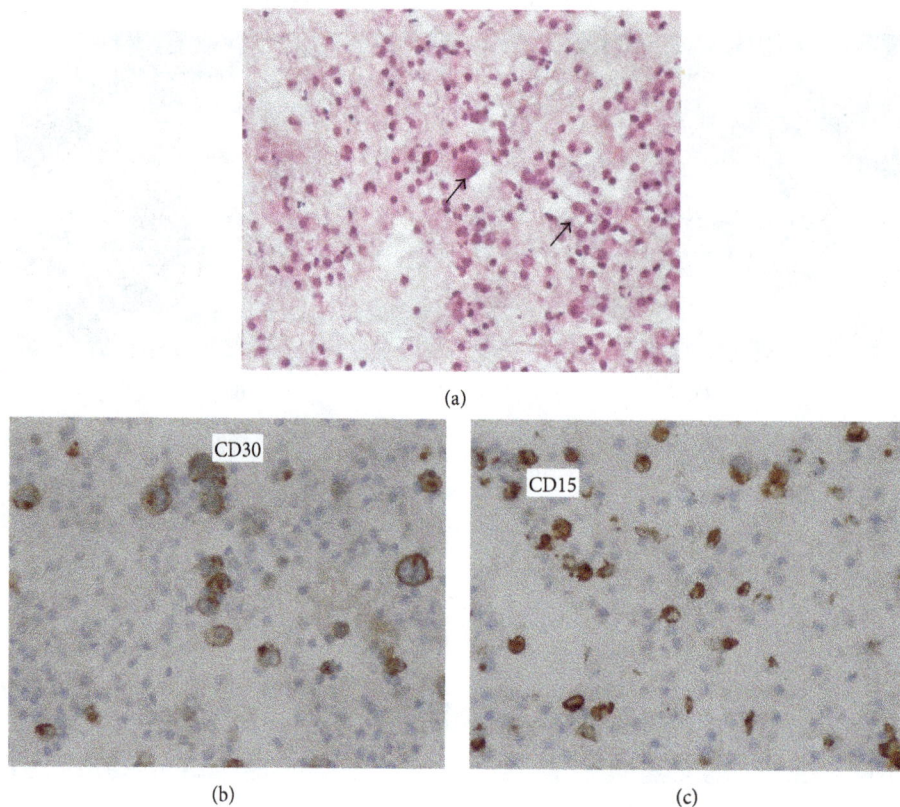

FIGURE 3: Histopathological examination of pleural fluid: cytological spreading showing atypical cells with cusped nuclei (arrows) on a background rich in neutrophils (magnification ×250) (a), immunocytochemistry expression of CD 30, and CD15 by tumor cells (b and c).

the rapidity of the treatment including early initiation of chemotherapy.

Conflict of Interests

The authors declare that there is no conflict of interests regarding the publication of this paper.

Acknowledgments

The authors would like to thank Professor Meryem Boubbou, Radiologist, Professor Azlarab Masrar and Professor Souad Benkirane, biologists, and Professor Fouad Kettani, pathologist, for their help in the management of this patient.

References

[1] J.-I. Henter, A. Horne, M. Aricó et al., "HLH-2004: diagnostic and therapeutic guidelines for hemophagocytic lymphohistiocytosis," *Pediatric Blood & Cancer*, vol. 48, no. 2, pp. 124–131, 2007.

[2] G. E. Janka, "Familial and acquired hemophagocytic lymphohistiocytosis," *European Journal of Pediatrics*, vol. 166, no. 2, pp. 95–109, 2007.

[3] A. Majluf-Cruz, R. Sosa-Camas, O. Pérez-Ramírez, A. Rosas-Cabral, F. Vargas-Vorackova, and J. Labardini-Méndez, "Hemophagocytic syndrome associated with hematological neoplasias," *Leukemia Research*, vol. 22, no. 10, pp. 893–898, 1998.

[4] Y. Allory, D. Challine, C. Haioun et al., "Bone marrow involvement in lymphomas with hemophagocytic syndrome at presentation: a clinicopathologic study of 11 patients in a Western institution," *The American Journal of Surgical Pathology*, vol. 25, no. 7, pp. 865–874, 2001.

[5] A.-R. Han, H. R. Lee, B.-B. Park et al., "Lymphoma-associated hemophagocytic syndrome: clinical features and treatment outcome," *Annals of Hematology*, vol. 86, no. 7, pp. 493–498, 2007.

[6] T. Celkan, S. Berrak, E. Kazanci et al., "Malignancy-associated hemophagocytic lymphohistiocytosis in pediatric cases: a multicenter study from Turkey," *Turkish Journal of Pediatrics*, vol. 51, no. 3, pp. 207–213, 2009.

[7] H. Kojima, N. Takei, H. Y. Mukai et al., "Hemophagocytic syndrome as the primary clinical symptom of Hodgkin's disease," *Annals of Hematology*, vol. 82, no. 1, pp. 53–56, 2003.

[8] F. Ménard, C. Besson, P. Rincé et al., "Hodgkin lymphoma-associated hemophagocytic syndrome: a disorder strongly correlated with Epstein-Barr virus," *Clinical Infectious Diseases*, vol. 47, no. 4, pp. 531–534, 2008.

[9] C. S. Chim and P. K. Hui, "Reactive hemophagocytic syndrome and Hodgkin's disease," *The American Journal of Hematology*, vol. 55, no. 1, pp. 49–50, 1997.

[10] M. Hagihara, M. Inoue, J. Hua, and Y. Iwaki, "Lymphocyte-depleted hodgkin lymphoma complicating hemophagocytic lymphohistiocytosis as an initial manifestation: a case report and review of the literature," *Internal Medicine*, vol. 51, no. 21, pp. 3067–3072, 2012.

27

The Value of Family History in Diagnosing Primary Immunodeficiency Disorders

Mohamed A. Hendaus,[1] **Ahmad Alhammadi,**[1,2] **Mehdi M. Adeli,**[2,3] **and Fawzia Al-Yafei**[4]

[1] Department of Pediatrics, Section of General Pediatrics, Hamad Medical Corporation, Doha, Qatar
[2] Weill Cornell Medical College, Doha, Qatar
[3] Department of Pediatrics, Allergy and Immunology Section, Hamad Medical Corporation, Doha, Qatar
[4] Department of Pediatrics, Endocrinology Section, Hamad Medical Corporation, Doha, Qatar

Correspondence should be addressed to Mehdi M. Adeli; madeli@hmc.org.qa

Academic Editor: Ozgur Cogulu

Eliciting proper family medical history is critical in decreasing morbidity and mortality in patients with primary immunodeficiency disorders (PIDs). Communities with a common practice of consanguinity have a high rate of PIDs. We are presenting 2 cases where digging deeply into the family medical history resulted in the diagnosis of Omenn syndrome, a possibly fatal entity if not managed in a reasonable period.

1. Introduction

Primary immunodeficiency disorders (PIDs) usually refer to various genetic disorders that disturb fundamental parts of the immune system resulting in flaws in function, differentiation, or both of these parts [1]. Early diagnosis of PID is crucial because often lifesaving interventions can be provided to decrease the rate of morbidity and mortality [2]. A major proportion of affected infants and children are offspring of consanguineous marriage; in addition, family medical history is very common in PID and it is an essential component in the diagnosis [3].

We are presenting two cases that show how crucial eliciting proper family medical history is in saving lives of infants and children with PID.

2. Case #1

A 3-month-old Pakistani female presented with generalized rash and failure to gain appropriate weight. The infant was born full term via normal spontaneous vaginal delivery. The initial family history was unremarkable except that parents are first degree cousins. The patient was admitted for failure to thrive workup. On examination, the vitals were appropriate for age. Anthropometric measurements were normal for age except the weight was below the 3rd percentile. The patient looked nontoxic, but thin. There was a generalized maculopapular rash with two bullae on the gluteal area. The rest of the examination was unremarkable. The rash disappeared on the second day of admission. Laboratory investigations showed hemoglobin of 6.6 g/dL, positive direct Coombs test, and positive occult blood.

The differential diagnosis was cow milk allergy, autoimmune hemolytic anemia, and sepsis.

We decided to transfuse the patient with packed red blood cells (PRBCs) due to severe anemia and premedicated the patient with diphenhydramine. Severe diffuse erythema and irritability developed and we had to discontinue the transfusion process. We reassessed the family medical history and the father mentioned that two older siblings passed away while receiving PRBC for the same condition. The new family medical history prompted us to broaden our laboratory investigation.

Her lab results showed white blood count (WBC) of 5400/uL, decreased absolute lymphocyte count (ALC) 2300/uL, increased immunoglobulin E (IgE) 213 Ku/L, IgA (98 mg/dL), and IgM (275 mg/dL). The lymphocyte subpopulation showed CD4 lymphopenia (212 cells/uL) and significant reduction in B cells (193 cells/uL) with normal NK cells count (1211 cells/uL); the majority of T cells receptors showed abnormal gamma/delta receptors, which can be seen in Omenn syndrome and hypomorphic RAGI/II mutation. In addition, the T cell function assay was abnormally low (below 15% of control). All of this confirmed the diagnosis of SCID variant.

3. Case #2

A 3-month-old Qatari female was admitted due to generalized rash, lymphadenopathy, and hepatosplenomegaly diagnosed by her pediatrician. The infant was born full term via normal spontaneous vaginal delivery. The initial family history was unremarkable except that parents are first degree cousins. On examination, the vitals were appropriate for age as well as the anthropometric measurements. There was a generalized maculopapular rash. In addition there were bilateral, nontender, nonerythematous axillary lymph nodes with diameter of 0.5 cm. The liver and spleen were palpable 3 cm below the costal margin. The rest of the examination was unremarkable. On further family medical history reassessment, it showed that both parents are carriers of Omenn syndrome and two siblings are affected by the disease.

Laboratory investigation showed that our patient had WBC of 9500/uL, lymphopenia (ALC: 600 cells/uL) with low T cells (7 cells/uL), very low both CD4 (4 cells/uL) and CD8 (2 cells/uL), absent B cells (0.00 cells/uL), and normal NK cells count (133 cells/uL) in the lymphocyte subpopulation; T cell function test showed no response to mitogens. In addition, the immunoglobulins levels showed low IgA (<5 mg/dL) and IgM (<4 mg/dL) with high IgE for age (2 Ku/L); all this confirmed the diagnosis of SCID variant.

Both cases were sent for bone marrow transplant (BMT) abroad due to the unavailability of those services in our institution.

4. Discussion

PIDs are acquired by different modes of inheritance [4]. Communities with a common practice of consanguinity, such as Iran, Saudi Arabia, Turkey, Morocco, Egypt, Kuwait, and Oman, have a high rate of PIDs [3]. In addition, autosomal recessive inheritance is not the only culprit in consanguineous marriage, but multifactorial factors play a role as well [5]. In infants and children with PID, a family history is positive in roughly 66% of all patients, with the highest rate in immune dysregulation (up to 100%) and phagocyte defects (92%) [3].

Family history is one of the components of the ten warning signs of PIDs as reported by Jeffrey Modell Foundation (JMF) [6]. Arkwright and Gennery studied the validity of these warning signs and found that family history is a strong identifier in PID [7]. Eliciting proper family history of PIDs is known to be crucial in avoiding delay in diagnosis and hence morbidity and mortality [8].

In a large study conducted by Rezaei et al., it was found that 65.6% of PID patients were the results of consanguineous marriages. Consanguinity was found to be 75.8% in combined immunodeficiency, 77.8% in cellular immunodeficiency, 72.5% in defects of phagocytic function, 58.6% in other immunodeficiencies, 54.1% in predominantly antibody deficiency, and 50% in complement deficiency [9].

Omenn syndrome is an autosomal recessive disorder that presents with lymphocytic infiltration of the gut, liver, spleen, and skin that results in skin changes similar to graft-versus-host disease; in addition, affected children present with diarrhea and failure to thrive [10].

The majority of mutations in Omenn syndrome are missense mutations in recombinase activating genes RAG1 and RAG2. Those mutations are usually detected on chromosome 11 [11, 12].

Children with Omenn syndrome usually present with hypogammaglobulinemia and elevated serum immunoglobulin E levels [10]. Moreover, affected children usually have absent B cells with present natural killers (NK) cells. The T lymphocytes count might be normal to high with variable distribution ratio of CD4+ : CD8+ subsets [13].

All children with Omenn syndrome have a high mortality rate in the first six months of age unless allogeneic haematopoietic stem cell transplantation is offered [10].

Our patients' parents perceived consanguinity and family medical history as unremarkable. Parent's perception might be different from the physician's. Moreover, people perceive family medical history differently and hence might be misleading. Hunt et al. stated that some individuals required a large number of affected relatives to perceive that they have a substantial family medical history [14].

Since family medical history could be lifesaving, some authors advocate for going one step further and interview additional family members, review death certificates, autopsy reports, and even review family members' medical reports [15].

Primary care physicians (PCPs) do not always elicit good family medical history and it is usually attributed to lack of time [16]. In addition, PCPs allot less than the suggested time to elicit family history information [15]. Other barriers, as perceived by PCPs, are lack of skills to take appropriate family medical history and counseling [17, 18] and lack of knowledge in the genetic field to merge up-to-date medical information in their practice [19]. Our team members reconsidered the initial elicited family medical history per patients' clinical course. More detailed history and definite determination by physicians were indispensable in the diagnoses of our patients.

5. Conclusion

Eliciting proper family medical history might be crucial in decreasing morbidity and mortality in infants and children. It is very important to educate communities that consanguineous marriage might be detrimental for the health of new generation. In addition, premarital counseling as well as newborn screening is recommended.

Conflict of Interests

The authors declare that there is no conflict of interests regarding the publication of this paper.

References

[1] N. Rezaei, F. A. Bonilla, K. Sullivan, E. de Vries, and J. S. Orange, "An introduction to primary immunodeficiency diseases," in *Primary Immunodeficiency Diseases*, N. Rezaei, A. Aghamohammadi, and L. D. Not-arangelo, Eds., pp. 1–38, Springer, Berlin, Germany.

[2] W. Al-Herz, M. E. Zainal, M. Salama et al., "Primary immunodeficiency disorders: survey of pediatricians in Kuwait," *Journal of Clinical Immunology*, vol. 28, no. 4, pp. 379–383, 2008.

[3] M. Ehlayel, A. Bener, and M. Abu Laban, "Effects of family history and consanguinity in primary immunodeficiency diseases in children in Qatar," *Open Journal of Immunology*, vol. 3, no. 2, pp. 47–53, 2013.

[4] J. M. Puck and R. L. Nussbaum, "Genetic principles and technologies in the study of Immune disorders," in *Primary Immunodeficiency Diseases: A Molecular and Genetic Approach*, H. D. Ochs, C. I. E. Smith, and J. M. Puck, Eds., pp. 16–26, Oxford University Press, New York, NY, USA, 2007.

[5] A. Bener, "Consanguineous marriages and their effect on common diseases in the Qatari population," in *Genetic Disorders in the Arab World: Qatar*, vol. 4, pp. 30–39, 2012, http://www.cags.org.ae/publications.html.

[6] Jeffrey Modell Foundation, 10 warning signs of primary immunodeficiency ichildren, 2009, http://www.info4pi.org/.

[7] P. D. Arkwright and A. R. Gennery, "Ten warning signs of primary immunodeficiency: a new paradigm is needed for the 21st century," *Annals of the New York Academy of Sciences*, vol. 1238, no. 1, pp. 7–14, 2011.

[8] E. Azarsiz, N. Gulez, N. Edeer Karaca, G. Aksu, and N. Kutukculer, "Consanguinity rate and delay in diagnosis in Turkish patients with combined immunodeficiencies: a single-center study," *Journal of Clinical Immunology*, vol. 31, no. 1, pp. 106–111, 2011.

[9] N. Rezaei, Z. Pourpak, A. Aghamohammadi et al., "Consanguinity in primary immunodeficiency disorders; the report from Iranian primary immunodeficiency registry," *American Journal of Reproductive Immunology*, vol. 56, no. 2, pp. 145–151, 2006.

[10] I. B. Elnour, S. Ahmed, K. Halim, and V. Nirmala, "Omenn's Syndrome: a rare primary immunodeficiency disorder," *Sultan Qaboos University Medical Journal*, vol. 7, no. 2, pp. 133–138, 2007.

[11] A. Villa, S. Santagata, F. Bozzi, L. Imberti, and L. D. Notarangelo, "Omenn syndrome: a disorder of RAG1 and RAG2 genes," *Journal of Clinical Immunology*, vol. 19, no. 2, pp. 87–97, 1999.

[12] M. A. Oettinger, B. Stanger, D. G. Schatz et al., "The recombination activating genes, RAG 1 and RAG 2, are on chromosome 11p in humans and chromosome 2p in mice," *Immunogenetics*, vol. 35, no. 2, pp. 97–101, 1992.

[13] J. V. Martin, P. B. Willoughby, V. Giusti, G. Price, and L. Cerezo, "The lymph node pathology of Omenn's syndrome," *The American Journal of Surgical Pathology*, vol. 19, no. 9, pp. 1082–1087, 1995.

[14] K. Hunt, C. Emslie, and G. Watt, "Lay constructions of a heart disease: potential for misunderstandings in the clinical encounter?" *The Lancet*, vol. 357, no. 9263, pp. 1168–1171, 2001.

[15] E. C. Rich, W. Burke, C. J. Heaton et al., "Reconsidering the family history in primary care," *Journal of General Internal Medicine*, vol. 19, no. 3, pp. 273–280, 2004.

[16] R. T. Acton, N. M. Burst, L. Casebeer et al., "Knowledge, attitudes, and behaviors of Alabama's primary care physicians regarding cancer genetics," *Academic Medicine*, vol. 75, no. 8, pp. 850–852, 2000.

[17] E. K. Watson, D. Shickle, N. Qureshi, J. Emery, and J. Austoker, "The "new genetics" and primary care: GPs' views on their role and their educational needs," *Family Practice*, vol. 16, pp. 420–425, 1999.

[18] A. Fry, H. Campbell, H. Gudmunsdottir et al., "GPs' views on their role in cancer genetics services and current practice," *Family Practice*, vol. 16, pp. 468–474, 1999.

[19] D. Bragg, D. Simpson, R. Treat, and R. Holloway, "The Genetics in Primary Care (GPC) Faculty Development Initiative Training Program: Final Evaluation Report," GPC External Evaluation Team from the Medical College of Wisconsin, 2002.

28

A Case of Polyarteritis Nodosa Associated with Vertebral Artery Vasculitis Treated Successfully with Tocilizumab and Cyclophosphamide

Kae Watanabe,[1] Dhanashree A. Rajderkar,[2] and Renee F. Modica[3]

[1]*Department of Pediatrics, University of Florida, 1600 SW Archer Road, Gainesville, FL 32608, USA*
[2]*Department of Radiology, University of Florida, Gainesville, FL 32608, USA*
[3]*Department of Pediatric Immunology, Rheumatology and Infectious Disease, University of Florida, Gainesville, FL 32608, USA*

Correspondence should be addressed to Renee F. Modica; modicar@peds.ufl.edu

Academic Editor: Nan-Chang Chiu

Pediatric polyarteritis nodosa is rare systemic necrotizing arteritis involving small- and medium-sized muscular arteries characterized by aneurysmal dilatations involving the vessel wall. Aneurysms associated with polyarteritis nodosa are common in visceral arteries; however intracranial aneurysms have also been reported and can be associated with central nervous system symptoms, significant morbidity, and mortality. To our knowledge extracranial involvement of the vertebral arteries has not been reported but has the potential to be deleterious due to fact that they supply the central nervous system vasculature. We present a case of a 3-year-old Haitian boy with polyarteritis nodosa that presented with extracranial vessel involvement of his vertebral arteries. After thorough diagnostic imaging, including a bone scan, ultrasound, Magnetic Resonance Imaging/Angiography, and Computed Tomography Angiography, he was noted to have vertebral artery vasculitis, periostitis, subacute epididymoorchitis, arthritis, and myositis. He met diagnostic criteria for polyarteritis nodosa and was treated with cyclophosphamide, methylprednisolone, and tocilizumab, which resulted in improvement of his inflammatory markers, radiographic findings, and physical symptoms after treatment. To the authors' knowledge, this is the first report of vertebral artery vasculitis in polyarteritis nodosa as well as successful treatment of the condition using the combination cyclophosphamide and tocilizumab for this condition.

1. Background

Polyarteritis nodosa (PAN), also known as Infantile Kawasaki's Disease (KD), is small- to medium-sized vasculitis affecting multiple organ systems throughout the body. It accounts for 3% of childhood vasculitis in the United States and, in the pediatric age group, the onset peaks at 9 years old [1]. The disease varies in its presentation from a relatively benign cutaneous form, which may resolve with minimal treatment, to a severe systemic form that can be associated with high morbidity and mortality. Initial presentation is nonspecific and may include fever, malaise, weight loss, myalgias, and arthralgias. It most frequently affects the vasculature of the skin, muscles, kidneys, and gastrointestinal tract [2–4]. Depending on the vasculature that is involved, the patient may present with hypertension, ischemic heart disease, testicular pain, abdominal pain, hematuria, or proteinuria [2–4]. However, intracranial involvement, although rare, has also been reported and can be associated with hemorrhage or stroke if ischemia or rupture occurs [5, 6]. Extracranial involvement, to our knowledge, has not been reported, but if it occurred it could have the potential to be deleterious leading to stroke or ischemic events. Laboratory markers of systemic inflammation are usually elevated but are nonspecific of the disease [2]. Diagnosis is made according to The European League Against Rheumatism (EULAR)/Pediatric Rheumatology European Society (PReS) or American College of Rheumatology (ACR) classification criteria for childhood PAN [7]. The major diagnostic factor is evidence of vasculitis either by angiography and/or biopsy. In a large series of adult patients with PAN, combined muscle and nerve biopsies in symptomatic patients provided histologic confirmation of vasculitis in 83% whereas isolated muscle biopsies demonstrated vascular inflammation in 65%. However, valuable diagnostic imaging modalities include selective Computed Tomography (CT), Magnetic Resonance Imaging (MRI), or conventional angiography, which may demonstrate findings consistent with medium or large vessel vasculitis without biopsy [8]. Bone scans have been used as a frequent modality in evaluating extremity pain in adult patients with PAN, which has detected periosteal inflammation even prior to periosteal reactions of the bone [9, 10].

Our case is a unique presentation of PAN, including symptoms of neck pain related to vertebral artery vasculitis and cervical myositis, which to our knowledge is the first case described in pediatric PAN. Evaluation with bone scans allowed for a noninvasive means of confirmation of periosteal inflammation, detection of clinically silent periosteal involvement, and resolution after treatment. The concomitant use of intravenous (IV) steroids, cyclophosphamide with tocilizumab, was a safe and effective treatment option for this case; however its usage needs further investigation in the pediatric PAN population [11].

2. Case Presentation

A 3-year-old Haitian boy presented to pediatric rheumatology clinic due to persistently elevated inflammatory markers for 9 months after treatment for suspected atypical KD. His past medical history is otherwise negative other than the initial diagnosis of atypical KD. He was born and raised in the United States without travel prior to his illness. He has neither developmental issues nor significant family history of rheumatic disease. The patient was diagnosed and treated for atypical KD at an outside hospital based upon initial presentation with tactile fevers of unclear duration, dry cracked lips, extremity changes, elevated inflammatory markers including C-reactive protein (CRP) (200–300 mg/L), Erythrocyte Sedimentation Rate (ESR) (>100 mm/h), and very mild ectasia of his coronary arteries without perivascular or vessel wall edema on his initial echocardiogram. He did lack other typical findings of KD including conjunctival injection, exanthema, cervical adenopathy, and thrombocytosis. At the time of presentation his pertinent laboratories showed CRP 219 mg/L, sodium 131 mmol/L, aspartate aminotransferase (AST)/alanine aminotransferase (ALT) 44/19 IU/L, albumin 2.5 g/dL, ferritin 190 mg/mL, white blood cell (WBC) $10(3)/\mu L$, and platelet count $180\ 10(3)/\mu L$. He also did present with hypochromic microcytic anemia (hemoglobin (Hgb) 5.6 g/dL) that required IV iron therapy and subsequently oral iron supplementation. The decision to treat for atypical KD was made due to his mild coronary artery ectasia, history of fevers, dry cracking lips, and extremity changes in spite of lack of thrombocytosis which is a common finding. His treatment included one dose of intravenous immunoglobulin (2 g/kg/dose) and low dose aspirin therapy (3–5 mg/kg/day). He was followed at cardiology clinic three months later and had a normal cardiac evaluation including normal echocardiogram without evidence of coronary artery ectasia, perivascular brightness, or abnormal tapering. He was noted

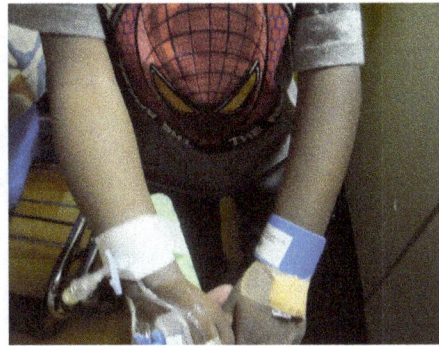

FIGURE 1: Comparison of right and left arm on physical exam. Right forearm notably enlarged compared to left. On palpation, bony enlargement and pain present circumferentially on right.

to have normal ventricular function and no pericardial effusion was noted. However, he continued to report intermittent tactile fevers without source and his laboratory evaluation showed persistently elevated CRP levels at 90 mg/L. His anemia improved (Hgb 9.8 g/dL) after oral iron therapy. Due to his persistent anemia, unclear diagnosis, and persistent inflammatory markers, he had a bone marrow biopsy and aspiration as well as hemoglobin electrophoresis that were normal. Six months after the initial presentation he developed epididymoorchitis, which was unresponsive to 4 weeks of oral antibiotic treatment with cephalexin. He continued to have persistently elevated ESR in the 90–100 (mm/hr) range at this duration, with CRP fluctuating between 51 and 90 mg/L. At their six-month cardiology appointment, the family reported that he was progressively more fatigued, developed a stiff neck, was shuffling gait, and was less active. He continued to have intermittent weekly subjective fevers. His outpatient evaluation by pediatric infectious diseases did not reveal a source of his fevers including negative blood cultures, T-spot TB test, treponemal Ab, rapid plasma reagin (RPR), Cytomegalovirus- (CMV-) polymerase chain reaction (PCR), Human Immunodeficiency Virus (HIV) Ab, Brucella Ag, hepatitis A, B, and C panel, and galactomannan. He was referred to pediatric rheumatology department for further evaluation 9 months after his initial presentation, diagnosis, and treatment for presumptive atypical KD.

At his initial pediatric rheumatology appointment, the patient's physical exam showed mild torticollis with preferential tilting of his head to the right, decreased and painful extension, flexion, and lateral rotation of his cervical spine. He also was noted to have tenderness, warmth, and bony hypertrophy involving the right forearm (Figure 1) but sparing the elbow joint with normal flexion, extension, supination, and pronation of the right elbow joint. He did not have peripheral arthritis on exam and his hip rotation was normal without pain. His gait was wide based and characterized by slight hip flexion, which was thought to be related to right epididymoorchitis. His right scrotum was enlarged to about 4 cm in length with tenderness, warmth, and erythema (Figure 2).

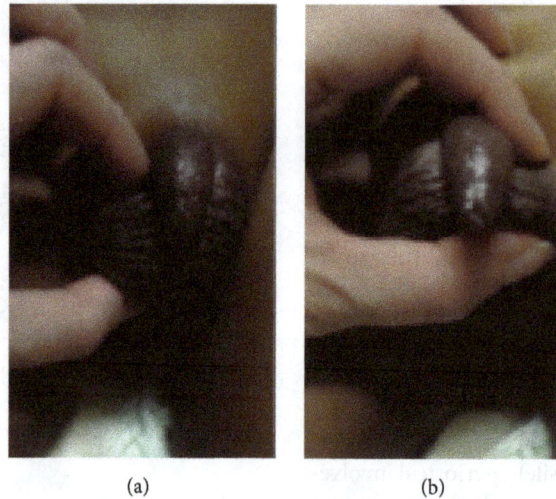

FIGURE 2: Comparison of left and right testicle on physical exam. Tender and warm right testis (a), approximately twice enlarged compared to left (b).

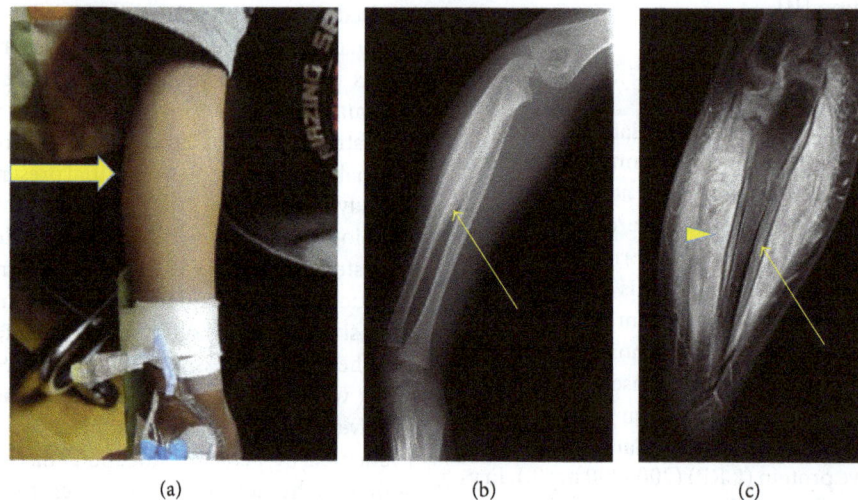

FIGURE 3: Physical findings and imaging of right arm at diagnosis. (a) Right forearm hypertrophy (yellow arrow). (b) Plain (lateral) radiograph of the right upper extremity revealing diffuse periosteal thickening of both the bones of the forearm (thin yellow arrow) without any focal lytic or sclerotic lesions. The extent and the degree of the involvement of the right ulna were marked as compared to the radius. (c) MRI T2 weighted images of the right forearm demonstrated marked diffuse, circumferential periosteal thickening involving the radius and ulna. Ulnar involvement (thin yellow arrow) was severe as compared with the radius. No focal osseous lesion was identified. Also notable was marked soft tissue involvement including the muscular compartment consistent with myositis (arrowhead).

X-rays and MRI of right forearm, MRI of neck, and Magnetic Resonance Angiography (MRA) of neck, chest and abdomen, and pelvis were recommended to evaluate ostitis, tenosynovitis, myositis, and systemic vasculitis, respectively. The right forearm X-ray showed periosteal thickening and right forearm MRI showed diffuse smooth circumferential periosteal reaction and thickening and enhancement of right ulna, as well as myositis (Figure 3). MRI of the neck showed notable adventitial inflammation of the vertebral arteries as well as irregularity and diffuse narrowing, with the left side involvement greater than the right side. There was focal area of superimposed short segment stenosis at C2-C3 with poststenotic dilatation on the left side. Myositis of the neck muscles was observed on the left side (Figure 4).

The MRA of his chest, abdomen, and pelvis were normal. MRA of forearm was not obtained. Due to the finding of chronic, stenotic vertebral artery vasculitis, he was admitted for additional workup and aggressive inpatient treatment.

During admission, his additional workup included consultation with neuroradiology who recommended CT Angiography of head and neck, which were obtained to further delineate his vasculitis especially as previous MRA did not include intracranial vessels. Bilateral vertebral artery vasculitis was confirmed by CT Angiography. Left vertebral

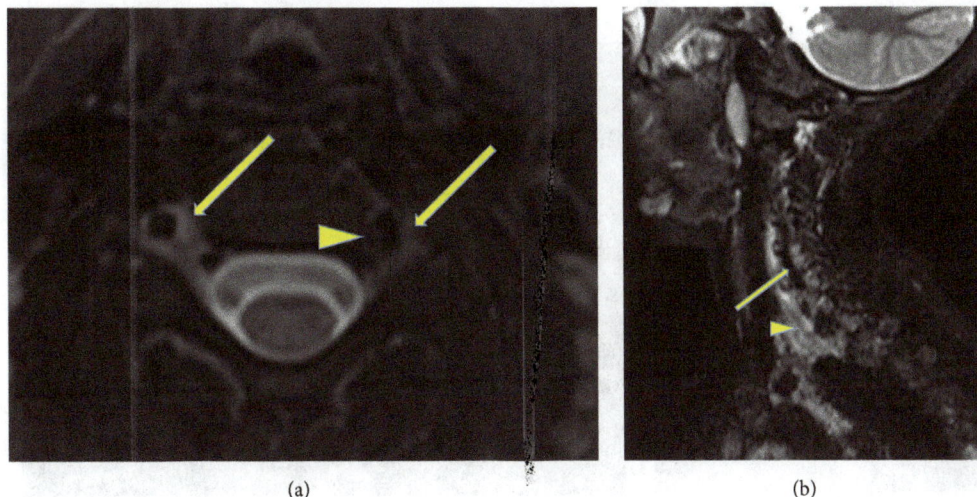

(a)   (b)

Figure 4: Imaging of cervical area at diagnosis. (a) Baseline MRI T2 weighted images showed moderate adventitial thickening of both the vertebral arteries at the level of C3 (thin yellow arrows) with adjacent soft tissue edema. There were focal areas of irregularity causing moderate stenosis on the left side (arrowhead). (b) Sagittal view of cervical MRI demonstrated poststenotic dilation of his left vertebral artery (arrow) and marked myositis (arrowhead).

artery showed stenosis at C2-C3 with poststenotic dilatation from C2 to basal skull. Due to the periosteal reaction of his right forearm, pediatric oncology and orthopedic oncology were consulted to evaluate the bony changes. The periosteal thickening was considered to be most likely a reaction from local myositis; therefore bone and muscle biopsies were deferred. Of note, the patient already did have a bone marrow biopsy done at the outside hospital, which was negative 2 months prior to his initial visit to pediatric rheumatology.

Pediatric urology was consulted due to his testicular enlargement and pain. Alfa fetal protein (AFP) and beta-human chorionic gonadotropin (HCG) tumor markers were obtained for concerns of scrotal enlargement, which were negative. Scrotal ultrasound (US) with Doppler (Figure 5) showed increased size of right epididymis and testis with increased vascularity, suggestive of inflammation; therefore testicular biopsy was deferred.

Bone scan was done to further evaluate his periostitis. There was diffuse increased uptake in the right forearm. Interestingly, in addition to the expected areas of increased activity, namely, the right forearm, few additional clinically occult areas also showed increased uptake. There was also diffuse uptake in the left forearm similar in the extent and activity and focal uptake was noted in right mid tibia (Figure 6).

Initially, the patient received scheduled intravenous ketorolac (0.5 mg/kg/dose every 6 hours) for his arthritis and myositis symptoms, which resulted in clinical improvement of his scrotal swelling as well as arm and neck pain. Additionally, his ESR and CRP also improved. Due to his extensive and chronic nature of his bilateral vertebral artery vasculitis, as well as the concern regarding the extracranial location of the vasculitis, he was initially treated with pulse methylprednisolone (30 mg/kg/dose daily × 3) and received one dose of infliximab (6 mg/kg) while inpatient. Subsequently

he received a total of 7 monthly doses of cyclophosphamide (500 mg/m^2) for his vasculitis and monthly tocilizumab for his vasculitis and arthritis with high dose oral steroid taper starting at 1 mg/kg daily (Figure 7). This aggressive, combined approach was decided due to the location and bilaterality of the vertebral artery vasculitis, as well as the chronicity of his symptoms and the presence of stenosis in order to circumvent life-threatening complications such as rupture or worsening stenosis in this critical area with limited ability to form collaterals. This treatment resulted in clinical improvement of his myositis, arthritis, ostitis, and epididymoorchitis as well as serologic improvement in his inflammatory markers and radiographic improvement in his vasculitis. Physical examination and follow-up imaging at 7 months after initiation of treatment showed resolution of his right forearm hypertrophy and near total resolution of periosteal reaction and myositis (Figure 8). Follow-up testicular exam and scrotal Doppler US showed normal appearing right testis and epididymis as well as normal vascularity of the right testis (Figure 9). Most importantly the focal residual irregularity of the wall of the vertebral arteries and adventitial thickening had markedly improved (Figure 10). Furthermore, on bone scan there was total response to the treatment with no abnormal residual activity (Figure 11).

3. Discussion

PAN is a rare systemic necrotizing arteritis involving small- and medium-sized muscular arteries with multisystem involvement making it challenging to diagnose. In case of being untreated or delayed treatment, PAN can be associated with significant morbidity and mortality. Childhood PAN has also been referred to as infantile KD or infantile PAN which are both on the spectrum of necrotizing vasculitis that can involve the coronary arteries, but the use of the term

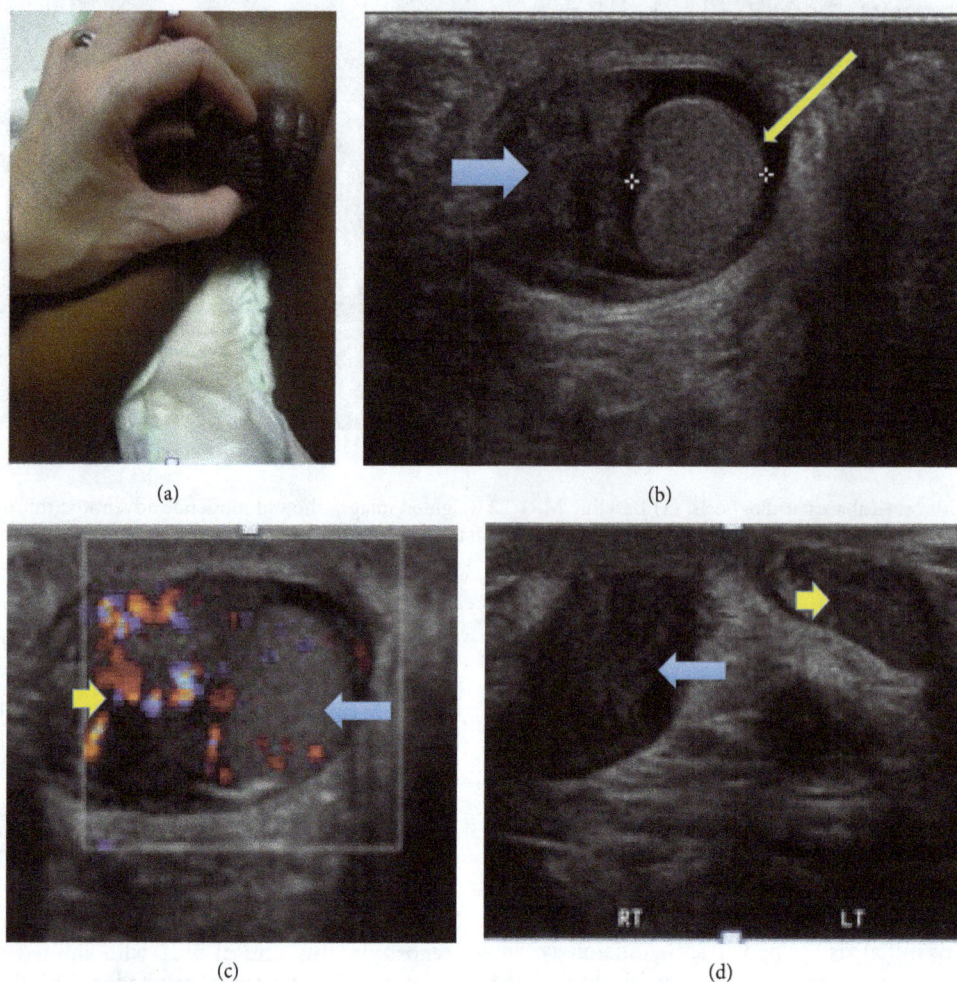

FIGURE 5: Physical exam and imaging of right testis at diagnosis. (a) Enlarged right testis. (b) Baseline ultrasound of the scrotum demonstrated enlarged right testis (thin yellow arrow) and epididymis (thick blue arrow). (c) Testicular Doppler showing hyperemic right testis (long blue arrow) and epididymis (short yellow arrow). (d) Right side testicle (long blue arrow) was estimated to be approximately twice the volume of the left (short yellow arrow).

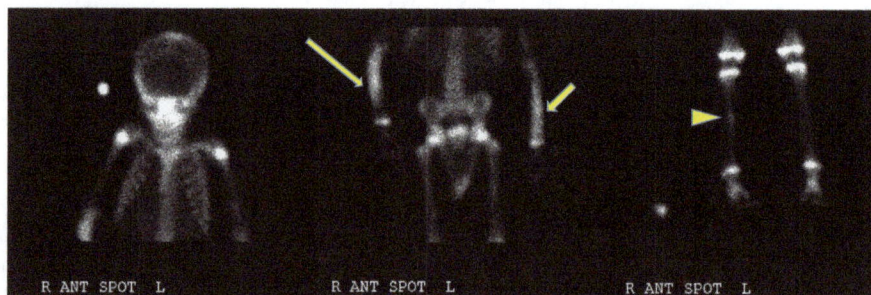

FIGURE 6: Bone scan at diagnosis. Bone scan: multifocal areas of uptake in the bilateral forearms most pronounced in the right ulna and radius (thin, long yellow arrow) as well as the left ulna and radius (thin short yellow arrow) and right proximal tibia (arrowhead). Gallium scan (not shown) obtained at this time demonstrated subtle increased uptake corresponding to the areas of increased activity on the bone scan, but the activity was less intense than the bone scan, supporting this to be inflammatory process. There was also soft tissue uptake in the right forearm.

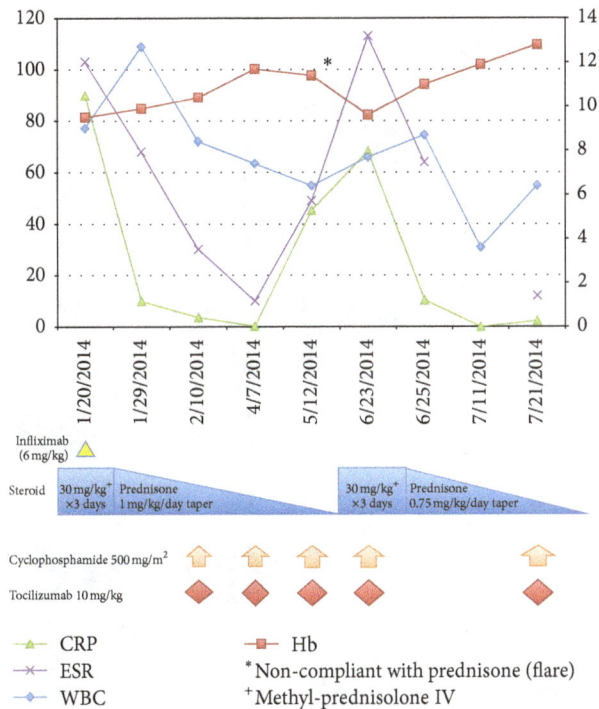

FIGURE 7: Summary of treatment course and laboratory parameters.

which could participate in the pathogenesis of periostitis [15]. In our case we had initially thought it was a secondary inflammation due to myositis that was localized in the same area, but it is hard to evaluate which came first. The patients right arm hypertrophy was not noted by the family or other treating physicians, possibly since it did not affect the patient's range of motion.

In several cases of PAN bone scan has been utilized for evaluation of extremity pain [9, 10, 13], which can be very useful in pediatric patients who may have difficultly in communicating pain level and location. In our case the muscle and bone biopsy were deferred and the patient met criteria of PAN with imaging studies and his other presenting symptoms. Obtaining periosteal histology may show evidence of necrotizing arteritis, although often the changes seen are nonspecific such as bone reabsorption and formation [14]. Cases with periostitis may or may not involve localized overlying cutaneous PAN lesions [14] which were absent in our patient. Bone scan may be a useful first-line examination in detecting subclinical and extra-articular involvement of inflammatory bone processes [9, 10, 13], especially in the pediatric population, as it is a low invasive test.

CNS involvement has been reported in up to 22% of cases of polyarteritis nodosa in the pediatric population, presenting with encephalopathy, focal deficits, stroke, and seizures [2–5]. The most common neuroradiological finding is focal ischemic areas, followed by intracranial hemorrhage with narrowing or occlusion of intracranial arteries on angiography [16]. There have been no reports on vertebral artery occlusion, which would be more common in large vascular arteritis including primary CNS angiitis, Takayasu Arteritis, and Giant Cell Arteritis, however our patient did not meet EULAR criteria [7]. Our patient did not present with neurologic symptoms. In patients with rheumatic disease, neck pain is often associated with arthritis, but in our case, we were able to diagnose radiographically cervical myositis and vasculitis as a contributing cause of neck pain. Due to the presence of chronic, bilateral vertebral artery vasculitis, with delayed treatment and focal stenosis, we decided to treat our patient more aggressively due to the potential deleterious effects of extracranial vascular injuries including further progression, stenosis, stroke, aneurysm formation, rupture, or hemorrhage [4, 5, 16, 17]. We believe that our treatment plan prevented intracranial progression and embolic/ischemic stroke. Collaterals were not observed in our patient, as the stenosis was less than 70%. Our initial aggressive approach included treatment with combination of high dose pulse corticosteroids, cyclophosphamide, and tocilizumab due to his vasculitis and arthritis. He did receive one initial dose of infliximab, which was available on the inpatient formulary for his arthritis and vasculitis.

Tocilizumab use has been described mainly in juvenile idiopathic arthritis, but in limited case reports, usage in Giant Cell Arteritis and Takayasu's Arteritis [11, 18] has shown benefit for treatment of vasculitis. The use of tocilizumab in PAN has not been approved by the United States Food and Drug Administration (FDA), but the blockage of IL-6 with tocilizumab has been used effectively to treat other forms of vasculitis [19, 20]. Furthermore in our case we had

infantile (which connotes < 1 year) is too restrictive and in our case this patient was older. The patient's coronary artery dilation resolved after one dose of IVIG and due to the latter development of more extensive symptoms of vertebral artery vasculitis, epididymitis, periostitis, and myositis, which are not typical of KD, we believe that his coronary artery dilation was likely part of his childhood PAN. Of note, a childhood onset of vasculopathy overlapping polyarteritis nodosa caused by a single gene defect in CECR1 (Cat Eye Syndrome Chromosome Region Candidate 1) resulting in deficiency of adenosine deaminase 2 has also been reported in families with autosomal recessive inheritance pattern [12]. Our patient was not tested for this condition at this time given lack of familial involvement but may be warranted in the future.

About 50% of children with newly diagnosed PAN present with musculoskeletal symptoms including joint, muscle, or limb pain [2]. Therefore, evaluation of periostitis, a more challenging diagnosis to make, is important in evaluating the extent of disease in addition to arthritis and myositis. Cases of periostitis and periosteal reactions in patients with PAN have been reported [9, 10, 13–15], but rarely in pediatrics. This finding may have clinically silent areas that can be detected by bone scan imaging modalities.

It has been stated that most periosteal reactions are found in long bones especially in the lower limb [13, 14]. In our case, his long bone involvement was his right ulna and radius as well as his right tibia and left radius and ulna, but these latter areas were clinically silent and notable on bone scan imaging only. Localized vasculitis is said to be responsible for local production of bone growth factors associated with hypoxia,

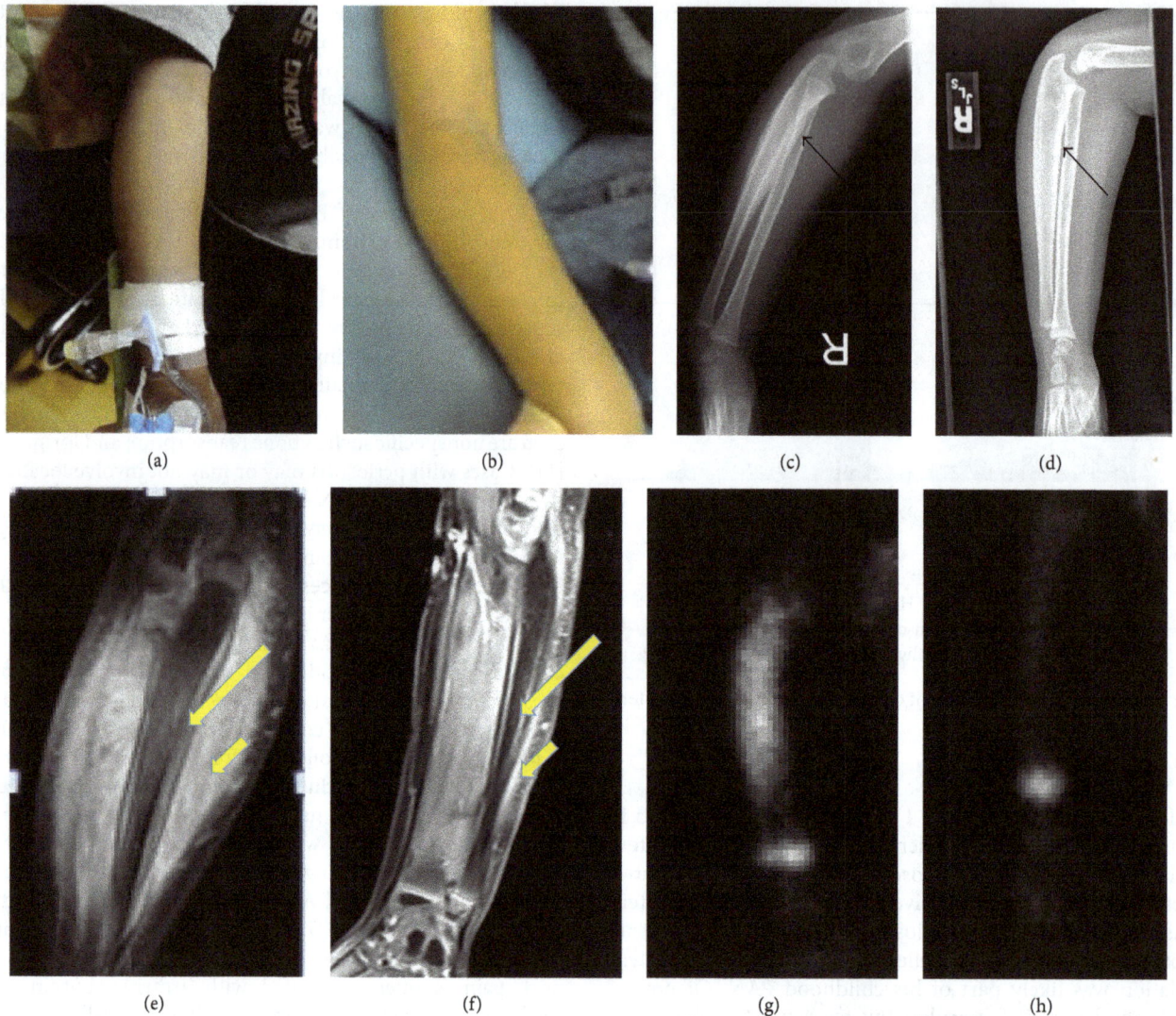

FIGURE 8: Comparison of right arm before and after treatment with exam and images. (a) Right arm before treatment. (b) Right arm after treatment showing resolution of right forearm hypertrophy. (c) Right arm X-ray before treatment. (d) Right arm X-ray after treatment: follow-up radiographs revealed near total resolution of the periosteal reaction (cf. thin blue arrows). (e) Right arm MRI before treatment. (f) Right arm MRI after treatment: follow-up MRI of the right forearm revealed resolution of periostitis (cf. long yellow arrows) and myositis (cf. short yellow arrows). (g) Right arm bone scan before treatment. (h) Right arm bone scan after treatment: follow-up revealed total resolution of the abnormal uptake in the forearm.

concomitant use of cyclophosphamide for his extracranial involvement. In spite of this combination of immunosuppressants, our patient has been infection-free during the 7 months of concomitant treatment and has not had common or severe adverse effects seen in tocilizumab such as upper respiratory infection, pharyngitis, diarrhea, increase in liver enzymes, hyperlipidemia, and neutropenia [18]. This concomitant use of tocilizumab, cyclophosphamide, and steroids has improved the systemic manifestations of vasculitis, myositis, arthritis, periostitis, and epididymoorchitis in our patient based on clinical exam, serologic markers, and follow-up imaging at 7 months. Future studies are recommended for the use of tocilizumab and combination therapy in PAN. For

our patient, follow-up imaging is planned to assess ongoing response to treatment.

4. Conclusion

Periostitis can be an initial presentation of PAN in the pediatric population. It may be clinically silent in some areas but could be helpful in differentiating PAN from other vasculitis. Bone scintigraphy may be utilized as a noninvasive modality to evaluate and monitor inflammation and response to treatment for periostitis. To our knowledge, we have also presented the first case of PAN presenting with vertebral artery dilatation and aneurysm development that

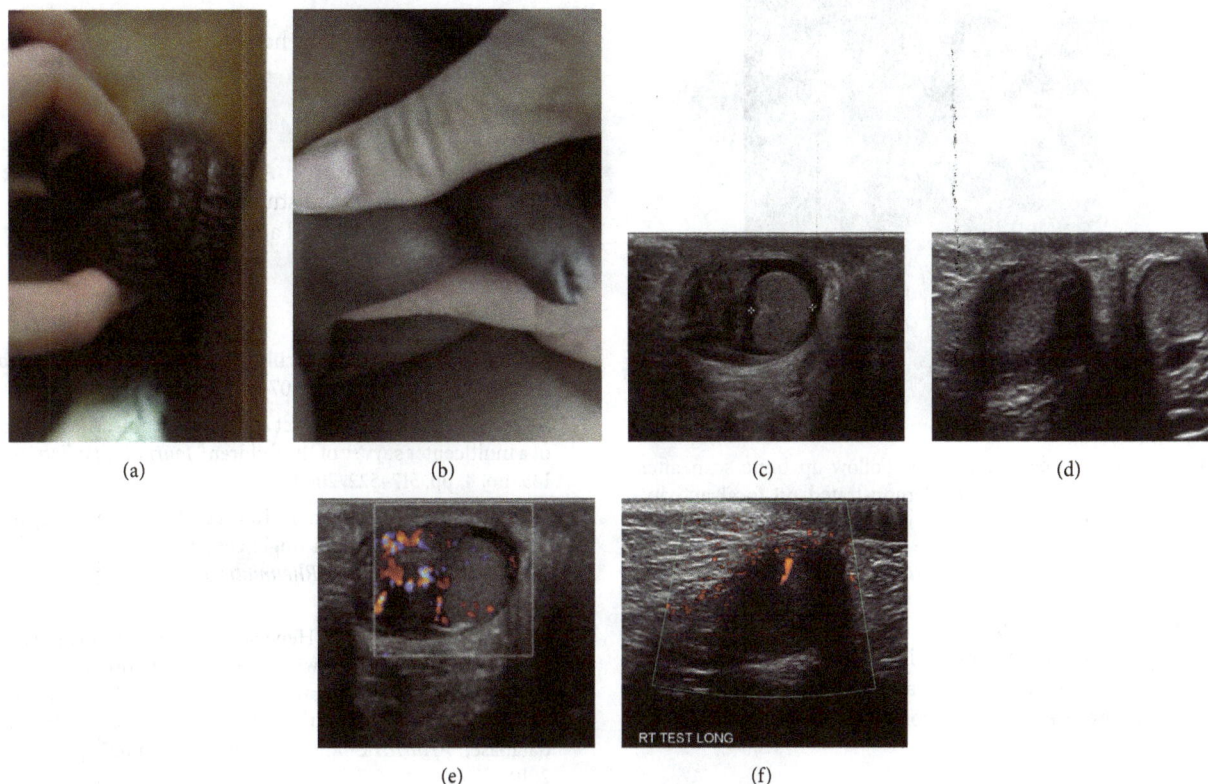

FIGURE 9: Comparison of right testes before and after treatment with exam and images. (a) Enlarged right testis before treatment, (b) normal sized right testis after treatment. Both testes (not shown) on follow-up exam were equal in size and volume. (c) Right testicular US before treatment. (d) Right testicular US after treatment: follow-up scrotal ultrasound demonstrated normal appearing right testis and epididymis with equal volume and size compared to left. (e) Right testicular Doppler before treatment shows hyperemia. (f) Right testicular Doppler after treatment shows normal Doppler flow.

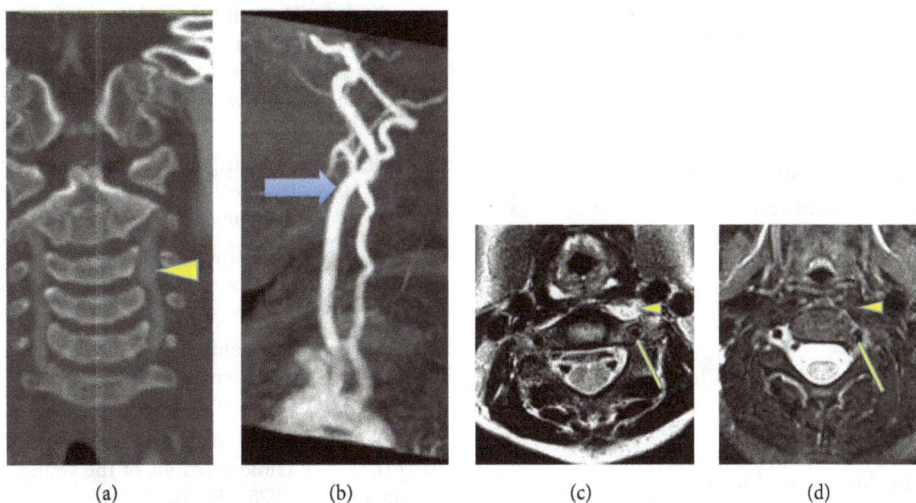

FIGURE 10: Neck imaging before and after treatment. (a) CTA coronal reformats demonstrating bilateral vertebral arteries prior to treatment. There is focal stenosis at C2-3 with poststenotic dilatation on the left side (arrowhead); the caliber of the right vertebral artery is maintained. (b) Left vertebral sagittal MRA after treatment demonstrating resolution of stenosis and poststenotic dilatation (thick blue arrow). (c) Axial MRI of cervical spine through C2 before treatment demonstrated marked adventitial thickening of bilateral vertebral arteries and focal stenosis at C2-C3 on the left side (arrow) and cervical myositis (arrowhead). (d) Posttreatment images demonstrated improvement in the adventitial thickening of bilateral vertebral arteries with improvement in the caliber of the artery at C2-3 (arrow). Note that there is complete resolution of muscular edema (arrowhead).

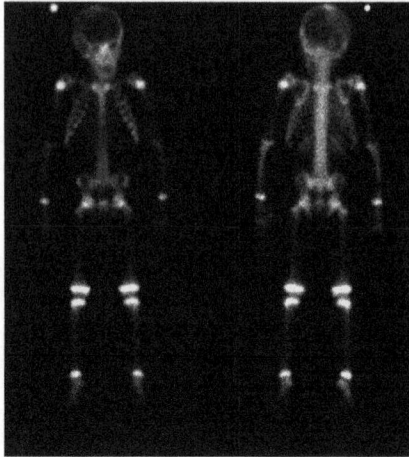

FIGURE 11: Posttreatment bone scan. Follow-up bone scan after the completion of the treatment demonstrated no focal activity, consistent with complete response to the therapy.

has responded to combination treatment with cyclophosphamide, glucocorticoids, and tocilizumab. Therapeutic trials are needed to determine the efficacy and use of tocilizumab in the treatment of PAN and in combination therapy.

Abbreviations

PAN: Polyarteritis nodosa
CNS: Central nervous system
KD: Kawasaki disease
MRI/A: Magnetic Resonance
         Imaging/Angiography (MRI/A)
EULAR: The European League Against
         Rheumatism
PReS: Pediatric Rheumatology European Society
ACR: American College of Rheumatology
IV: Intravenous
CRP: C-reactive protein
ESR: Erythrocyte Sedimentation Rate
AST: Aspartate aminotransferase
ALT: Alanine aminotransferase
WBC: White blood cell
RPR: Rapid plasma reagin
CMV: *Cytomegalovirus*
HIV: Human Immunodeficiency Virus
PCR: Polymerase chain reaction
AFP: Alfa fetal protein
HCG: Human chorionic gonadotropin
US: Ultrasound
FDA: Food and Drug Administration.

Consent

Written informed consent was obtained from the patient for publication of this case report and any accompanying images.

Conflict of Interests

The authors declare that they have no competing interests.

Authors' Contribution

Kae Watanabe, Dhanashree A. Rajderkar, and Renee F. Modica conceptualized the study and wrote the paper. All authors revised the paper and approved the final version.

References

[1] P. F. Weiss, "Pediatric vasculitis," *Pediatric Clinics of North America*, vol. 59, no. 2, pp. 407–423, 2012.

[2] S. Ozen, J. Anton, N. Arisoy et al., "Juvenile polyarteritis: results of a multicenter survey of 110 children," *Journal of Pediatrics*, vol. 145, no. 4, pp. 517–522, 2004.

[3] D. Eleftheriou, M. J. Dillon, K. Tullus et al., "Systemic polyarteritis nodosa in the young: a single-center experience over thirty-two years," *Arthritis and Rheumatism*, vol. 65, no. 9, pp. 2476–2485, 2013.

[4] C. Pagnoux, R. Seror, C. Henegar et al., "Clinical features and outcomes in 348 patients with polyarteritis nodosa: a systematic retrospective study of patients diagnosed between 1963 and 2005 and entered into the French Vasculitis Study Group database," *Arthritis & Rheumatism*, vol. 62, no. 2, pp. 616–626, 2010.

[5] K. Toyoda, K. Tsutsumi, T. Hirao et al., "Ruptured intracranial aneurysms in pediatric polyarteritis nodosa: case report," *Neurologia Medico-Chirurgica*, vol. 52, no. 12, pp. 928–932, 2012.

[6] J. C. Takahashi, N. Sakai, K. Iihara et al., "Subarachnoid hemorrhage from a ruptured anterior cerebral artery aneurysm caused by polyarteritis nodosa. Case report," *Journal of Neurosurgery*, vol. 96, no. 1, pp. 132–134, 2002.

[7] S. Ozen, A. Pistorio, S. M. Iusan et al., "EULAR/PRINTO/PRES criteria for Henoch-Schönlein purpura, childhood polyarteritis nodosa, childhood Wegener granulomatosis and childhood Takayasu arteritis: Ankara 2008. Part II: final classification criteria," *Annals of the Rheumatic Diseases*, vol. 69, no. 5, pp. 798–806, 2010.

[8] J. Hernández-Rodríguez, M. A. Alba, S. Prieto-González, and M. C. Cid, "Diagnosis and classification of polyarteritis nodosa," *Journal of Autoimmunity*, vol. 48-49, pp. 84–89, 2014.

[9] S. Sanges, N. Le Gouellec, E. Nedeva, and G. Petyt, "Bilateral femoral periostitis revealing *polyarteritis nodosa*," *BMJ Case Reports*, 2013.

[10] W. B. G. MacDonald and M. P. Blake, "Periostitis and localized myositis in polyarteritis nodosa," *Clinical Nuclear Medicine*, vol. 29, no. 11, pp. 703–705, 2004.

[11] D. Eleftheriou, M. Melo, S. D. Marks et al., "Biologic therapy in primary systemic vasculitis of the young," *Rheumatology*, vol. 48, no. 8, pp. 978–986, 2009.

[12] P. N. Elkan, S. B. Pierce, R. Segel et al., "Mutant adenosine deaminase 2 in a polyarteritis nodosa vasculopathy," *The New England Journal of Medicine*, vol. 370, no. 10, pp. 921–931, 2014.

[13] P. Carron, I. E. A. Hoffman, L. De Rycke et al., "Case number 34: relapse of polyarteritis nodosa presenting as isolated and localised lower limb periostitis," *Annals of the Rheumatic Diseases*, vol. 64, no. 8, pp. 1118–1119, 2005.

[14] D. J. Short and M. Webley, "Periosteal new bone formation complicating juvenile polyarteritis nodosa," *Journal of the Royal Society of Medicine*, vol. 77, no. 4, pp. 325–327, 1984.

[15] L. M. Astudillo, F. Rigal, B. Couret, and E. Arlet-Suau, "Localized polyarteritis nodosa with periostitis," *Journal of Rheumatology*, vol. 28, no. 12, pp. 2758–2759, 2001.

[16] J. M. Provenzale and N. B. Allen, "Neuroradiologic findings in polyarteritis nodosa," *American Journal of Neuroradiology*, vol. 17, no. 6, pp. 1119–1126, 1996.

[17] M. B. Pritz, "Aneurysms of the anterior inferior cerebellar artery," *Acta Neurochirurgica*, vol. 120, no. 1-2, pp. 12–19, 1993.

[18] R. Gurion and N. G. Singer, "Tocilizumab in pediatric rheumatology: the clinical experience," *Current Rheumatology Reports*, vol. 15, no. 7, article 338, 2013.

[19] M. Murakami and N. Nishimoto, "The value of blocking IL-6 outside of rheumatoid arthritis: current perspective," *Current Opinion in Rheumatology*, vol. 23, no. 3, pp. 273–277, 2011.

[20] L. Iannetti, R. Zito, S. Bruschi et al., "Recent understanding on diagnosis and management of central nervous system vasculitis in children," *Clinical and Developmental Immunology*, vol. 2012, Article ID 698327, 9 pages, 2012.

29

Tuberculous Dactylitis: An Uncommon Presentation of a Common Infection

G. Nayantara Rao,[1] Jayasri Helen Gali,[2] and S. Narasimha Rao[1]

[1]Department of Pediatrics, Apollo Institute of Medical Sciences and Research, Hyderabad 500096, India
[2]Department of Pulmonology, Apollo Institute of Medical Sciences and Research, Hyderabad 500096, India

Correspondence should be addressed to G. Nayantara Rao; nayantara.dr@gmail.com

Academic Editor: Abraham Gedalia

Tuberculous dactylitis is an unusual form of osteoarticular tuberculosis involving the short tubular bones of hands and feet, which is uncommon beyond six years of age. We report the case of a fifteen-year-old adolescent boy who was diagnosed with tuberculous dactylitis, involving contralateral hand and foot. His diagnosis was delayed due to lack of suspicion of this rare entity. The report also examines the diagnostic difficulties faced by clinicians in arriving at an appropriate diagnosis.

1. Introduction

Tuberculous infection of metacarpals, metatarsals, and phalanges of hands and feet is known as tuberculous dactylitis. Eighty-five percent of the patients are younger than six years of age [1] and data relating to tuberculous dactylitis among adolescents is scarce. To the best of our knowledge, simultaneous involvement of both the limbs in a child above six years of age is extremely rare and has been hardly reported.

2. Case Report

A fifteen-year-old adolescent boy initially presented with a dull aching pain followed by a swelling over the dorsum of his right foot. After a fortnight, he noticed a painful swelling on the dorsum of his left hand, which gradually progressed over the last six months. Initially, he was taken to a general practitioner after a month of his presenting complaints, for which he was prescribed analgesics for pain and oral antibiotics (a combination of amoxicillin and clavulanic acid) for a period of 10 days suspecting a pyogenic infection, but to no avail. However, the swelling persisted only to increase in size, forming an abscess. The child consulted another doctor after 3 months, where both the abscesses were incised and drained leading to discharging sinuses. The pain persisted despite the treatment causing restricted movements of the fingers and toes. Finally, he was brought to our Outpatient Department, where we admitted him to our ward. On carefully probing into the history, the parents told us that the child's grandfather was diagnosed with pulmonary tuberculosis and was taking treatment for the same for 5 months. However, the child had no history of fever, cough, night sweats, loss of weight, or trauma.

Local examination revealed an oval shaped swelling of 4 cm * 2 cm over the right 1st metatarsal bone with a discharging sinus and another swelling over the left 2nd metacarpal bone of 2 cm * 1 cm. Both swellings were hard and fixed to the underlying bone. There was tenderness and local rise of temperature on palpation. Movements were restricted at the left proximal interphalangeal joint of the index finger and the right great toe. There was no lymphadenopathy. Systemic examination was unremarkable.

Complete laboratory investigations were done which revealed a haemoglobin of 10.5 g/dL, total leukocyte count of 11,600/mm^3, and an ESR of 90 mm/hr, and Mantoux test was strongly positive (20 mm). Chest radiograph was normal. Open biopsy specimen for histopathological examination taken from the 1st metatarsal of right foot revealed a caseating granulomatous inflammation consistent with tuberculosis, but staining for mycobacterium was negative. Radiograph of the left hand showed a diffuse thickening of 2nd metacarpal with subperiosteal new bone formation

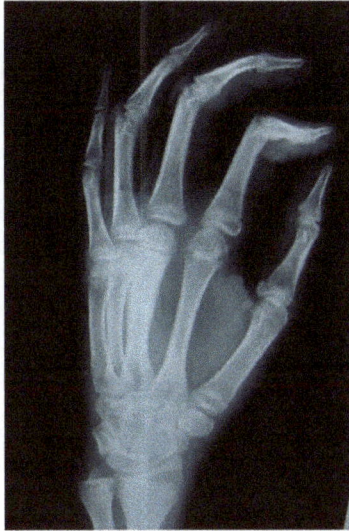

FIGURE 1: Radiograph of left hand (lateral view), showing cortical thickening and expansion of third metacarpal predominantly involving diaphysis with subperiosteal reaction.

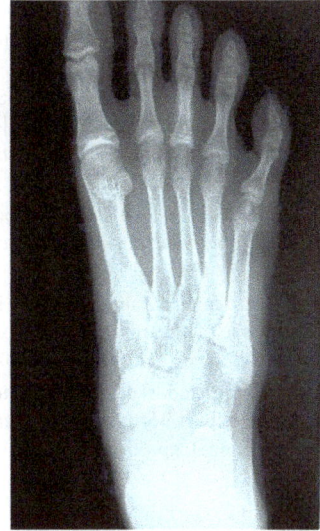

FIGURE 2: Radiograph of right foot (AP view), showing irregular destruction of proximal phalanx of 3rd toe and cortical thickening of 4th metatarsal with solid periosteal reaction.

(Figure 1). Radiograph of the right foot showed central cystic lesion with diffuse thickening of metatarsal bone and proximal phalanx of the great toe (Figure 2). Based on all these features, a probable diagnosis of tuberculous dactylitis was established and antitubercular therapy was initiated, which consisted of a four-drug regimen (Isoniazid, Rifampicin, Pyrazinamide, and Ethambutol) for a period of two months and two-drug regimen (Isoniazid and Rifampicin) for four months as per the guidelines of Revised National Tuberculosis Control Program in India (DOTS Category 1). The child responded well to the treatment within 8–10 weeks. On follow-up, there was a substantial reduction in the size of the swelling, restoration of the finger and toe movements, and healing of the sinus within 4-5 months.

3. Discussion

In childhood tuberculosis, the time between infection and development of symptomatic disease is very short. Without an adequate treatment, the risk of progression to active disease has been estimated to be higher in children (24% in 1–5 years of age) and increases again in adolescence (15%). Therefore, children are more prone to develop extrapulmonary tuberculosis [2].

The diagnostic delay in this child is attributed to

(i) Lack of high index of suspicion and poor awareness among the clinicians.

(ii) Nonspecific clinical manifestations.

(iii) Simultaneous involvement of both the limbs (usually bones of the hand are more commonly involved) [3].

(iv) Presentation at an unusual age (uncommon beyond 6 years of age, once the epiphyseal centres are well established).

(v) Absence of concomitant pulmonary involvement.

(vi) Paucibacillary nature of the lesion [4].

Therefore, a conglomeration of findings from careful history taking and physical examination supported with appropriate diagnostic work-up should form the basis of a prompt diagnosis of tuberculous dactylitis. As *Mycobacterium tuberculosis* does not produce proteolytic enzymes that can destroy the cartilage, there is potential for preservation of good function when early diagnosis is made [5]. Even in an endemic country like India where tuberculosis is rampant, the diagnosis is missed or often delayed as in this case, particularly due to usual absence of stigmata of pulmonary tuberculosis ending up with potentially fatal consequences. One must be vigilant while dealing with the pathology of short tubular bones of hands and feet, as various conditions like benign and malignant tumors, noninfectious granulomatous disease, sickle cell dactylitis, endocrinopathies, metabolic disorders, pyogenic and fungal osteomyelitis, Brodie's abscess, syphilitic dactylitis, brucellosis, and actinomycosis can mimic and resemble tuberculous dactylitis [6, 7].

However, it should be remembered that tuberculosis can present in the most unusual form and in least expected sites, so the budding clinicians are reminded of the importance of early diagnosis of this rare form of an ancient disease.

Conflict of Interests

The authors declare that there is no conflict of interests regarding the publication of this paper.

References

[1] R. Salimpour and P. Salimpour, "Picture of the month. Tuberculous dactylitis," *Archives of Pediatrics and Adolescent Medicine Journal*, vol. 151, no. 8, pp. 851–852, 1997.

[2] E. D. Carrol, J. E. Clark, and A. J. Cant, "Non-pulmonary tuberculosis," *Paediatric Respiratory Reviews*, vol. 2, no. 2, pp. 113–119, 2001.

[3] D. Sunderamoorthy, V. Gupta, and A. Bleetman, "TB or not TB: an unusual sore finger," *Emergency Medicine Journal*, vol. 18, no. 6, pp. 490–491, 2001.

[4] A. Panchonia, C. V. Kulkarni, R. Meher, and S. Mandwariya, "Isolated tuberculous dactylitis [Spina ventosa] in a 9 year old boy—a rare entity," *International Journal of Basic and Applied Medical Sciences*, vol. 2, 52, no. 20, p. 55, 2012.

[5] L. J. Nelson and C. D. Wells, "Global epidemiology of childhood tuberculosis," *The International Journal of Tuberculosis and Lung Disease*, vol. 8, no. 5, pp. 636–647, 2004.

[6] L. Maruschke, T. Baumann, H. Zajonc, and G. Herget, "Monostotic fibrous dysplasia of the middle phalanx of the hand," *Journal of Medical Cases*, vol. 4, no. 5, pp. 318–322, 2013.

[7] F. O. A. Hassan, "Tuberculous dactylitis pseudotumor of an adult thumb: a case report," *Strategies in Trauma and Limb Reconstruction*, vol. 5, no. 1, pp. 53–56, 2010.

30

Use of Scrambler Therapy in Acute Paediatric Pain:
A Case Report and Review of the Literature

Sabrina Congedi,[1,2] **Silvia Spadini,**[1,2] **Chiara Di Pede,**[1,2]
Martina Ometto,[1,2] **Tatiana Franceschi,**[1,2] **Valentina De Tommasi,**[1,2]
Caterina Agosto,[1,2] **Pierina Lazzarin,**[1,2] **and Franca Benini**[1,2]

[1]*Department of Women's and Children's Health, University of Padua, 3 Giustiniani Street, 35128 Padua, Italy*
[2]*Pediatric Pain and Palliative Care Service, University of Padua, 59 Ospedale Civile Street, 35121 Padua, Italy*

Correspondence should be addressed to Franca Benini; benini@pediatria.unipd.it

Academic Editor: Juan Manuel Mejía-Arangurè

We report our clinical experience on the effect of Scrambler Therapy (ST) for a child with acute mixed pain refractory to pharmacological treatment. ST, recently proposed as an alternative treatment for chronic neuropathic pain in adults, is a noninvasive approach to relieve pain, by changing pain perception at brain level. It is safe and has no side effects. Further research is needed to assess its efficacy for acute pain and for paediatric population.

1. Introduction

Scrambler Therapy (ST) is a noninvasive and fully automated medical device for pain treatment, approved by the Food and Drug Administration (FDA). It provides cutaneous electrostimulation with surface electrodes placed surrounding the pain area, in order to replace "pain" signals with "no-pain" signals. It has been used in adults to treat chronic pain, mainly neuropathic pain (postherpetic neuralgia, spinal cord stenosis, and chemotherapy-induced peripheral neuropathy) [1–6] and untreatable cancer pain [6–10]. Here, we report our clinical experience using ST in a situation never experimented before: acute pain treatment in a paediatric patient.

2. Methods

We used Calmare MC5A device (Figure 1) in a 12-year-old girl with acute neuropathic pain admitted to Hospice and Palliative Care Unit, University of Padua, Italy, in September 2015. According to literature best practice and after locating the pain area (Figure 3), we treated our patient with this medical device for 4 consecutive days with 45-minute daily sessions, attaching 4 electrodes (Figure 4).

Pain measures were performed before and after each treatment, using the numeric rating scale (NRS) [11]. We monitored pain intensity for 4 weeks after discharge.

3. Case Presentation

We present the case of a 12-year-old Caucasian female affected by minimal change congenital myopathy, diagnosed when she was 7 years old. She required night time noninvasive mechanical ventilation for a chronic hypercapnic respiratory failure and "Obstructive Sleep Apnea Syndrome" (OSAS), in a restrictive lung disease background. She was able to walk without supports and was independent in all "Activity of Daily Living" (ADL) and "Instrumental Activities for Daily Life" (IADL). She had a severe cervical-dorsal scoliosis. The girl had a history of osteoblastoma of talus bone in the left foot, surgically treated with success at the age of 6 years. She was in therapy with vitamin D.

The girl was admitted to the Paediatric Unit of a peripheral hospital (Italy) for an acute scapular pain which started

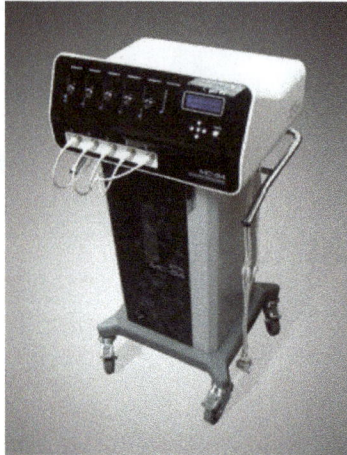

FIGURE 1: Calmare MC-5A (http://www.lifeepistemeitalia.it/calmare-mc-5a/dati-tecnici/).

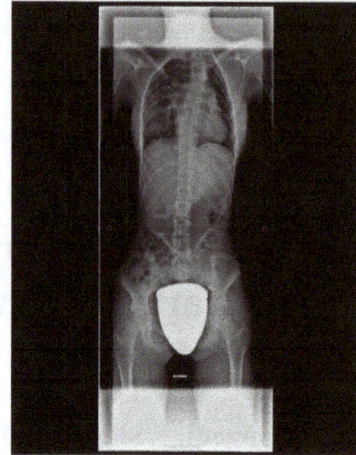

FIGURE 2: Chest radiograph (CXR) image. CXR shows a left cervical and right dorsal scoliosis with left deviation of sternum.

36 h earlier. No previous events of acute pain were reported in her medical history. Pain had started suddenly, causing the interruption of normal activities. It was localized in the interscapular area, with irradiation to the right shoulder. Pain was described as compressive, at first pulsing, and then continuous, with nocturnal awakenings. She denied trauma or stress. Before hospital admission, the girl was treated with topic diclofenac, oral ibuprofen (correct dosage for age), and osteopathic therapy, without benefit. She referred to pain increase and paresthesia appearance (without radicular distribution) in the right upper arm, so she was admitted to the peripheral hospital. At admission, her pain intensity was 8/10 (NRS pain score). Laboratory evaluation did not reveal alterations of phlogosis markers nor any other anomalies. HSV1/2 serology was negative. Rachis and right shoulder radiography and chest MRI were performed and fractures or malignant lesions were excluded. She was treated with acetaminophen (10 mg/kg × 3/day, p.o.) and ibuprofen (10 mg/kg × 3/day, p.o.) without benefit, so a therapy with ketorolac (0.8 mg/kg × 2/day e.v.) and diazepam (0.05 mg/kg/day) was performed.

After 7 days of pharmacological treatment, pain was reduced but still present (from 8/10 to 5/10). The patient was transferred to our Paediatric Pain and Palliative Care Unit, in Padua. At admission, she was suffering. She reported a continuous and compressive pain of 5/10 intensity. It was localized in the interscapula area, with irradiation to cervical region and lateral chest wall bilaterally; no shoulder and arm irradiation nor paresthesias were present. Pain intensity was exacerbated by standing and sitting and reduced by lying down.

On examination, she presented a myopathic face, nasal tone vocalization, left cervical and right dorsal scoliosis with left deviation of sternum (Figure 2), and bilateral scapulas alata. Generalized muscle weakness and hypotonia were observed. At inspection, contracture and edema of right paravertebral musculature were evident, with no heat to the touch. Pain was accentuated by acupressure of cervical and T3–T9 dorsal spinal apophysis and palpation (on the right side) of trapezium, elevator scapulae, rhomboid

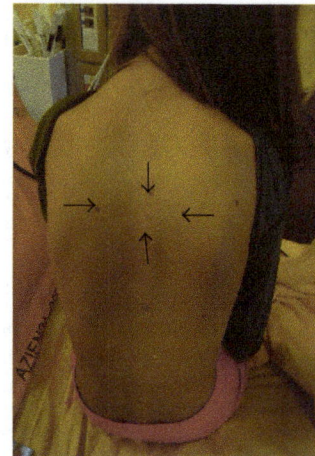

FIGURE 3: Patient's painful area.

(bilaterally, but greater on the right side), and big serratus anterior muscles. Tactile, pain, and thermal sensibilities were preserved. A psychological pain in our patient was excluded by a psychological assessment by psychologist of our Paediatric Pain and Palliative Care Unit.

On the basis of clinical history and physical examination, a mixed acute pain, both nociceptive and neuropathic, was diagnosed. Damage in the musculoskeletal apparatus can explain the somatic painful component and consequently the partial and temporary symptom control with painkillers. This alteration induced the nervous system involvement probably through a nervous branch compression by muscular contracture and edema.

Therapy with ketorolac (0.8 mg/kg × 2/die) and lorazepam (0.7 mg/die) was continued. Acetaminophen (10 mg/kg e.v.) was required twice in the first 24 h of hospitalization because pain was much severe (7-8/10). On the 2nd day of hospitalization, she started Scrambler Therapy. We set up a 45-minute daily treatment session for 4 consecutive days,

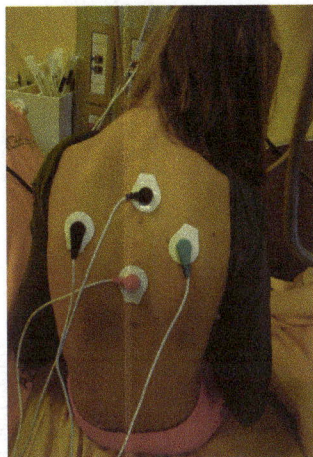

FIGURE 4: Sites where electrodes were attached.

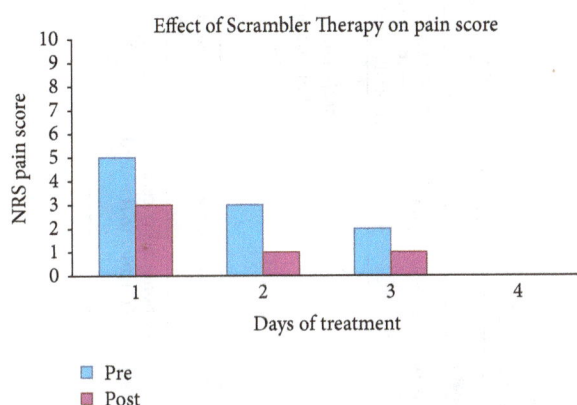

FIGURE 5: Effect of Scrambler Therapy on pain score during days of treatment.

at the same time and provided by the same trained nurse. No side effects were observed.

Before the beginning of treatment and after positioning of electrodes, NRS score was 5/10 and after the first session it was 3/10. Next sessions were followed by marked improvement of pain: after the fourth treatment, NRS score was 0/10 (Figure 5). Following pain reduction, drugs were progressively reduced and then prescribed at need. No other treatment sessions were performed, because the patient was discharged after 6 days of hospitalization, with resolution of acute pain (0/10 NRS). We evaluated her pain control by phone. Pain intensity was investigated 1 week and 4 and 8 weeks after discharge: the patient referred to no pain.

4. Review of the Literature

We carried out PubMed search of literature using the following key word "Scrambler Therapy" and 16 items were obtained [1–8, 10–17]. When picking age filters and choosing the category "children", no article was found. Moreover, evaluating the articles found and their references, there was no evidence about the use of this medical device for acute pain treatment (Table 1).

The first available study was conducted on 11 patients with pancreatic cancer: 9 stopped drug therapy thanks to ST [7]. Sabato et al. [2] conducted a prospective study recruiting 226 patients with intense drug resistant neuropathic pain; they were treated with Scrambler Therapy: 1 to 6 sessions of 5 treatments (about 30 min). This study highlighted the efficacy of the new medical device, thanks to a significant score pain reduction after therapy (80% patients: pain relief >50%) [2]. A smaller sample ($n = 52$) suffering from chronic neuropathic pain was treated with ST obtaining lower pain scores after the 10th session. Moreover, at one month, the mean VAS score was reduced from 8 to 0.7 points (−91%) [4]. In the study by Smith et al. [1], 16 adult patients with chemotherapy-induced peripheral neuropathy were successfully treated with ST; 1 h daily treatment for 10 days reduced the pain score of 59% (5.81 ± 1.11 to 2.38 ± 1.82) and 9 patients had no residual pain [1]. Similar results were obtained by Pachman et al. [3]. They reported the effect of ST on 37 patients with chemotherapy-induced peripheral neuropathy: there was a reduction in pain score of 53% from baseline after a 10-day treatment [3].

Results by Ricci et al. [9] support the use of ST to treat both cancer-derived pain and non-cancer-derived pain (a lower pain score was obtained for about 80 patients) [9]. A third study [6] reported the effect of ST on 39 patients complaining of cancer related pain. The authors concluded that a 45-minute daily treatment with ST for 10 days is effective in pain alleviation [6]. The most recent paper on ST in cancer pain was published by Notaro et al. [8]. This study was conducted on 25 patients with pain induced by bone and visceral metastases; all participants had a pain relief ≥50% [8].

Two case series have been published. Park et al. [10] reported the treatment results of using ST in three cancer patients with intractable pain and good results were obtained [10]. A work was published by Ko et al. [5] on the effect of ST on postherpetic neuralgia. They reported 3 cases and have shown that ST can be a good option for this type of pain [5]. Recently, Moon et al. [12] published a multicentre analysis on 147 patients from 3 medical centres with neuropathic, nociceptive, and mixed pain. They used ST with different setting sessions, obtaining low success rate (38.1% patients had a pain relief ≥50%) [12]. In PubMed research, we found a recent randomized controlled trial: Pachman et al. [14] performed double-blinded RCT analyzing 30 patients with chronic low back pain. 15 patients were treated with ST: 47% showed improvement (>50% reduction of "worst" pain score to 3-week follow-up), 33% showed partial improvement (30–49% reduction), and in 20% pain scores were reduced by 20–29%. Pain scores were significantly different between groups at 1-week and 3-week follow-up visit [13].

5. Discussion

Thanks to our literature research, we can assess two different and important aspects: (i) no data are available in literature about the use of ST in children and (ii) there is no information concerning treatment of acute pain by this device.

The mechanism of Scrambler Therapy is not clear, but Marineo et al. [4] suggested that electrical stimulus by electrodes gives "no-pain" information to peripheral receptors;

TABLE 1: Some papers available in literature on Scrambler Therapy.

Source	Type of study	Subjects	Pain etiologies and causes	Therapy session data	Effects on pain
Marineo (2003) [7]	Prospective	11 adult patients; mean age: 63.5 y.	Cancer related pain	45-minute daily treatment for 10 consecutive days.	9 (81.8%) of the patients suspended painkillers within the first 5 applications.
Sabato et al. (2005) [2]	Prospective	226 adult patients.	Neuropathic pain	1–6 cycles of 5 treatments (each treatment 30 min).	80.09% patients: pain relief >50%; 10.18% partially responders (pain relief 25–49%) and 9.73% of no responders (pain relief <24% or VAS >3).
Smith et al. (2010) [1]	Prospective	16 adult patients; mean age: 58.6 y.	Chemotherapy-induced peripheral neuropathy	60-minute daily treatment for 10 consecutive days.	64% chemotherapy-induced peripheral neuropathy pain score reduction from start to the end (10th day) of the study.
Ricci et al. (2012) [9]	Prospective	73 adult patients; mean age: 66 y.	Cancer-derived pain and non-cancer-derived pain	30-minute daily treatment for 10 consecutive days.	Pain score decreased by 74% at 10th day of treatment.
Marineo et al. (2012) [4]	Prospective and randomized trial	52 adult patients were randomized; ST group $n = 26$; mean age: 56.	Chronic neuropathic pain	45-minute daily treatment for 10 consecutive days.	At one month, the mean VAS score was reduced from 8 to 0.7 points (−91%) and from 8.1 to 5.8 (−28%) in the control group.
Ko et al. (2013) [5]	Case series: 3	3 patients: 70–75 y.	Postherpetic neuralgia	50 minutes daily for 10 consecutive days.	After treatment, pain decreased by 50%.
Park et al. (2013) [10]	Case series: 3	3 patients: 49–56 y.	Cancer pain	40 minutes daily for 10 consecutive days.	After ST, pain decreased by 50% or more.
Coyne et al. (2013) [6]	Prospective	39 adult patients; mean age 56.5 y.	Cancer pain syndromes and chronic chemotherapy-induced peripheral neuropathy	45-minute daily treatment for 10 consecutive days.	Pain scores reduced from 6.6 before treatment to 4.5 at 14 days, 4.6, 4.8, and 4.6 at 1, 2, and 3 months.
Moon et al. (2015) [12]	A multicentre analysis	147 adult patients; mean age: 37.6 y.	Neuropathic, nociceptive, and mixed pain	A minimum of either 3 therapies on consecutive days or 5 therapies overall.	38.1% patients: ≥50% pain relief.
Starkweather et al. (2015) [13]	Double-blinded, randomized controlled trial	30 adult patients were randomized; ST group $n = 15$; mean age: 42.5.	Low back pain	30-minute sessions were administered over 10 working days or until the participant reported no pain.	In the Calmare group, 47% participants had a >50% reduction in the "worst" pain score from baseline to the 3-week follow-up visit; 33% participants had a 30–49% reduction, and 20% had a 20–29% reduction.
Pachman et al. (2015) [3]	Prospective	37 adult patients; mean age: 58 y.	Chemotherapy-induced peripheral neuropathy	30-minute daily treatment for 10 consecutive days.	53% reduction in pain score from baseline to day 10.
Notaro et al. (2015) [8]	Prospective	25 patients; mean age: 62.	Pain induced by bone and visceral metastases and refractory to standard therapies	30/40-minute daily treatment for 10 consecutive days.	100%: ≥50% pain relief.

C-fibers and Aδ fibers lead the stimulus to the central nervous system that receives it and reduces pain symptoms. During ST, patients can refer nonpain sensations in the pain area, such as pressure and itching [4].

The ST success is strongly operator-dependent: health professionals decide where to place electrodes and how to regulate stimulation intensity. Correct use of this medical device requires fitting and education; our professionals had a specific training. The procedure for ST starts with a clear identification of the pain area. After this, electrodes are attached along the dermatome of the pain area, not on pain sites. There are a total of five paired sets of electrodes, to treat up to 5 or more painful areas. After every treatment, before starting the next one, it is necessary to evaluate the pain areas again: the painful area can change and electrodes must be attached in a different way. After the placement of electrodes, electrical stimuli are applied. Intensity is gradually increased to the maximum value tolerated by the patient. This stimulus must not cause any additional pain or discomfort. "No-pain" information appropriate for the patient must be searched, modulating the 16 types of action potential, pulse rate from 43 to 52 Hz, phase duration from 0.7 to 10 seconds, and amplitude. The maximum current density is $0.0002009 \, W/cm^2$ and amperage (A) is 3.50–5.50 mA [4]. We used ST according to literature best practice [4].

In our experience, we observed an interesting aspect about stimulus intensity. Previous papers reported that subsequent treatments were usually started at the highest tolerated setting from the previous session and increased, as tolerated [1, 4]. However, in our case, we did not confirm this habitual practice. After the first day, each treatment started at the previous highest intensity but we had to reduce it immediately, because pain or discomfort was present. Our patient undergoing Scrambler Therapy experienced immediate pain alleviation and the latest NRS pain scores were lower: 0/10 (Figure 5).

Pain decreased by 80–100% and similar results were observed in other papers [1, 4, 14].

No pain was recorded after 1, 4, and 8 weeks. In agreement with Marineo's work [4], the effect of Scrambler Therapy persists thanks to remodulation that occurs in the periphery and central nervous system or in the calcium channels of the synapses, which become the main target for treating neuropathic pain. The patient feels the sensation in all the dermatome and not only in the points of electrode application, suggesting the spreading of signals along nervous transmissions [18].

In our case, ST was used to treat acute pain in a child. Different experiences are reported about ST use and all of these concern adult population. No paediatric patients have been reported to be treated with ST. Moreover, this case report suggests an effective use of this medical device to treat acute pain: this aspect has never been investigated. Acute pain starts suddenly, its localization is well defined, and it serves as a warning of disease or a threat to the body. The duration is less than few weeks and it reduces with healing. Acute pain is very common in hospitalized children: 84–86% of children have pain [6, 18].

We defined our patient pain as mixed: nociceptive and neuropathic. Pain can be neuropathic, nociceptive, or mixed, and clinical evaluation is the current "gold standard" to achieve a diagnosis of pain [19, 20]. Pain arising from activation of peripheral nerve endings by tissue injury is a nociceptive pain. Neuropathic pain derives by a disease or lesion of the somatosensory system [19].

In literature, there are papers regarding the positive effects of ST on neuropathic and somatic pain [3].

We reduced analgesic drugs during Scrambler treatment, because there was a reduction in our patient's pain score, such as that reported by Park et al. [10].

Positive effects of ST on daily and weekly activities of patients affected by neuropathy symptoms are demonstrated by Pachman et al. [3]. After the 4th day of treatment, thanks to resolution of pain, our child slowly started dancing again.

6. Conclusions

Scrambler Therapy is a noninvasive medical device and has no side effects. Our clinical experience supports the efficacy of ST for acute pain treatment in children. More research is necessary to realize a specific protocol for evaluating the effect of ST therapy in this population and for this type of pain.

Conflict of Interests

The authors declare they have no conflict of interests regarding the publication of this paper.

References

[1] T. J. Smith, P. J. Coyne, G. L. Parker, P. Dodson, and V. Ramakrishnan, "Pilot trial of a patient-specific cutaneous electrostimulation device (MC5-A Calmare®) for chemotherapy-induced peripheral neuropathy," *Journal of Pain and Symptom Management*, vol. 40, no. 6, pp. 883–891, 2010.

[2] A. F. Sabato, G. Marineo, and A. Gatti, "Scrambler therapy," *Minerva Anestesiologica*, vol. 71, no. 7-8, pp. 479–482, 2005.

[3] D. R. Pachman, B. L. Weisbrod, D. K. Seisler et al., "Pilot evaluation of Scrambler therapy for the treatment of chemotherapy-induced peripheral neuropathy," *Supportive Care in Cancer*, vol. 23, no. 4, pp. 943–951, 2015.

[4] G. Marineo, V. Iorno, C. Gandini, V. Moschini, and T. J. Smith, "Scrambler therapy may relieve chronic neuropathic pain more effectively than guideline-based drug management: results of a pilot, randomized, controlled trial," *Journal of Pain and Symptom Management*, vol. 43, no. 1, pp. 87–95, 2012.

[5] Y. K. Ko, H. Y. Lee, and W. Y. Lee, "Clinical experiences on the effect of scrambler therapy for patients with postherpetic neuralgia," *Korean Journal of Pain*, vol. 26, no. 1, pp. 98–101, 2013.

[6] P. J. Coyne, W. Wan, P. Dodson, C. Swainey, and T. J. Smith, "A trial of Scrambler therapy in the treatment of cancer pain syndromes and chronic chemotherapy-induced peripheral neuropathy," *Journal of Pain and Palliative Care Pharmacotherapy*, vol. 27, no. 4, pp. 359–364, 2013.

[7] G. Marineo, "Untreatable pain resulting from abdominal cancer: new hope from biophysics?" *Journal of the Pancreas*, vol. 4, no. 1, pp. 1–10, 2003.

[8] P. Notaro, C. A. Dell'Agnola, A. J. Dell'Agnola, A. Amatu, K. B. Bencardino, and S. Siena, "Pilot evaluation of scrambler therapy for pain induced by bone and visceral metastases and refractory to standard therapies," *Supportive Care in Cancer*, 2015.

[9] M. Ricci, S. Pirotti, E. Scarpi et al., "Managing chronic pain: results from an open-label study using MC5-A Calmare® device," *Supportive Care in Cancer*, vol. 20, no. 2, pp. 405–412, 2012.

[10] H. S. Park, W. K. Sin, H. Y. Kim et al., "Scrambler therapy for patients with cancer pain—case series," *Korean Journal of Pain*, vol. 26, no. 1, pp. 65–71, 2013.

[11] M. McCaffery and A. Beebe, *Pain: Clinical Manual for Nursing Practice*, Mosby, Maryland Heights, Mo, USA, 1989.

[12] J. Y. Moon, C. Kurihara, J. P. Beckles, K. E. Williams, D. E. Jamison, and S. P. Cohen, "Predictive factors associated with success and failure for Calmare (Scrambler) therapy: a multicenter analysis," *Clinical Journal of Pain*, vol. 31, no. 8, pp. 750–756, 2015.

[13] A. R. Starkweather, P. Coyne, D. E. Lyon, R. K. Elswick, K. An, and J. Sturgill, "Decreased low back pain intensity and differential gene expression following Calmare®: results from a double-blinded randomized sham-controlled study," *Research in Nursing and Health*, vol. 38, no. 1, pp. 29–38, 2015.

[14] D. R. Pachman, J. C. Watson, and C. L. Loprinzi, "Therapeutic strategies for cancer treatment related peripheral neuropathies," *Current Treatment Options in Oncology*, vol. 15, no. 4, pp. 567–580, 2014.

[15] R. K. Ghatak, S. N. Nandi, A. Bhakta, G. C. Mandal, M. Bandyopadhyay, and S. Kumar, "Prospective study of application of biological communication (cybernatics) in management of chronic low back pain—a preliminary report," *Nepal Medical College Journal*, vol. 13, no. 4, pp. 257–260, 2011.

[16] D. Fallon and B. P. Hallenborg, "A simple and versatile fear-conditioning chamber requiring no shock scrambler," *Physiology and Behavior*, vol. 5, no. 1, pp. 129–130, 1970.

[17] C. Compagnone and F. Tagliaferri, "Chronic pain treatment and scrambler therapy: a multicenter retrospective analysis," *Acta BioMedica*, vol. 86, no. 2, pp. 149–156, 2015.

[18] D. Harrison, C. Joly, C. Chretien et al., "Pain prevalence in a pediatric hospital: raising awareness during Pain Awareness Week," *Pain Research and Management*, vol. 19, no. 1, pp. e24–e30, 2014.

[19] S. P. Cohen and J. Mao, "Neuropathic pain: mechanisms and their clinical implications," *British Medical Journal*, vol. 348, Article ID f7656, 2014.

[20] R. Freynhagen, R. Baron, U. Gockel, and T. R. Tölle, "painDETECT: a new screening questionnaire to identify neuropathic components in patients with back pain," *Current Medical Research and Opinion*, vol. 22, no. 10, pp. 1911–1920, 2006.

31

Unexplained Neonatal Cardiorespiratory Collapse at Five Minutes of Age

Sona Zaleta, Sarah Miller, and Prashant Kumar

Department of Paediatrics, Timaru Public Hospital, Timaru 7910, New Zealand

Correspondence should be addressed to Sarah Miller; sarah217miller@gmail.com

Academic Editor: Denis A. Cozzi

We report a case in which a term neonate suffered cardiorespiratory collapse at five minutes of age following an uncomplicated delivery and Apgar score of eight at one minute. Following prolonged cardiopulmonary resuscitation, the infant recovered well with no neurological deficit. Although sudden and unexpected postnatal collapse has been extensively described, this case does not fulfil its definition criteria. It provides a diagnostic challenge for clinicians and to the best of our knowledge is the first report of unexplained cardiorespiratory collapse at five minutes of age. The case serves as a timely reminder that cord gas analysis is recommended in all cases of potential fetal compromise and that Apgar scores should be used with caution as a predictor of neurological sequelae.

1. Introduction

Apgar scores assess the clinical state and physiological transition of a newborn infant [1]. Typically scores improve between one, five, and ten minutes of age [1]. Cases in which Apgar scores decline are rare. We report a challenging case in which a term neonate, with a one-minute Apgar score of eight, experienced a rapid, unexpected cardiorespiratory collapse at five minutes of age. Prolonged resuscitation resulted in a successful outcome whereby at sixteen weeks the patient has no neurological complications. Although sudden and unexpected postnatal collapse (SUPC) has been previously described, this case does not fulfil its definition criteria. To our knowledge, it is the first reported case of unexplained cardiorespiratory collapse as early as five minutes of age.

2. Case Presentation

A 2700 g female was born at term to a fit and well 38-year-old primigravida mother following an uncomplicated in vitro fertilisation (IVF) pregnancy. Ventouse delivery was performed in the operating theatre due to suboptimal progress in the second stage of labour and a nonreassuring cardiotocography (CTG) trace. Policy at our hospital dictates that there must be a paediatric consultant present at every emergency delivery, together with a consultant anaesthetist and obstetrician.

Whilst delivery was uncomplicated, fresh meconium was noted following delivery of the head. One-minute Apgar score was eight. At three minutes, intramuscular vitamin K was given. The patient was pink and moving spontaneously but intermittently grunting. Continuous positive airways pressure (CPAP) with room air was therefore initiated. At five minutes she became white with no respiratory effort and absent heart sounds. Immediate resuscitation was commenced by the paediatric consultant and accompanying team, including intubation, cardiac compression, and administration of three doses of adrenaline via an umbilical venous catheter. There was no evidence of meconium at intubation. Chest rise and breath sounds were noted following intubation with assisted ventilation, and expiratory carbon dioxide was confirmed via a colorimetric end-tidal carbon dioxide monitor. Intermittent positive pressure ventilation (IPPV) with 100% oxygen was initiated. Further help, in the form of an additional experienced paediatric consultant and senior paediatric nurse practitioner, was summoned during the resuscitation.

Cardiac compression continued for 15 minutes until return of heart beat. Five minutes following this, the patient began gasping and respirations normalised. Oxygen

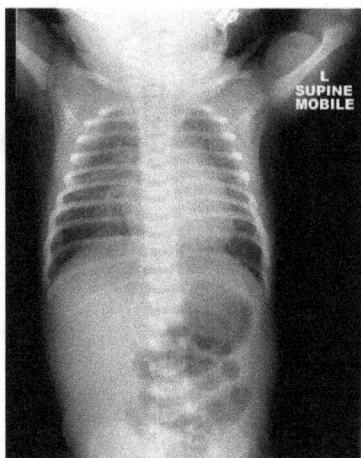

FIGURE 1: Chest X-ray and abdominal X-ray at two hours of age. The endotracheal tube tip is in the right main bronchus and was withdrawn 15–20 mm. The cardiothalamic silhouette is normal and lung and pleural spaces are clear. No pneumothorax is seen. The umbilical venous catheter lies to the right of the midline at T10.

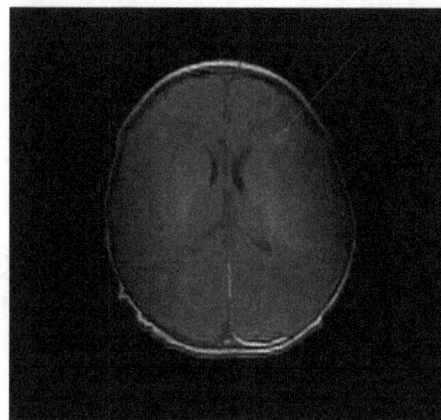

FIGURE 2: Magnetic resonance imaging demonstrating a 1–1.5 cm focal area of parenchymal abnormality in the left frontal lobe anterolaterally, appearances of which are consistent with infarction.

saturations improved to 100%. CPAP via endotracheal tube was commenced and inspired oxygen weaned to room air. Cardiovascular examination was normal with no abnormalities seen on cardiac monitoring. Bloods demonstrated haemoglobin 129 g/L, white count 23.8×10^9/L, platelets 311 $\times 10^9$/L, sodium 136 mmol/L, potassium 2.8 mmol/L, urea 5.2 mmol/L, creatinine 128 μmol/L, and glucose 12.8 mmol/L. Liver function tests, magnesium, phosphate, calcium, and c-reactive protein were unremarkable. No cord gas had been taken. Initial umbilical venous blood gas at 90 minutes of age demonstrated a pH 7.03, pCO2 28.8 mmHg, pO2 55.9 mmHg, HCO3 7.5 mmol/L, BE −23.2 mmol/L, and lactate 16.19 mmol/L. The profound metabolic acidosis normalised over 24 hours with supportive management only. IV antibiotics were administered and continued for 24 hours, however blood cultures were negative and chest X-ray showed no collapse or consolidation (Figure 1). Due to a rapid recovery, cerebral spinal fluid was not obtained.

By 150 minutes, the patient was displaying spontaneous limb movements, normal grasp and gag reflexes, symmetrical eye movements, and good tone. At four hours she was successfully extubated. Head ultrasound at 24 hours detected no abnormality. She did not receive head cooling. Over subsequent days, she exhibited normal behaviour and established feeding well. There were no signs of encephalopathy or seizures. Magnetic resonance imaging (MRI) at seven days showed a small amount of subdural blood, common following ventouse delivery, and a small focal left frontal lobe infarct (Figure 2). There was no evidence of hypoxic ischaemic injury or congenital brain anomaly. Guthrie testing was normal. Placental histology was unremarkable and no pathogens were isolated on maternal genital swabs.

At sixteen-week follow-up there are no developmental, behavioural, or feeding concerns. The patient has no dysmorphic features and systems examination remains unremarkable.

3. Discussion

The complex physiological transition from the intrauterine to extrauterine environment can be a dangerous period for the neonate. 90% complete the transition independently, with approximately 10% requiring some intervention and 1% demanding extensive resuscitation [2]. Multisystem organ adaptation to the extrauterine environment is recorded using Apgar scores, which enable clinicians to rapidly assess an infant's physiological condition and the need for medical intervention [1, 3, 4]. Typically, scores improve between one, five, and ten minutes of age [1]. There is limited literature of cases in which Apgar scores fall. Our case is novel in this regard, particularly as the patient displays no neurological sequelae.

To the best of our knowledge, there are no previously reported cases of unexplained cardiorespiratory collapse at five minutes. Multiple differential diagnoses have been considered and excluded. Sudden and unexpected postnatal collapse (SUPC) is well reported and describes infants with a normal Apgar score at five minutes who collapse unexpectedly in cardiorespiratory extremis [5]. Incidence is between 0.03 and 0.08/1000 live births and risk factors include primiparous mothers, skin to skin contact, and prone positioning [5, 6]. Given the patient's Apgar scores of eight at one minute and zero at five minutes, our case does not meet SUPC criteria.

This case provided a diagnostic challenge for the clinicians involved. Airway causes of collapse cannot explain how the patient independently established regular and spontaneous respirations at one minute of age nor explain her complete and rapid recovery. A septic screen was negative and chest imaging excluded both pneumothorax and pleural effusion. Grunting followed by rapid cardiovascular collapse due to transient tachypnoea of the newborn appears improbable given how rapidly ventilator support was weaned. There was no maternal drug history to suggest neurological and subsequent respiratory depression. The small frontal infarct is an unlikely cause of the patient's collapse. Cardiac disease is an unconvincing diagnosis in view of normal cardiac monitoring and a normal cardiovascular examination. Specific metabolic, genetic, endocrine, or neurological diagnoses are unlikely given normal Guthrie testing, rapid recovery period, and the patient's normal neurology and development at sixteen weeks. We therefore hypothesise that cardiorespiratory collapse may have occurred due to an unknown anomaly during the physiological stress of fetal-neonatal transition. Instrumental delivery was performed due to a nonreassuring CTG and one can speculate that cord gas analysis may have aided diagnosis. This case therefore acts as a reminder that although no current consensus exists regarding umbilical cord blood acid-base analysis, multiple colleges recommend that it is performed in all caesarean or instrumental deliveries, where indication is potential fetal compromise [7].

Finally, considerable literature discusses the use of Apgar scores for predicting mortality, neurological development, asphyxia, and cognitive function. Apgar scores are an accurate predictor of mortality; however, their use in the prediction of long term neurological outcome is inappropriate, particularly where encephalopathy and seizures are absent [1, 3, 4, 8, 9]. This case provides further evidence that clinicians should not rely on Apgar scores to predict neurological outcomes.

Key Points

(i) To the best of our knowledge this is the first reported case of sudden, unexplained, and unexpected cardiorespiratory collapse at five minutes of age.

(ii) This case serves as a timely reminder that cord gas analysis is recommended in all cases of potential fetal compromise and that Apgar scores should be used with caution as a predictive tool for subsequent neurological sequelae.

(iii) Well-performed cardiopulmonary neonatal resuscitation can lead to good outcomes. It is essential that all clinicians ensure that they remain up to date with the latest resuscitation guidelines so that they have the necessary skills to perform high quality resuscitation.

Conflict of Interests

The authors declare that there is no conflict of interests regarding the publication of this paper.

References

[1] V. Apgar, "A proposal for a new method of evaluation of the newborn infant," *Current Researches in Anesthesia and Analgesia*, vol. 32, no. 4, pp. 260–267, 1953.

[2] J. Kattwinkel, J. M. Perlman, K. Aziz et al., "Part 15: Neonatal resuscitation: 2010 American Heart Association Guidelines for Cardiopulmonary Resuscitation and Emergency Cardiovascular Care," *Circulation*, vol. 122, no. 3, pp. S909–S919, 2010.

[3] ACOG Committee on Obstetric Practice, American Academy of Pediatrics, and Committee of Fetus and Newborn, "ACOG committee opinion. Number 333: the Apgar score," *Obstetrics & Gynecology*, vol. 107, no. 5, pp. 1209–1212, 2006.

[4] S. R. Leuthner and U. G. Das, "Low Apgar scores and the definition of birth asphyxia," *Pediatric Clinics of North America*, vol. 51, no. 3, pp. 737–745, 2004.

[5] J. Becher, M. Ashworth, J. Bell et al., *Guidelines for the Investigation of Newborn Infants Who Suffer a Sudden and Unexpected Postnatal Collapse in the First Week of Life: Recommendations from a Professional Group on Sudden Unexpected Postnatal Collapse*, Wellchild, London, UK, 2011.

[6] E. Herlenius and P. Kuhn, "Sudden unexpected postnatal collapse of newborn infants: a review of cases, definitions, risks, and preventive measures," *Translational Stroke Research*, vol. 4, no. 2, pp. 236–247, 2013.

[7] Royal College of Obstetricians and Gynaecologists, Royal College of Midwives, Royal College of Anaesthetists, Royal College of Paediatrics, and Child Health, *Safer Childbirth. Minimum Standards for the Organisation and Delivery of Care in Labour. Report of Joint Working Party*, vol. 46, RCOG Press, London, UK, 2007.

[8] B. M. Casey, D. D. McIntire, and K. J. Leveno, "The continuing value of the Apgar score for the assessment of newborn infants," *The New England Journal of Medicine*, vol. 344, no. 7, pp. 467–471, 2001.

[9] D. J. Harrington, C. W. Redman, M. Moulden, and C. E. Greenwood, "The long-term outcome in surviving infants with Apgar zero at 10 minutes: a systematic review of the literature and hospital-based cohort," *American Journal of Obstetrics and Gynecology*, vol. 196, no. 5, pp. 463.e1–463.e5, 2007.

32

Clostridium sordellii as a Cause of Fatal Septic Shock in a Child with Hemolytic Uremic Syndrome

Rebekah Beyers,[1] **Michael Baldwin,**[2] **Sevilay Dalabih,**[1] **and Abdallah Dalabih**[1]

[1] *Department of Child Health, University of Missouri, 400 Keene Street, Columbia, MO 65201, USA*
[2] *Department of Molecular Microbiology and Immunology, University of Missouri, Columbia, MO 65201, USA*

Correspondence should be addressed to Abdallah Dalabih; dalabiha@missouri.edu

Academic Editor: Giovanni Montini

Clostridium sordellii is a toxin producing ubiquitous gram-positive anaerobe, mainly associated with trauma, soft tissue skin infections, and gynecologic infection. We report a unique case of a new strain of *Clostridium sordellii* (not present in the Center for Disease Control (CDC) database) infection induced toxic shock syndrome in a previously healthy two-year-old male with colitis-related hemolytic uremic syndrome (HUS). The patient presented with dehydration, vomiting, and bloody diarrhea. He was transferred to the pediatric critical care unit (PICU) for initiation of peritoneal dialysis (PD). Due to increased edema and intolerance of PD, he was transitioned to hemodialysis through a femoral vascular catheter. He subsequently developed severe septic shock with persistent leukocytosis and hypotension, resulting in subsequent death. Stool culture confirmed Shiga toxin producing *Escherichia coli 0157:H7*. A blood culture was positively identified for *Clostridium sordellii*. *Clostridium sordelli* is rarely reported in children; to our knowledge this is the first case described in a pediatric patient with HUS.

1. Introduction

Clostridium sordellii is a toxin producing ubiquitous gram-positive rod anaerobe, mainly associated with trauma, soft tissue skin infections, and gynecologic infection [1]. It is known to cause a severe shock syndrome characterized by a leukemoid reaction and significant capillary leak [2]. It has a characteristically high mortality rate, approaching 70% in previously healthy individuals [3]. It is rarely described in children and rarely isolated from the blood. It has been previously reported to cause sepsis and omphalitis in children [4], but never in association with other infections. We describe the case of a toxic shock syndrome caused by a new strain of *Clostridium sordellii* in a previously healthy two-year-old male, with acute *Escherichia coli 0157:H7* positive hemolytic uremic syndrome.

2. Clinical Presentation

A previously healthy two-year-old male was admitted to the general pediatric floor with a two-day history of abdominal pain, vomiting, and diarrhea. The diarrhea was initially watery and became bloody at the time of admission. Vital signs and laboratory values on admission were normal except for white blood cells (WBCs) of $25.9\,10^3/\mu L$ (83% neutrophils and 7% bands). His hemoglobin was 14.8 g/dL and platelets were $427\,10^3/\mu L$, and initial BUN and creatinine were 17 and 0.3 mg/dL, respectively. Abdominal ultrasound showed no abnormal findings.

The following day he had decreased urine output, elevated blood pressure, lower extremity and eyelid edema, and fever of 38.5°C. Vital signs and laboratory values at that time revealed tachycardia and elevated WBCs $34.6\,10^3/\mu L$ (61% neutrophils and 20% bands); hemoglobin dropped to 10.8 g/dL and platelets to $43\,10^3/\mu L$. LDH level was 1319 unit/L and C3 and C4 were 76 and <9 mg/dL, respectively (normal values for a 2-year-old male are as follows: C3 = 80–170 mg/dL and C4 = 14–44 mg/dL). The peripheral smear showed toxic granulations and megakaryocytes and schistocytes. Abnormal electrolytes at that time were serum sodium of 131 mmol/L, potassium of 4.8 mmol/L, and elevated serum creatinine (0.9 mg/dL). Urine output had decreased from 3 cc/kg/hour to 1.3 cc/kg/hour. A presumptive diagnosis of hemolytic uremic syndrome (HUS) was made and he was transferred to the pediatric critical care unit (PCCU) for further management. Repeated stool studies and blood cultures were obtained upon transfer to the PCCU. A chest radiograph showed hazy bilateral airspace opacities and small right pleural effusion. Upon admission to the PCCU a peritoneal dialysis (PD) catheter (Covidien, Dublin) was inserted, and a 3 lumen (5 French/12 cm) central line (Cook Medical, IN) was placed in the left femoral vein. Next day in the PCCU the fever recurred and the peritoneal dialysis catheter became nonfunctional. The blood culture from the day before became positive for gram-positive rods, growing in anaerobic media. A new culture was repeated before starting antibiotics and the patient was started on cefepime and piperacillin-tazobactam for empiric coverage. At that time vancomycin was avoided due to impaired renal function. The stool culture and toxin testing from the day of admission was also reported positive for Shiga toxin producing *Escherichia coli 0157:H7*.

In the following few hours the patient became progressively oliguric, with increasing serum creatinine level to 1.6 mg/dL and persistent hypotension. Laboratory values at day 2 in the PCCU showed WBC $56.7\,10^3/\mu L$ (29% neutrophils, 28% bands), Hgb 13.2 g/dL, and platelets of $26\,10^3/\mu L$. Due to altered mental status he was emergently intubated and after insertion of a right side 11.5 French femoral hemodialysis catheter hemodialysis was started. Due to the hypotension and acidosis (lactate level of 15 mmol/L) the patient was started on epinephrine and dopamine infusions (peak infusion rates of 15 mcg/kg/minute of dopamine and 0.1 mcg/kg/minute of epinephrine). He continued to be hemodynamically unstable, so a stress dose of hydrocortisone was administered. Clindamycin was added for empiric treatment of toxin production. Throughout the day, the patient continued to be hypotensive not responsive to fluid resuscitation or inotropic medications. Within 36 hours of admission to the PCCU hypotension persisted and toxic shock syndrome worsened; shortly after that, the patient arrested and was pronounced dead.

The repeated stool culture was also noted to be positive for *E. coli 0157:H7* and tested positive for Shiga toxin. Abdominal and pleural fluid cultures did not grow any organisms. Final blood culture identification was *Clostridium sordellii*. This identification was confirmed from 2 blood cultures 24 hours apart in the hospital laboratory and a plated sample was forwarded to an expert at the state laboratory. Repeated manual identification confirmed *Clostridium sordellii* (Table 1). When the samples of the bacteria were sent to the CDC, the center examined the samples and reported that this was a new strain of *Clostridium sordellii* not currently present in the CDC database.

3. Materials and Methods

3.1. Cell Cytotoxicity of Culture Supernatants. Vero cells were either left untreated (control) or incubated with various dilutions of sterile culture filtrates in medium containing fetal cell serum (FCS) for 2 hours at 37°C. Morphological changes

TABLE 1: The list of the biochemical tests on the panel.

Substrates	Abbreviations	Organism reaction
p-Nitrophenyl-β-D-galactopyranoside	BGAL	Negative
p-Nitrophenyl-α-D-galactopyranoside	AGAL	Negative
bis-p-Nitrophenyl-phosphate	BPO4	Negative
p-Nitrophenyl-N-acetyl-β-D-glucosaminide	NGLU	Negative
p-Nitrophenyl-α-D-glucopyranoside	AGL	**Positive**
o-Nitrophenyl-β-D-glucopyranoside	BGL	Negative
p-Nitrophenyl-phosphate	PO4	Negative
p-Nitrophenyl-α-L-fucopyranoside	AFU	**Positive**
p-Nitrophenyl-α-D-mannopyranoside	MNP	Negative
L-Leucine-β-naphthylamide	LEU	Negative
DL-Methionine-β-naphthylamide	MET	Negative
L-Lysine-β-naphthylamide (alkaline)	LYB	Negative
Substrates	Abbreviations	Negative
L-Lysine-β-naphthylamide (acid)	LYA	Negative
Glycylglycine-β-naphthylamide	GGLY	Negative
Glycine-β-naphthylamide	GLY	Negative
L-Proline-β-naphthylamide	PRO	**Positive**
L-Arginine-β-naphthylamide	ARG	Negative
L-Pyrrolidonyl-β-naphthylamide	PYR	Negative
L-Tryptophan-β-naphthylamide	TRY	Negative
3-Indoxyl phosphate	IDX	Negative
Trehalose	TRE	Negative
Urea	URE	**Positive**
Indole	IND	**Positive**
Nitrate	NIT	Negative

This set of biochemical reactions was compared to the MicroScan Database for *Clostridia* species. The result for this set of positive and negative biochemical reactions was consistent with a 99.99% probability of *Clostridium sordellii*.

of intoxicated cells were directly analyzed in wells using an inverted microscope equipped with a DIC prism (Figure 1).

3.2. PCR Analysis of Sordellilysin Expression in C. sordellii. Oligonucleotides (Integrated DNA Technologies Inc.) (Forward primer = 5′-GTACATATCCAGGAGCATTACAAC-3′; Reverse primer = 5′-CCACCATTCCCAAGCAAG-ACCTGT-3′) were designed to amplify sordellilysin based on the reported sequence of perfringolysin O [5]. PCR was performed using *Pfu* high fidelity polymerase (Agilent Genomics) and appropriate cycling conditions. Products were separated via agarose gel electrophoresis and compared with corresponding products from *C. sordellii* ATCC9714 (Figure 2).

3.3. Detection of Large Clostridial Toxins via Inhibitory Antibodies. Certain toxigenic isolates of *C. sordellii* produce toxins that are very similar to the toxins of *C. difficile*.

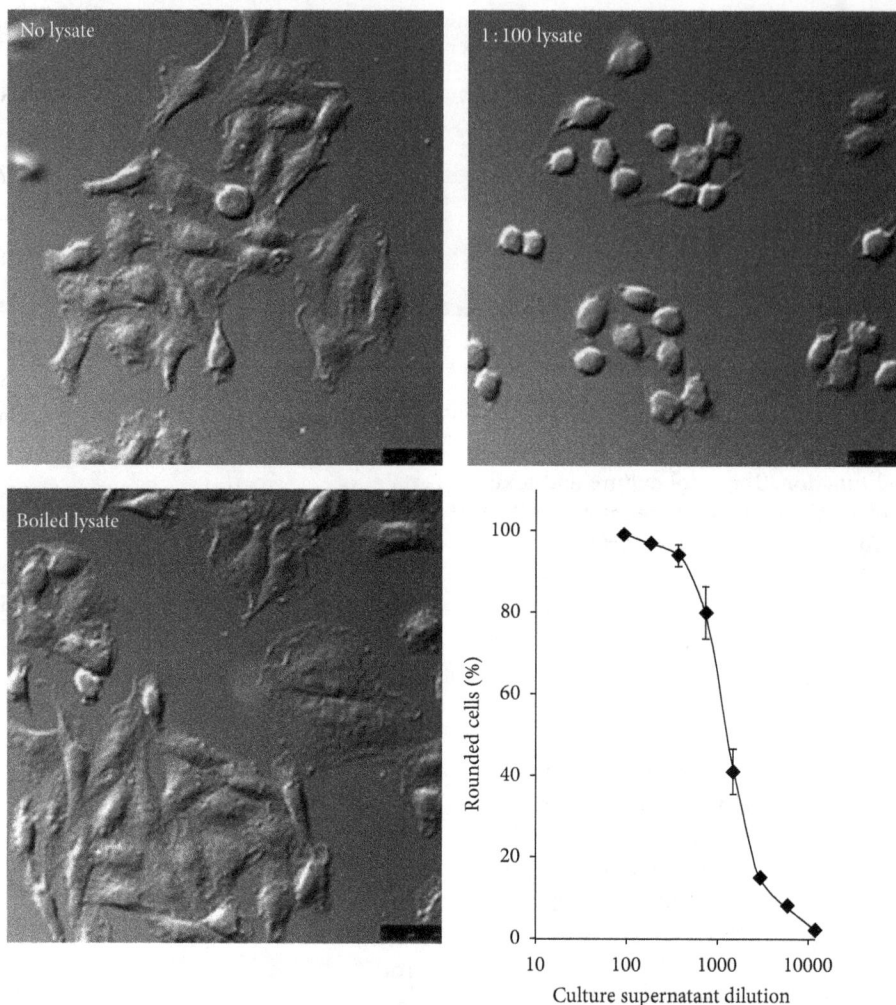

FIGURE 1: Supernatant cytotoxicity of *Clostridium sordellii* isolate. Culture supernatant (48 h) C. sordellii was incubated with an ~50% confluent Vero cell monolayer in a 96-well plate in a total of 100 μL per well and observed for 2 hr for cytopathic effects (CPE). Pictures shown are representative of a routine cell treatment with the indicated supernatant dilution, and cells were observed at a magnification of ×40. As a negative control, culture supernatant was heated to 90°C for 10 min and cooled prior to addition to cells. The degree of cytopathic effect was plotted against the relative dilution of the culture supernatant and is representative of eight independent trials.

The hemorrhagic toxin (toxin HT) of *C. sordellii* is very similar to toxin A whereas the lethal toxin (toxin LT) is very similar to toxin B. Antibodies against the *C. difficile* toxins neutralize the toxins HT and LT of *C. sordellii*, and antibodies against toxins HT and LT neutralize toxins A and B. To confirm the absence of HT or LT expression in our *C. sordellii* isolate a *C. difficile* Toxin/Antitoxin Kit (Techlab, VA) was used in conjunction with a Vero cell culture cytotoxicity assay in accordance with the manufacturer's instructions. In brief, serial dilutions of culture supernatants from *C. difficile* 630, *C sordellii* ATCC9714, and *C. sordellii* isolate XXX (our study) were mixed with either control or antitoxin antibodies prior to incubation within monolayers of Vero cells. Vero cells were monitored for up to 24 hr for cell rounding and visually scored. As expected, antitoxin antibodies effectively neutralized the toxin activity present in culture supernatants from *C. difficile* and *C. sordellii* ATCC9714, but not from *C. sordellii* isolate XXX.

4. Discussion

Clostridium sordellii is a spore forming gram-positive rod anaerobe found commonly in soil and the intestinal tract of mammals. Infections with *Clostridium sordellii* are mainly associated with trauma and medically induced abortions. It has been noted to be highly lethal in previously healthy individuals. It has been more recently described in normal term deliveries and heroin users [6]. There are over 40 different strains of *C. sordellii* and not all are toxin producing. Seven different exotoxins have been identified to be produced by *C. sordellii*, the two most virulent being lethal toxin and hemorrhagic toxin. These toxins are related to the large clostridial cytotoxin family, which affect cell signaling and are responsible for the characteristic leukemoid reaction and severe capillary leakage associated with *C. sordellii* infection [6]. Lethal toxin causes cell necrosis and edema secondary to increased vascular permeability. Hemorrhagic toxin has

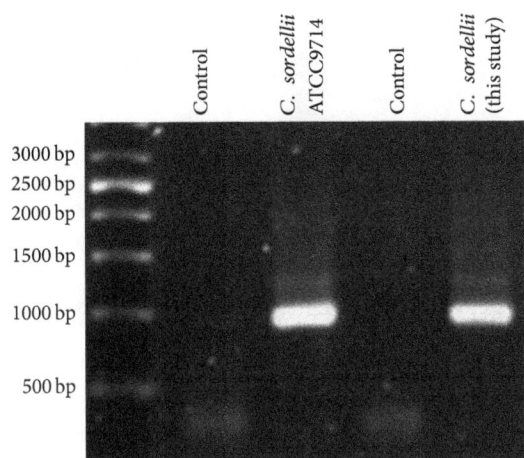

FIGURE 2: Analysis of sordellilysin in *Clostridium sordellii* isolates. Primers designed to amplify cholesterol dependent cytolysins (*cdc*) based on the reported sequence of perfringolysin O (*pfo*) were included in PCR reactions for each *C. sordellii* isolate. Amplification products were separated by 0.8% agarose gel electrophoresis and visualized via ethidium bromide staining. Lanes are designated by the strain names of each isolate in the figure. *C. sordellii* ATCC9714 was used as a positive control from sordellilysin expression.

been noted to be directly cytotoxic *in vivo* studies [7]. The toxins have been known to directly depress cardiac output and systemic vascular resistance [6].

The initial absence of fever is a characteristic finding and often persists throughout the course of the illness. Severe symptoms of resistant hypotension and tachycardia follow quickly. Laboratory findings include leukocytosis, thrombocytosis, elevated hematocrit, and significant hypoalbuminemia. The leukocytosis is usually profound, often exceeding 75,000 and with a remarkable left shift, which we observed in our patient. Leukocytosis is also known to be a poor prognostic factor in HUS and highly associated with fatality in *C. sordellii* infection [6]. Pleural effusion and pulmonary edema are common and associated with capillary leakage and profound hypoalbuminemia [4]. *Clostridium sordellii* infection not only carries a high mortality rate but is also associated with very rapid progression of the disease, with death occurring most commonly within 2–6 days of initial infection. In many reported cases, onset of severe hypotension and shock occurred within hours of symptom onset as in our case [4]. The rapid progression of the sepsis makes the infection difficult to identify and treat; our patient's blood culture identification was only available after the child had already died. Penicillin, tetracycline, and clindamycin have been tested *in vivo* for their efficacy in treatment. Clindamycin may have the added effect of decreasing toxin effect [5]. Treatment is mainly supportive in regard to hypotension and cardiovascular strain.

Although *C. sordellii* infection is relatively rare, there is suspicion that it is underreported, particularly in critically ill patients, due to its rapid progression and fastidious nature [6, 7]. A high index of suspicion, rapid initiation of treatment, and increased early identification would be key to decrease

mortality associated with this organism. This case is unique in that *C. sordellii* infection has not been extensively described in children; isolation of *C. sordellii* from the blood is rare and to our knowledge has not been described in association with HUS. Although the exact source of *Clostridium sordellii* infection in this case is unknown, development of *C. sordellii* sepsis caused by translocation through the GI tract has been suspected in adult patients with comorbidities [6]. Hunley et al. had suggested that diarrhea associated HUS comprises a clinical entity which appears to predispose to a traumatic *C. septicum* infection, where acidic and anaerobic conditions in the diseased colon favor *C. septicum* invasion [8].

This could explain the mechanism of the suggested bacterial translocation in our patient. Clinicians should be aware of the possibility of clostridial infection in the presence of gastrointestinal pathology and hemodynamic instability, considering *Clostridia* and broadening the antibiotic coverage early on in the course might be lifesaving.

Abbreviations

HR: Heart rate
WBCs: White blood cells
PCCU: Pediatric critical care unit
PD: Peritoneal dialysis
CDC: Center for Disease Control
FCS: Fetal cell serum
CPE: Cytopathic effects
HUS: Hemolytic uremic syndrome.

Conflict of Interests

The authors declare that there is no conflict of interests regarding the publication of this paper.

References

[1] R. Chaudhry, N. Verma, T. Bahadur, P. Chaudhary, P. Sharma, and N. Sharma, "*Clostridium sordellii* as a cause of constrictive pericarditis with pyopericardium and tamponade," *Journal of Clinical Microbiology*, vol. 49, no. 10, pp. 3700–3702, 2011.

[2] K. Grimwood, G. A. Evans, S. T. Govender, and D. E. Woods, "*Clostridium sordellii* infection and toxin neutralization," *Pediatric Infectious Disease Journal*, vol. 9, no. 8, pp. 582–585, 1990.

[3] D. M. Aronoff, "*Clostridium novyi*, *sordellii*, and *tetani*: mechanisms of disease," *Anaerobe*, vol. 24, pp. 98–101, 2013.

[4] M. J. Aldape, A. E. Bryant, and D. L. Stevens, "*Clostridium sordellii* infection: epidemiology, clinical findings, and current perspectives on diagnosis and treatment," *Clinical Infectious Diseases*, vol. 43, no. 11, pp. 1436–1446, 2006.

[5] D. E. Voth, O. V. Martinez, and J. D. Ballard, "Variations in lethal toxin and cholesterol-dependent cytolysin production correspond to differences in cytotoxicity among strains of *Clostridium sordellii*," *FEMS Microbiology Letters*, vol. 259, no. 2, pp. 295–302, 2006.

[6] D. L. Stevens, M. J. Aldape, and A. E. Bryant, "Life-threatening clostridial infections," *Anaerobe*, vol. 18, no. 2, pp. 254–259, 2012.

[7] A. Abdulla and L. Yee, "The clinical spectrum of *Clostridium sordellii* bacteraemia: two case reports and a review of the literature," *Journal of Clinical Pathology*, vol. 53, no. 9, pp. 709–712, 2000.

[8] T. E. Hunley, M. D. Spring, T. R. Peters, D. R. Weikert, and K. Jabs, "Clostridium septicum myonecrosis complicating diarrhea-associated hemolytic uremic syndrome," *Pediatric Nephrology*, vol. 23, no. 7, pp. 1171–1175, 2008.

Ophthalmic Treatment and Vision Care of a Patient with Rare Ring Chromosome 15: A Case Report

Lidia Puchalska-Niedbał,[1] Stanisław Zajączek,[2] Elżbieta Petriczko,[3] and Urszula Kulik[1]

[1] Department of Ophthalmology, Pomeranian Medical University, Aleja Powstaców Wielkopolskich 72, 70-111 Szczecin, Poland
[2] Cytogenetic Unit, Department of Pathology, Pomeranian Medical University, Aleja Powstaców Wielkopolskich 72, 70-111 Szczecin, Poland
[3] Department of Paediatrics, Endocrinology, Diabetology, Metabolic Disorders and Cardiology, Pomeranian Medical University, Aleja Powstaców Wielkopolskich 72, 70-111 Szczecin, Poland

Correspondence should be addressed to Lidia Puchalska-Niedbał; lidianiedbal@tlen.pl

Academic Editor: Ozgur Cogulu

The Aim. Ring chromosome 15 is a very rare genetic abnormality with a wide spectrum of clinical findings. Up to date, about 50 cases have been documented, whereas no reports on ophthalmological treatment of such patients have been published. The aim of this study is not only to describe a new patient, but also, for the first time, to present the results of nonoperative management of divergent strabismus. *Material and Methods.* We present an amblyopic patient with 46,XX, r(15) karyotype: treated conservatively for exotropia of 60 prism diopters. The management consisted of refractive and prismatic correction, eye occlusion, and orthoptic exercises between the age of 15 months and 8 years. *Results.* The deviation angle of exotropia was decreased to 10 prism diopters, the visual acuity improved to 1.0 in both eyes (Snellen chart) and the fixation pattern was normal. The prisms enabled permanent symmetrical stimulation of the retina, which lead to a development of normal single binocular vision (Maddox test, filter test, and synoptophore tests). *Conclusions.* Parental karyotype was normal; the analysis of a three-generation pedigree has shown no genetic abnormalities or pregnancy losses so the child's karyotype anomaly was classified as *de novo that is* a single occurrence of this type of chromosomal disorder in this family. Strabismus in ring chromosome 15 patients is a difficult condition to manage, although success may be achieved.

1. Introduction

Ring chromosome 15 r(15) is a rare anomaly both in "pure" and in mosaic forms [1]; so far, only ~50 cases were described [2], and only three cases so far have been reported in prenatal diagnosis [2–4] and just one with a twenty-year cytogenetic and molecular followup [5]. Previous studies showed that ring chromosome 15 results in a varied and unspecific phenotype [6, 7]. However, a recurrent form has been characterized by growth deficiency, mental retardation, and characteristic dysmorphic features. Diagnosis has been problematic as similar clinical findings have also been noted in patients with other syndromes [2, 4, 8].

The purpose of this case study is to present for the first time the state of visual acuity and formation of normal binocular vision in the squinting eye with initial eccentric fixation and amblyopia by means of long-term conservative treatment [9]. As far as we know, there have been no previous reports published on ophthalmic treatment and vision care among ring chromosome 15 patients.

2. Case Study

A 15-month-old girl was referred to the pediatric outpatient department and the clinic of ophthalmology for treatment of divergent strabismus of the right eye. The girl underwent treatment between the age of 15 months and 8 years.

Her medical history revealed that she was born at term from a 5th uneventful pregnancy and delivery (10 points on the Apgar score), with a weight of 2900 g (10–25 percentile), length of 49 cm (50 percentile), and a normal head circumference of 33 cm (10 percentile). The girl is a daughter of healthy, unrelated parents. Her mother is 37 years old and 172 cm tall (+1.0 SD) and her father is 29 years old and 188 cm tall (+1.4

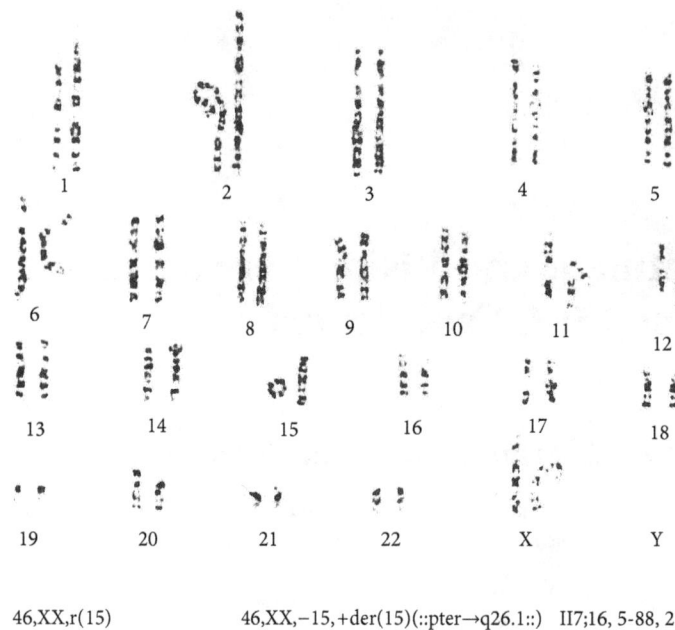

46,XX,r(15)   46,XX,−15,+der(15)(::pter→q26.1::)   II7;16, 5-88, 2

FIGURE 1: The karyotype of 46,XX, r(15) pattern.

SD). The girl has four older healthy siblings; three sisters—17 years old with a height of 180 cm (+2.3 SD), 14 years old with a height of 175 cm (+2.2 SD), and 12 years old with a height of 164 cm (+1.7 SD). Her only brother is 7 years old with a height of 130 cm (+1.3 SD). During the neonate period she was diagnosed with atrial septum defect type II, which was corrected at the age of 12 months. At the age of 3 months the girl was also qualified for orthopedic treatment due to equinovarious feet. At 15 months, because of the dysmorphic features and growth retardation, she was diagnosed in the department of pediatric endocrinology and department of clinical genetics.

Cytogenetic analyses from 72 hr lymphocyte cultures showed pathological karyotype: mos 45,XX-15[4%]/46,XX,-15,+der(15)(::pter->q26.1::)[96%]. Parental karyotype is normal and according to the parents, the karyotype anomaly was classified as *de novo* (Figure 1). The analysis of a three-generation pedigree has shown no genetic abnormalities or pregnancy losses.

During the first clinical examination at the age of 15 months, extreme short stature was noticed—the girl was 66 cm (−5.6 SD); her weight was also very low: 7 kg (<3 percentile) and her BMI was 15.9 kg/m^2. A detailed examination revealed several dysmorphic features: hypertelorism, high-broad nasal bridge, short hands and feet, and divergent strabismus (Figures 2(a) and 2(b)). Detailed neuropediatric consultation revealed psychomotor development delay, hypotonia, and a speech development delay; hyperactivity was not noticed. Liver and renal function and anatomy were normal. The imaging of the central nervous system yields normal results. Bone age—assessed according to the Greulich-Pyle method—was 12 months delayed.

In hormonal tests no abnormalities were detected. Thyroid status as well as adrenal hormones was normal. Growth hormone stimulation tests showed normal results (maximal GH peak in L-DOPA test was 11.8 ng/mL; maximal peak in Clonidine test was 15.3 ng/mL). IGF-1 (198 ng/mL at the age 2 years and 11 months) and IGFBP-3 (5.2 ug/mL) [normal range 0.9–4.3 ug/mL] levels were normal. Because of extreme short stature rhGH therapy was introduced at the age of 3 years with the initial dose of 0.035 mg/kg/d. The result of the 1st year of therapy was an increase in growth velocity by 6 cm. Screening for inborn metabolism disorders with the use of GC-MS method showed no abnormalities.

At initial visit (at 15 months of age) the patient presented with signs of amblyopia in the right eye by fixation pattern, hypermetropia of +3.50 diopters (D) in both eyes, and intermittent right eye exotropia of 60 prism diopters (PD) at distance and near in the primary position as well as convergence insufficiency. A dilated fundus exam showed no abnormalities.

Initial management included spectacle correction +1,0 D and 25 PD each eye, nonsquinting eye occlusion (conventional occlusion) for 2 hours per day, and simultaneous undercovering, as well as daily convergence exercises. The lack of parental consent for strabismus operation left conservative treatment as the only option, which proved to be a challenge. At the age of 4 years the best corrected visual acuity (BCVA) was 0.22 OD and 0.33 OS. Remarkable progress in the treatment was seen in the eighth year of therapy governed by the patient's own efforts. The prisms enabled permanent symmetrical stimulation of the retina which leads to the development of normal single binocular vision (Maddox test, filter test, and synoptofor tests). In this case study, the final

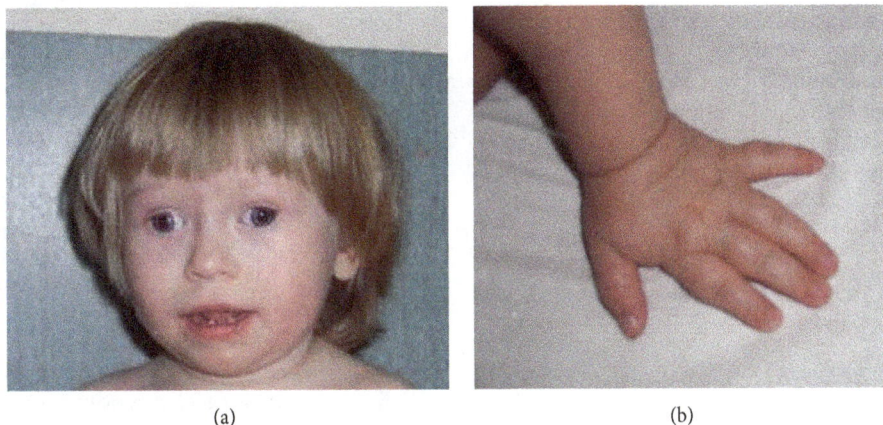

FIGURE 2: (a) Dysmorphic features of the patient, big exotropia. (b) Fifth finger clinodactyly.

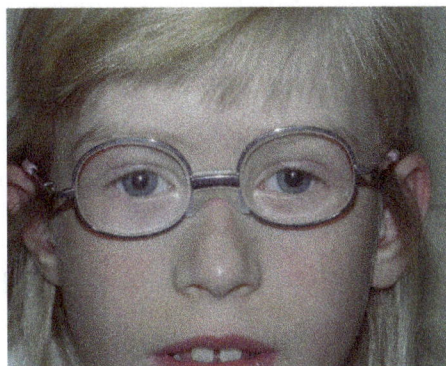

FIGURE 3: Facial features at age 8 years. Result of ophthalmological treatment: parallel position of the eyeball with final correction OD 5PD, OS 5PD.

correction OD 5PD, OS 5PD led to achievement of normal single binocular vision and improvement of visual acuity (1.0 OD/OS) (Figure 3).

3. Discussion

The etiology and pathogenic pathways for developing r(15) are not completely understood. All ring chromosomes are formed by a loss of the terminal fragment of the chromosome and a break-point junction to the terminal region of the short arm of the same chromosome. In this scenario, the size of lost fragment and haploinsufficiency of the missed genes determine the clinical features. Because nearly all of the patients present with loss of different span of the terminal chromosome fragments, determining common genotype-phenotype correlation is impossible. They present with unspecific features, classified by Fryns et al. [10] and Kosztolanyi et al. [11, 12] as the so called "ring phenotype." Our patient showed in first years of life the clinical features resembling Silver-Russel phenotype (growth deficit, microcephaly, triangular face with typical dysmorphic signs). It is probably due to a loss of one copy of the IGFR-1 gene (Insuline-Like Growth Factor Recepror 1). IGF- like receptor mutations are discussed

as one of the main factors influencing the pathogenesis of Silver—Russell Syndrome, mainly characterized by growth deficit [13].

Ring chromosomes in general but particularly r(15) may be unstable structures and in some cases may be lost or duplicated in some cells during embryonic differentiations resulting in new mosaic cell lines; such mechanism could be present in our patient as we observed a monosomy 15 cell line without r(15) in small number of cells [14]. The risk of having next child with pathology increases with mother's age (>age 35) and continues to increase with each year of life. Parental karyotype was normal, and no genetic abnormalities found in siblings consolidate us in a single occurrence of this type of chromosomal disorder in this family.

According to the original report of Jacobsen [1], congenital malformations in ring chromosome 15 patients included eye anomalies (e.g., macular defects, hyperopia, strabismus and heterochromia), ear abnormalities (e.g., dysplastic ears and hearing loss), café-au-lait macules, and cardiac anomalies [2, 6, 7]. Of the genes mapped to distal 15q (http://www.ncbi.nlm.nih.gov/mapview), none have been directly implicated in the etiology of human strabismus. Literature search showed no data in regard to ophthalmologic treatment in children diagnosed with r(15). As far as we know, abovementioned case of achieving normal single binocular vision and improving visual acuity has been presented for the first time.

Delayed psychomotor development and difficult contact with the child certainly had an impact on the length of ocular treatment. As previously mentioned, in this r(15) case study the ophthalmological findings included exotropia and deep amblyopia. Spherical correction of hyperopia and prismatic lenses were utilized to correct the strabismus angle in order to achieve symmetrical stimulation of both retinas at distance and near. At the beginning of therapy, the first given spectacles were purposely of less prismatic value then the angle of squint. Knowing that if we wanted to completely correct the deviation of the eye we would have to prescribe full prism correction, and they would worsen the already poor visual acuity. Therapy has prolonged to several years due to general complications of the congenital defects (typical for ring15) and ocular disorders (strabismus instability, abnormal fixation pattern, deep amblyopia, and convergence insufficiency). An optimistic attitude of both the ophthalmologists and the parents, as well as the cooperation of many specialists in treating such a difficult ring chromosome 15 patient resulted in an optimal positive ocular result.

Abbreviations

BCVA: Best corrected visual acuity
BMI: Body mass index
D: Diopters
GH: Growth hormone
IGF-1:   Insulin-like growth factor 1
IGFBP-3:   Insulin-like growth factor binding protein 3
L-DOPA: L-3,4-Dihydroxyphenylalanine
OD: Right eye
OS: Left eye
r(15):   Ring chromosome 15
rhGH: Recombinant human growth hormone
PD: Prism diopters.

Consent

Written informed consent was obtained from the parent of the patient for publication of this case report. A copy of the written consent is available for review by the Editor of this journal.

Conflict of Interests

The authors have no conflict of interests regarding the publication of this paper.

Authors' Contribution

Dr. Puchalska-Niedbał conceptualized and designed the study, drafted the initial paper, and approved the final paper as submitted; Dr. Petriczko conceptualized and designed the study, reviewed and revised the paper, and approved the final paper as submitted; Dr. Zajączek conducted the final analyses, critically reviewed the paper, and approved the final paper as submitted; Dr. Kulik reviewed and revised the paper and approved the final paper as submitted.

References

[1] P. Jacobsen, "A ring chromosome in the 13–15 group associated with microcephalic dwarfism, mental retardation and emotional immaturity," *Herediatias*, vol. 55, pp. 188–191, 1966.

[2] I. A. Glass, K. A. Rauen, E. Chen et al., "Ring chromosome 15: characterization by array CGH," *Human Genetics*, vol. 118, no. 5, pp. 611–617, 2006.

[3] Y.-H. Liu, S. D. Chang, and F.-P. Chen, "Increased fetal nuchal fold leading to prenatal diagnosis of ring chromosome 15," *Prenatal Diagnosis*, vol. 21, no. 12, pp. 1031–1033, 2001.

[4] E. Hatem, B. R. Meriam, D. Walid, M. Adenen, G. Moez, and S. Ali, "Molecular characterization of a ring chromosome 15 in a fetus with intra uterine growth retardation and diaphragmatic hernia," *Prenatal Diagnosis*, vol. 27, no. 5, pp. 471–474, 2007.

[5] R. S. Guilherme, V. D. F. A. Meloni, S. S. Takeno et al., "Twenty-year cytogenetic and molecular follow-up of a patient with ring chromosome 15: a case report," *Journal of Medical Case Reports*, vol. 6, article 283, 2012.

[6] M. G. Butler, A. B. Fogo, D. A. Fuchs, F. S. Collins, V. G. Dev, and J. A. Phillips III, "Brief clinical report and review: two patients with ring chromosome 15 syndrome," *American Journal of Medical Genetics*, vol. 29, no. 1, pp. 149–154, 1988.

[7] E. W. Roback, A. J. Barakat, V. G. Dev, M. Mbikay, M. Chretien, and M. G. Butler, "An infant with deletion of the distal long arm of chromosome 15 (q26.1 → qter) and loss of insulin-like growth factor 1 receptor gene," *American Journal of Medical Genetics*, vol. 38, no. 1, pp. 74–79, 1991.

[8] M. Werner, Z. Ben-Neriah, S. Silverstein, I. Lerer, Y. Dagan, and D. Abeliovich, "A patient with Prader-Willi syndrome and a supernumerary marker chromosome r(15)(q11.1–13p11.1)pat and maternal heterodisomy," *American Journal of Medical Genetics*, vol. 129, no. 2, pp. 176–179, 2004.

[9] T. Baranowska-George, *Traitement du Strabisme References Particulieres a la Methode de Szczecin*, Sylwjana, Szczecin, Poland, 1995.

[10] J. P. Fryns, J. Timmermans, F. D'Hondt, B. François, L. Emmery, and H. van den Berghe, "Ring chromosome 15 syndrome," *Human Genetics*, vol. 51, no. 1, pp. 43–48, 1979.

[11] G. Kosztolanyi, "Does "Ring Chromosome" exist? An analysis of 207 case reports on patients with Ring Autosome," *Human Genetics*, vol. 75, no. 2, pp. 174–179, 1987.

[12] G. Kosztolanyi, K. Mehes, and E. B. Hook, "Inherited ring chromosomes: an analysis of published cases," *Human Genetics*, vol. 87, no. 3, pp. 320–324, 1991.

[13] T. Tamura, T. Tohma, T. Ohta et al., "Ring chromosome 15 involving deletion of the insulin-like growth factor 1 receptor gene in a patient with features of Silver-Russell syndrome," *Clinical Dysmorphology*, vol. 2, no. 2, pp. 106–113, 1993.

[14] R. J. McKinlay Gardner, G. R. Sutherland, and L. G. Shaffer, *Chromosome Abnormalities and Genetic Counselling*, Oxford University Press, New York, NY, USA, 2012.

34

Kawasaki Disease with Retropharyngeal Edema following a Blackfly Bite

Toru Watanabe

Department of Pediatrics, Niigata City General Hospital, 463-7 Shumoku, Chuo-ku, Niigata 950-1197, Japan

Correspondence should be addressed to Toru Watanabe; twata@hosp.niigata.niigata.jp

Academic Editor: Nan-Chang Chiu

We describe a patient with Kawasaki disease (KD) and retropharyngeal edema following a blackfly bite. An 8-year-old boy was referred to our hospital because of a 3-day-history of fever and left neck swelling and redness after a blackfly bite. Computed tomography of the neck revealed left cervical lymph nodes swelling with edema, increased density of the adjacent subcutaneous tissue layer, and low density of the retropharyngeum. The patient was initially presumed to have cervical cellulitis, lymphadenitis, and retropharyngeal abscess. He was administered antibiotics intravenously, which did not improve his condition. The patient subsequently exhibited other signs of KD and was diagnosed with KD and retropharyngeal edema. Intravenous immunoglobulin therapy and oral flurbiprofen completely resolved the symptoms and signs. A blackfly bite sometimes incites a systemic reaction in humans due to a hypersensitive reaction to salivary secretions, which may have contributed to the development of KD in our patient.

1. Introduction

Kawasaki disease (KD) is a systemic vasculitis that predominantly affects children ≤5 years of age [1, 2]. Children with KD typically have an acute onset of fever, followed by signs of mucosal inflammation and vasodilatation that evolve over the first week of the illness. Although the cause of KD remains unclear, it is thought that the immune system is activated by infectious or environmental triggers in genetically susceptible hosts [3]. Controversy exists regarding the mechanism of immune system activation, but recent studies suggest that T cell activation is important in determining the susceptibility and severity of KD [3]. Various viral and bacterial pathogens have been postulated as triggers for the development of KD, but no single pathogen has been confirmed to be an etiologic agent [4]. Thus, KD represents a stereotyped, pathologic immune response to one or a variety of environmental or infectious triggers [3].

Blackflies (Simuliidae) are small flies that have a characteristic hump-back appearance [5]. A blackfly bite usually causes local pain, swelling, and redness, while systemic symptoms, such as malaise, fever, leukocytosis, and lymphadenitis, develop in some patients due to a delayed hypersensitivity reaction to blackfly salivary secretions [5, 6]. KD following a blackfly bite has never been reported. We describe a patient with KD and retropharyngeal edema following a blackfly bite.

2. Case Presentation

An 8-year-old boy complained of left neck pain soon after a blackfly bite on his left neck. Because the patient had a high-grade fever and left neck erythema and swelling the next day, he was referred to his family physician 4 days after the blackfly bite. He was diagnosed with bacterial lymphadenitis and was transferred to our hospital. The boy had bronchial asthma since 2 years of age and was treated with inhaled steroid therapy; he also had allergies to mites, cedars, and cats.

On admission, the patient was febrile with a body temperature of 40.8°C and left neck pain. The physical examination revealed left cervical erythema and lymph node swelling with tenderness (Figure 1). Laboratory studies revealed leukocytosis (white blood cell count = 17,700/μL), elevated C-reactive protein (CRP; 12.20 mg/dL [reference range, 0.01–0.31 mg/dL]), serum aspartate aminotransferase (171 IU/L), and serum alanine aminotransferase levels (152 IU/L), and

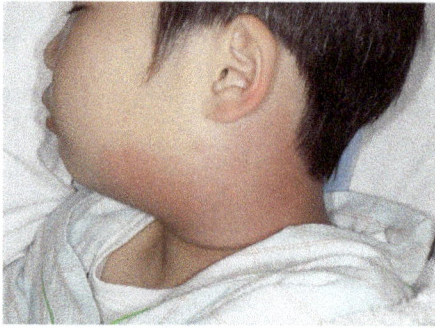

FIGURE 1: A photograph showing wide spreading left cervical erythema and lymph node swelling.

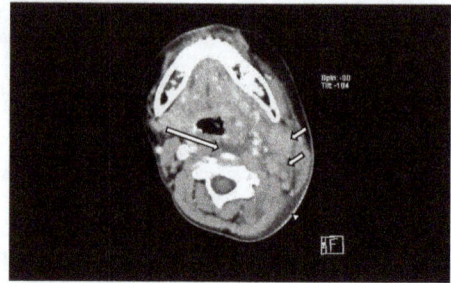

FIGURE 2: Postcontrast computed tomography of the neck showing left cervical lymph nodes swelling (arrow) with edema and increased density of adjacent subcutaneous tissue layer (arrowhead), and retropharyngeal low density without ring enhancement (long arrow).

hyponatremia (sodium = 132 mEq/L). Serum potassium, chloride, creatinine, uric acid, amylase, and blood urea nitrogen levels were all normal. The serum antistreptolysin O titer was within the normal ranges. A urinalysis revealed 2 + protein, 4 + acetone, 2 + occult blood, 5–9 red blood cells per high-power field, and a few granular casts per low-power field. Postcontrast computed tomography of the neck (Figure 2) revealed left cervical lymph nodes swelling with edema, increased density of the adjacent subcutaneous tissue layer, and low density of the retropharyngeum without ring enhancement. The patient was initially presumed to have cervical cellulitis, lymphadenitis, and a retropharyngeal abscess caused by a bacterial infection secondary to the blackfly bite. Intravenous ceftriaxone was begun after obtaining 2 blood samples, a throat swab, and an aspirate from the subcutaneous cervical neck lesion for bacterial cultures. His condition did not improve and no pathogens were isolated in the bacterial culture samples. The patient subsequently exhibited conjunctival hyperemia, truncal exanthema, a strawberry tongue, and palmar erythema over the ensuing 2 days and was diagnosed with KD and retropharyngeal edema. An echocardiography revealed no coronary arterial lesions. Intravenous immunoglobulin therapy (IVIG; 2 g/kg/dose) for 1 day and oral administration of flurbiprofen (4 mg/kg per day) resulted in rapid improvement of the KD signs, left cervical lesion, and abnormal laboratory test results. The patient exhibited membranous desquamation of the fingers on the 14th day of the present illness. He remains well without coronary artery abnormalities 6 months after the onset of the present illness.

3. Discussion

Although extremely rare, systemic vasculitis after an insect bite has been reported and includes Henoch-Schönlein purpura after undetermined insect bites [7, 8], serum sickness-like syndrome due to mosquito bites [9], and multisystemic leukocytoclastic vasculitis following a centipede bite [10]. It is suggested that a hypersensitivity response to the insect bite induces leukocytoclastic vasculitis in these patients [8, 9].

Our patient developed KD after a blackfly bite. A blackfly bite usually causes local pain, swelling, and redness; however, the bite can also cause a systemic reaction (blackfly fever)

that precipitates headaches, fever, nausea, vomiting, malaise, and generalized lymphadenopathy [11, 12]. Blackfly salivary secretions contain a wide range of physiologically active molecules that can induce local immunomodulation and anticoagulation and local and systemic hypersensitivity reactions in humans [13]; however, patients with severe blackfly hypersensitivity reactions have rarely been reported. Orange et al. [14] reported a patient with recurrent episodes of presumed cellulitis after blackfly bites who subsequently developed two episodes of delayed hypersensitivity reactions to these bites, including Guillain-Barré syndrome (GBS) and nephrotic syndrome (NS). Because immune systems, especially T cells, play a major role in the development of both GBS [15] and NS [16], a blackfly bite may induce systemic T cell activation in some susceptible humans. Likewise, recent data suggest that T cell activation is important in determining the susceptibility and severity of KD [4]. In addition, NS has also been reported in some patients with KD [17]. Therefore, systemic T cell activation due to a blackfly bite may have contributed to the development of KD in our patient.

The diagnosis of KD is important because it implies a specific therapeutic choice of IVIG. Our patient was initially presumed to have a retropharyngeal abscess secondary to a blackfly bite on the findings of cervical CT. A retropharyngeal abnormality mimicking a retropharyngeal abscess on CT is occasionally seen in patients with KD and is generally thought to be edema [18]. Although the precise pathophysiology of retropharyngeal edema in KD is unclear, clinical findings, operative details, sterile culture results, and the responses to intravenous immunoglobulin treatment suggest that the mechanism is an intense inflammatory response [18]. Because most patients with KD and retropharyngeal edema are initially misdiagnosed as having a retropharyngeal abscess, such patients frequently have a delayed diagnosis of KD and undergo unnecessary antibiotic treatment and/or pharyngeal aspiration [19]. Nomura et al. [20] recently reported that clinical symptoms of dysphagia and neck pain and neck CT findings, including a ring enhancement and mass effect of retropharyngeal lesions, occurred significantly more frequently in patients with retropharyngeal abscesses than in KD patients with retropharyngeal edema. Because delayed diagnosis of KD may lead to the development of cardiovascular complications, careful attention to clinical manifestations and close analyses of neck CT imaging in patients with retropharyngeal abnormalities are necessary to avoid a delayed diagnosis of KD [20].

In summary, we have reported a patient with KD and retropharyngeal edema following a blackfly bite. Although the precise pathogenesis remains unclear, hypersensitivity reactions against blackfly salivary secretions, especially systemic T cell activation, may have contributed to the development of KD in our patient.

Consent

Written informed consent was obtained from a parent of the patient for publication of this case report.

Conflict of Interests

The author declares that there is no conflict of interests regarding the publication of this paper.

References

[1] T. Kawasaki, F. Kosaki, S. Okawa, I. Shigematsu, and H. Yanagawa, "A new infantile acute febrile mucocutaneous lymph node syndrome (MLNS) prevailing in Japan," *Pediatrics*, vol. 54, no. 3, pp. 271–276, 1974.

[2] J. C. Burns and M. P. Glodé, "Kawasaki syndrome," *The Lancet*, vol. 364, no. 9433, pp. 533–544, 2004.

[3] R. P. Sundel and R. E. Petty, "Kawasaki disease," in *Textbook of Pediatric Rheumatology*, J. T. Classidy, R. M. Laxer, and C. B. Lindsley, Eds., pp. 505–520, Saunders, Philadelphia, Pa, USA, 2011.

[4] R. Scuccimarri, "Kawasaki Disease," *Pediatric Clinics of North America*, vol. 59, no. 2, pp. 425–445, 2012.

[5] T. B. Erickson and A. Márquez Jr., "Arthropod envenomation and parasitism," in *Wilderness Medicine*, P. S. Auerbach, Ed., pp. 925–954, Elsevier, San Diego, Calif, USA, 6th edition, 2012.

[6] G. E. Gaillard, R. Schellin, and A. D. Larkin, "Blood sucking black fly (Simulidae) treatment with alum precipitated pyradine extract," *Annals of Allergy*, vol. 26, no. 3, pp. 138–144, 1968.

[7] D. M. Burke and H. L. Jellinek, "Nearly fatal case of Schönlein-Henoch syndrome following insect bite," *American Journal of Diseases of Children*, vol. 88, no. 6, pp. 772–774, 1954.

[8] G. Sharan, R. K. Anand, and K. P. Sinha, "Schönlein-Henoch syndrome after insect bite," *British Medical Journal*, vol. 1, no. 5488, p. 656, 1966.

[9] P. Gaig, P. Garcia-Ortega, E. Enrique, A. Benet, B. Bartolome, and R. Palacios, "Serum sickness-like syndrome due to mosquito bite," *Journal of Investigational Allergology and Clinical Immunology*, vol. 9, no. 3, pp. 190–192, 1999.

[10] A. Soylu, S. Kavukçu, B. Erdur, K. Demir, and M. A. Türkmen, "Multisystemic leukocytoclastic vasculitis affecting the central nervous system," *Pediatric Neurology*, vol. 33, no. 4, pp. 289–291, 2005.

[11] S. Borah, S. Goswami, M. Agarwal et al., "Clinical and histopathological study of Simulium (blackfly) dermatitis from North-Eastern India—a report," *International Journal of Dermatology*, vol. 51, no. 1, pp. 63–66, 2012.

[12] J. G. Demain, "Papular urticaria and things that bite in the night," *Current Allergy and Asthma Reports*, vol. 3, no. 4, pp. 291–303, 2003.

[13] P. Chattopadhyay, D. Goyary, S. Dhiman, B. Rabha, S. Hazarika, and V. Veer, "Immunomodulating effects and hypersensitivity reactions caused by Northeast Indian black fly salivary gland extract," *Journal of Immunotoxicology*, vol. 11, no. 2, pp. 126–132, 2014.

[14] J. S. Orange, L. A. Song, F. J. Twarog, and L. C. Schneider, "A patient with severe black fly (Simuliidae) hypersensitivity referred for evaluation of suspected immunodeficiency," *Annals of Allergy, Asthma and Immunology*, vol. 92, no. 2, pp. 276–280, 2004.

[15] M. M. Dimachkie and R. J. Barohn, "Guillain-Barré syndrome and variants," *Neurologic Clinics*, vol. 31, no. 2, pp. 491–510, 2013.

[16] W. G. Couser, "Basic and translational concepts of immune-mediated glomerular diseases," *Journal of the American Society of Nephrology*, vol. 23, no. 3, pp. 381–399, 2012.

[17] T. Watanabe, "Kidney and urinary tract involvement in Kawasaki disease," *International Journal of Pediatrics*, vol. 2013, Article ID 831834, 8 pages, 2013.

[18] E. W. Langley, D. K. Kirse, C. E. Barnes, W. Covitz, and A. K. Shetty, "Retropharyngeal edema: an unusual manifestation of kawasaki disease," *Journal of Emergency Medicine*, vol. 39, no. 2, pp. 181–185, 2010.

[19] M. E. Cavicchiolo, P. Berlese, S. Bressan et al., "Retropharyngeal abscess: an unusual presentation of Kawasaki disease. Case report and review of the literature," *International Journal of Pediatric Otorhinolaryngology Extra*, vol. 7, no. 4, pp. 179–182, 2012.

[20] O. Nomura, N. Hashimoto, A. Ishiguro et al., "Comparison of patients with Kawasaki disease with retropharyngeal edema and patients with retropharyngeal abscess," *European Journal of Pediatrics*, vol. 173, no. 3, pp. 381–386, 2014.

35

A Rare Case of Neonatal Complicated Appendicitis in a Child with Patau's Syndrome

Valentina Pastore and Fabio Bartoli

Pediatric Surgery Unit, Medical and Surgical Sciences Department, University of Foggia, Viale Pinto 1, 71122 Foggia, Italy

Correspondence should be addressed to Valentina Pastore; valentinapastore1427@gmail.com

Academic Editor: Denis A. Cozzi

Neonatal appendicitis is a rare condition with high mortality rate. Signs and symptoms are often nonspecific, imaging modalities are not always diagnostic, and preoperative diagnosis is difficult with subsequent delay and complications. Its pathophysiology may be different from appendicitis in older children and comorbidities can be found. We report a case of a female neonate with Patau's syndrome, intestinal malrotation, and Fallot tetralogy in whom perforated appendix, probably occurring during fetal period due to vascular insufficiency, was found at laparotomy.

1. Introduction

Despite the fact that acute appendicitis is a common diagnosis and is the most common indication for urgent abdominal surgery in children, it is very rare in neonates and shows a high mortality rate, which remains as high as 34% especially in perforated cases [1]. Incidence has been reported to be 0.04–0.2% and male neonates with prematurity or comorbidities (Hirschsprung disease, cystic fibrosis, cardiac defects, tracheoesophageal fistula, and inguinal hernias) are more often affected [2, 3]. Overall, during the last century, about 100 cases have been described [1] and, given its rarity and nonspecific signs and symptoms, preoperative diagnosis is quite difficult with subsequent delay and complications. We report a case of a female neonate with Patau's syndrome, intestinal malrotation, and Fallot tetralogy in whom perforated appendix was found at laparotomy.

2. Case Presentation

A female baby, born at 39-week gestation by cesarean section to a second gravid mother with an uncomplicated prenatal history, weighing 2850 gr, was admitted to NICU immediately after birth due to dysmorphia (hands claw and bilateral microphthalmia and aplasia cutis). White blood cell count and CRP were normal, abdomen was palpable, and she suffered only from a slight respiratory distress. In the suspect of a karyotypic abnormality, a cardiac ultrasonography with Doppler was done and a picture compatible with Fallot tetralogy was found. Abdominal US and X-ray showed no evidence of free air and only a slight peritoneal effusion. Chest X-ray was normal. Head MR showed thinning of *corpus callosum*. Three days after admission, general clinical conditions worsened with tachycardia, fever, and abdominal distension. Baby refused food and bile-stained vomiting started. White blood cell count was 17.6×10^3 U/L (neutrophil 77%) and CRP was elevated. The renal function tests were within normal limits. Antibiotic and supporting therapy were started and, in the suspect of bowel intussusception, an abdominal US was done. No ecographic typical signs (apart from a perivesical fluid collection) were found. Then, the baby underwent a barium enema, which showed a bowel malrotation. This was considered the reason of the acute abdomen and a laparotomy was immediately started. Surgical findings included bowel malrotation, dilated small bowel coated with purulent exudates, gangrenous appendicitis with perforation near the tip, and turbid fluid in the peritoneal cavity (Figure 1). Furthermore, there were strong adhesions around the appendix. Ladd's procedure, appendectomy, and toilet of the peritoneal cavity were done. Histological examination of the appendix showed that the lumen was filled with

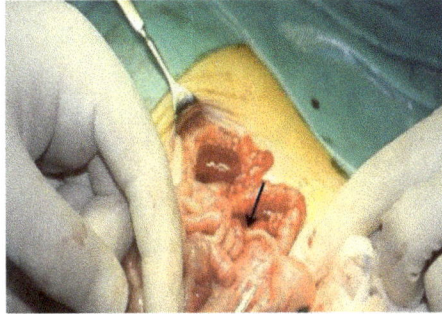

FIGURE 1: Appendix with perforation near the tip.

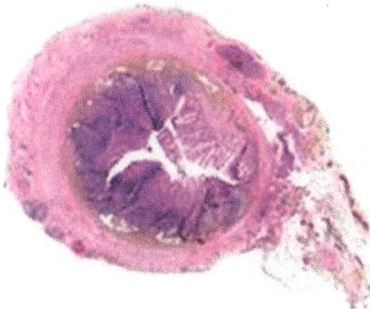

FIGURE 2: Histological examination of the appendix showing concretions, dense fibrinosuppurative infiltrate, and transmural granulation at the site of perforation.

concretions with dense fibrinosuppurative infiltrate and tranmural granulation at the site of perforation (Figure 2). Postoperative management was regular: antibiotic and supporting therapy were continued, Patau's syndrome was confirmed as result of karyotype examination, clinical conditions remained stable, and feeding started three days after surgery. White blood cell count switched back to standard rate, CRP normalized, and no changes on cardiac US appeared. Surgical procedure for correction of Fallot syndrome was scheduled but two months after birth the baby suffered from a sepsis due to Klebsiella pneumoniae and she suddenly died.

3. Discussion

Neonatal appendicitis is a very rare condition, with no more than 100 cases described over the last century and high mortality and perforation rates [1]. The low incidence can be due to different factors such as the presence of a fetal form of the appendix (funnel shaped with wide opening into the cecum), a liquid diet, recumbent posture, and rare infections [4]. Its pathophysiology may be different from appendicitis in older children and authors think that it could be considered as a localized form of NEC (especially in otherwise healthy neonate) [5], a *morbus sui generis* [6], or that it could be secondary to comorbidities such as Hirschprung disease, cardiac anomalies, tracheoesophageal fistula, cystic fibrosis, or infective diseases (cytomegalovirus and chorioamnionitis) [3]. Since signs and symptoms are nonspecific, a preoperative diagnosis is very difficult and most of neonates have been

diagnosed intraoperatively. In fact, all the authors emphasize the difficulty of diagnosis considering both the nonspecific signs and symptoms and the rarity of the disease at this age [2, 7]. Generally, the babies affected may show irritability, distressed breathing, wriggling, swelling of the scrotum, a right lower quadrant palpable mass, abdominal distension, bilious vomiting, erythematous rash over the abdominal wall, and also anorexia, fever, and leukocytosis [3]. As the signs and symptoms are not characteristic, the incidence of perforation is high and is a significant factor in determining the prognosis. Other reasons are to be found in thin appendiceal wall and indistensible cecum. Furthermore, a relatively small undeveloped and functionally nonexistent omentum and small size of the peritoneal cavity allow a more rapid and diffuse contamination and little physiological reserve and are important factors contributing to this high morbidity and mortality rate associated with peritonitis in infants [8]. In the neonate we report, Patau's syndrome was diagnosed based on chromosome testing after a suspected clinical examination. Patau's syndrome, or trisomy 13, affects 1 : 10000–21700 live births and presents abnormalities of nervous system, musculoskeletal, cutaneous, and urogenital and cardiac systems. Evaluation of symptoms and signs was very difficult and in fact, having excluded intussusception (negative abdominal US and barium enema) and believing she could suffer from an acute abdomen due to bowel malrotation, laparotomy was done about 12 hours after diagnostic examinations. We found bowel malrotation but the acute abdomen was due to the perforated appendix with secondary peritonitis. Retrospectively examining the signs we had found before surgery, we think that, even if the clinical conditions worsened three days after birth, peritoneal effusion shown on abdominal US made few hours after birth could have been considered an initial sign. Furthermore, at laparotomy, there were strong adhesions around the appendix and these can justify a pre- or perinatal perforation and negative preoperative abdominal US and barium enema. About the possible aetiologies of appendiceal perforation in our patient, the most probable could be the vascular insufficiency (considered a major cause of perforation) which might have induced poor circulation before the onset of symptoms [3, 9]. Surgical approach was the standard Ladd's procedure, classical appendectomy, and peritoneal toilet without intraoperative complications. Postoperative course was uneventful strictly considering the surgical management and the baby started feeding three days after surgery. Postoperative laboratory findings were normal and clinical conditions remained stable. However, Patau's syndrome carries a high mortality rate with more than 89% of the children dying before hospital discharge and comfort care is the treatment of choice for most of them [10]. In fact, about two months after surgery, our baby became septic, not responsive to antibiotic therapy, and she suddenly died. In conclusion, acute appendicitis is a rare condition in neonates and is rarely diagnosed preoperatively because symptoms are not specific. Delay in diagnosis carries a high perforation and complication rate, also because diagnostic examinations are not always comprehensive, even if we believe that in our patient perforation occurred during fetal period. In order to reduce mortality, in doubtful cases, appendicitis should also be considered in the differential diagnosis especially in neonates with comorbidities.

Conflict of Interests

The authors declare that they have no conflict of interests.

References

[1] K. L. Schwartz, E. Gilad, D. Sigalet, W. Yu, and A. L. Wong, "Neonatal acute appendicitis: a proposed algorithm for timely diagnosis," *Journal of Pediatric Surgery*, vol. 46, no. 11, pp. 2060–2064, 2011.

[2] R. A. Khan, P. Menon, and K. L. N. Rao, "Beware of neonatal appendicitis," *Journal of Indian Association of Pediatric Surgeons*, vol. 15, no. 2, pp. 67–69, 2010.

[3] T. Jancelewicz, G. Kim, and D. Miniati, "Neonatal appendicitis: a new look at an old zebra," *Journal of Pediatric Surgery*, vol. 43, no. 10, pp. e1–e5, 2008.

[4] G. R. Schorlemmer and C. A. Herbst Jr., "Perforated neonatal appendicitis," *Southern Medical Journal*, vol. 76, no. 4, pp. 536–537, 1983.

[5] M. van Veenendaal, F. B. Plötz, P. G. J. Nikkels, and N. M. A. Bax, "Further evidence for an ischemic origin of perforation of the appendix in the neonatal period," *Journal of Pediatric Surgery*, vol. 39, no. 8, pp. e11–e12, 2004.

[6] D. Stiefel, T. Stallmach, and P. Sacher, "Acute appendicitis in neonates: complication or morbus sui generis?" *Pediatric Surgery International*, vol. 14, no. 1-2, pp. 122–123, 1998.

[7] Y. A. Khan, K. Zia, and N. S. Saddal, "Perforated neonatal appendicitis with pneumoperitoneum," *APSP Journal of Case Reports*, vol. 4, pp. 21–22, 2013.

[8] M. E. Ruff, W. M. Southgate, and B. P. Wood, "Radiological case of the month: neonatla appendicitis with perforation," *The American Journal of Diseases of Children*, vol. 145, no. 1, pp. 111–112, 1991.

[9] A. Karaman, Y. H. Çavuşoğlu, I. Karaman, and O. Çakmak, "Seven cases of neonatal appendicitis with a review of the English language literature of the last century," *Pediatric Surgery International*, vol. 19, no. 11, pp. 707–709, 2003.

[10] Eunice Kennedy Shriver National Institute of Child Health and Human Development Neonatal Research Network, "Mortality and morbidity of VLBW infants with trisomy 13 or trisomy 18," *Pediatrics*, vol. 133, pp. 226–235, 2014.

36

A Case Study of Intractable Vomiting with Final Diagnosis of Neuromyelitis Optica

Rachel Bramson[1,2] and Angela Hairrell[1]

[1]College of Medicine, Texas A&M Health Science Center College of Medicine, Bryan, TX 77807, USA
[2]Family Medicine, Scott and White University Clinic, College Station, TX 77845, USA

Correspondence should be addressed to Rachel Bramson; bramson@medicine.tamhsc.edu

Academic Editor: Denis A. Cozzi

This case study presents a patient living in a suburban/rural community who received appropriate referral to secondary and tertiary care for nausea and vomiting, accompanied by waxing and waning neurological symptoms, yet proved difficult to diagnose. This patient is presented to draw attention to a rare neurological disorder which should be included in the differential diagnosis of nausea and vomiting with some key neurological complaints, even in the absence of physical findings.

1. Introduction

When a previously healthy adolescent presents with nausea and vomiting, the most common diagnoses are viral gastroenteritis or pyelonephritis. Vague waxing and waning neurological symptoms in an adolescent may be attributed to stress or developmental issues. Here we present a patient living in a suburban/rural community who received appropriate referral to secondary and tertiary care, yet proved difficult to diagnose. This patient is presented to draw attention to a rare neurological disorder which should be included in the differential diagnosis of nausea and vomiting with some key neurological complaints, even in the absence of physical findings. Physical findings may develop late in the course of the disease making a heightened index of suspicion important for early diagnosis and treatment.

2. Patient Presentation

The patient is a 17-year-old African-American female, multisport athlete in 11th grade in a rural high school. She is the second of four children and lives at home with her parents and two siblings. She gets Bs and Cs in school and is extremely well-liked by teachers and fellow students. She presented to Urgent Care with abdominal pain, nausea, and vomiting with a 19 lb. unintentional weight loss over a three-month period and BMI of 20. Her past medical history revealed normal development, immunizations being up to date, and pyelonephritis at age 14 for which she was hospitalized. She had no past surgeries and no history of alcohol, tobacco, or drug use. Her parents and siblings are healthy.

3. Clinical Findings

On initial presentation, the patient appeared healthy with no notable physical findings. She was discharged on Zofran and a clear liquid diet. On a follow-up two days later she had mild epigastric tenderness on physical exam and described a problem with shaky hands and back pain radiating into the right leg off and on, worse when she runs. The neurological exam was normal. CBC and CMP were normal with the exception of low WBC 3400 and sodium 134. TSH was low normal (0.5). On Beck's Anxiety Inventory she scored 11 (mild), and on Beck's Depression Inventory she scored 1 (negative).

4. Timeline

Due to the protracted course of this patient's illness and workup, Table 1 details her visits and care over a three-month period. The following is a brief summary of her clinical presentation.

TABLE 1: Timeline of presentation and diagnosis.

Date	Chief complaint/history	Consultant	Diagnostic study	Findings and treatment
9/7/2014 Urgent care visit	(i) Vomiting (ii) Unintentional weight loss	Primary care		Prescribing ondansetron and follow-up with PCP for weight loss
9/9/2014 PCP follow-up office visit	(i) Gastritis (ii) Weight loss (iii) Orthostatic hypotension (iv) Intermittent right lower back pain with radiation into the right leg	Primary care	(i) Beck's Anxiety and Depression Inventory (ii) CBC, CMP (iii) Lipid Panel (iv) TSH	(i) Mild anxiety (ii) No depression (iii) All labs normal (iv) Normal reflexes, muscle tone, coordination
9/11/2014 ER visit	(i) Vomiting (ii) Dehydration (iii) Weight loss		(i) Chest X-ray (ii) CBC, CMP (iii) Urine pregnancy test and UA (iv) ESR (v) CRP	(i) All normal, except low prealbumin at 18 and sodium 136 (ii) Given IV fluids (iii) Discharged on promethazine for vomiting and nausea
9/14–9/22/2014 Community hospital admittance with same day transfer to children's hospital	(i) Intractable vomiting (ii) Weight loss (iii) Hypertension (iv) 5-day history of hiccoughs		Right upper quadrant ultrasound	Small amount of gall bladder sludge, no gallstones
			CT abdomen pelvis with contrast	Normal
		Pediatric GI	EGD	(i) *H. Pylori* gastritis, biopsy diagnosis (ii) Triple therapy was initiated, changed to IV due to persistent nausea and vomiting, completed
		Pediatric nephrology	Colonoscopy with biopsies	No abnormalities
			Urine VMA, Renal ultrasound	Both normal
		Pediatric nutrition		(i) 15% weight loss in 3 months (ii) 27th percentile weight for age (iii) 32nd percentile stature for age
		Neurology		Normal strength, tone, movement

TABLE 1: Continued.

Date	Chief complaint/history	Consultant	Diagnostic study	Findings and treatment
		Discharge Diagnosis: H. pylori gastritis *medication:* Triple therapy for *H. pylori*: clonidine patch, pantoprazole, sucralfate		
9/28–10/4/2014 ER visit/transfer to children's hospital	(i) Pancreatitis (ii) Hypertension *History*: 2 fleeting episodes of blurry vision, lightheadedness, pain, itching on left side of face since 9/25, syncope on 9/24, 10-second loss of consciousness, difficulty following commands	Pediatric neurology Pediatric GI Pediatric nephrology *Discharge diagnosis:* Dehydration, abdominal pain, intractable vomiting, syncope, *H. pylori* infection, neuropathic left facial pain (worsened on gabapentin, so stopped) *Medication:* Clonidine patch 0.1 mg/24 hr weekly, pantoprazole 40 mg 2x daily, sucralfate 1 g 2x daily prn, ondansetron 8 mg 2x daily prn	(i) Brain CT (ii) Brain MRI EGD with biopsy for emesis Echo	(i) Both Normal (ii) Normal strength, tone, movement (iii) PT consult for instability in ambulation (i) Gastric nodularity, *H. pylori* positive (ii) Lipase 465–1498, Lactic acid 2.7 elevated Normal
10/6/2014 PCP follow-up from hospitalization	(i) Pancreatitis (ii) Hypertension *History*: lower extremity weakness, numbness in fingers, hyperesthesia of the face and head, shaking episodes, feeling cold, mom reports symptoms worsening, had "seizure" in hospital		(i) Lipase (ii) West Nile IGG and IGM (iii) ESR (iv) TSH Neurological exam	(i) Physical exam: normal reflexes, no cranial nerve deficits, normal muscle tone, decreased sensation in extremities (ii) Labs normal except elevated lipase (277) (iii) Cold intolerance (iv) Spells (v) Urgent referral to neurology (i) Cranial nerves intact (ii) Sensation intact (iii) Bilateral upper and lower extremities (iv) Right upper extremity strength 5/5 (v) Left upper extremity strength 4/5 (vi) Pronator drift (vii) Bilateral lower extremities 4/5 (viii) Gait weak on left side
10/7–9/2014 Office visit with pediatric neurology resulting in hospitalization at children's hospital	*History*: shaking episodes since 9/27 affecting head and upper extremities, occur randomly, last seconds with no postictal confusion, pins and needles sensation affecting entire face and left arm, itching and burning of left face with hyperpigmentation, weakness requiring wheelchair	Pediatric neurology, pediatric GI, adolescent medicine, neurosurgery	Continuous 24-hr. Video EEG EMG and Nerve conduction study (i) Ceruloplasmin (ii) Vitamin D (iii) Cortisol (iv) Lipase (v) ANA profile (vi) Entrovirus	Normal in awake, drowsy, sleeping states; 7 episodes with no EEG correlate Normal (i) Low (ii) Low (iii) Normal (iv) Elevated lipase (771) (v) Negative (vi) Negative

TABLE 1: Continued.

Date	Chief complaint/history	Consultant	Diagnostic study	Findings and treatment
				Discharge Diagnosis: (i) Left-sided upper and lower extremity weakness (ii) Spells *Medications:* Vitamin D deficiency, hydrocortisone cream, ondansetron, sucralfate, vitamin D, multivitamin, ranitidine
10/18/2014 PCP f/u hospitalization	(i) Pain in bilateral upper extremities, chest, low back (ii) Shaking		Lipase	(i) Almost normal (126) (ii) Myalgias (iii) Parasthesias (iv) Spells (v) Tremors (vi) Hypertension (vii) Urgent referral to pediatric neurology
10/23/2014 Pediatric neurology	(i) Pain in bilateral upper extremities, chest, low back (ii) Shaking	Pediatric neurology	(i) MRI whole spine, with and without contrast (performed on 11/3) (ii) Neurological exam	(i) Tremors (ii) Parasthesias (face, arms, trunk, legs) (iii) Nonspecific muscle tenderness, possible weakness (iv) Reflexes normal, downgoing plantar Muscle normal bulk, tone, strength (v) Decreased cold face to T4, decreased pinprick face to toes. (vi) Recent history of pancreatitis
10/29/2014 pediatric GI f/u hospitalization	Intractable vomiting	Pediatric GI	Serum copper	Normal
11/4/2014 PCP follow-up	MRI results		(i) MRI cervical spine (ii) MRI thoracic spine, lumbar spine, sacrum, coccyx	(i) 4×3 cystic dilation of the central canal from C5 to T2 (ii) Increased signal in the medulla oblongata and C2 to C5, relative expansion of the cervical spinal cord (iii) Syringomyelia (iv) Normal
11/7/2014 pediatric neurosurgery	Abnormal cervical spine MRI *History:* decreased activity due to neck pain, difficulty starting urination, hand tremor, weakness in all extremities, numbness and tingling in left leg	Pediatric neurosurgery	Neurological exam	(i) Abnormal reflexes, increased muscle tone, clonus in both feet, spastic gait (ii) No muscle atrophy, no cranial nerve or sensory deficit, normal position and vibration sense, normal coordination (iii) Possible multilevel spinal cord tumor (iv) Referred to 2nd children's hospital neurosurgery

TABLE 1: Continued.

Date	Chief complaint/history	Consultant	Diagnostic study	Findings and treatment
				(i) CSF positive for neuromyelitis optica (NMO), WBC 18, RBC 3, gram stain culture negative, IgG index 0.6, oligoclonal bands negative, ACE 1.1, NMDA receptor antibody negative; seropositive for NMO.
				(ii) Extensive cervical spine longitudinal myelitis; confluent ill-defined, partly enhancing, abnormal intramedullary signal from pontomedullary junction through the lower cervical cord. No optic nerve abnormality.
11/16–25/2014 ER visit and hospitalization at a second children's hospital	Possible multilevel spinal cord tumor	Child neurology	(i) Lumbar puncture (ii) MRI cerv. spine	(iii) Dystonia
				(iv) Tegretol 300 mg 3x daily
				(v) 2 days of IV IG
				(vi) 5-day course of IV methylprednisone, discharged on prednisone taper
		Discharge diagnosis: (i) Neuromyelitis optica (NMO) (ii) Cervical myelopathy (iii) Dystonia		
12/3/2014 Follow-up with pediatric neurology				(i) Neuromyelitis optica (NMO) (ii) Cervical myelopathy (iii) Secondary Paroxysmal Kinesigenic Dyskinesia (PKD) (iv) Start Cellcept with slow increase to goal of 1000 mg BID
1/22/2015 Follow-up with PCP	(i) Neuromyelitis optica (ii) Cervical myelopathy			(i) Weight gain since November of 34 lb (ii) Taking mycophenolate, carbamazepine, prednisone (iii) Referral to ophthalmology for baseline evaluation and ongoing care

Two days after her initial presentation, she presented to the emergency room with vomiting and dehydration. Bloodwork and chest X-ray were unremarkable except for low prealbumin. She was treated with IV fluids and discharged on promethazine to relieve the nausea and vomiting. Three days later, she presented with intractable vomiting and a five-day history of hiccoughs. She was admitted to the local hospital and transferred the same day to the regional children's hospital. She was discharged eight days later with a biopsy-proven diagnosis of *H. pylori* gastritis and hypertension having had multiple imaging studies, upper and lower endoscopy, and renal and nutrition consultation for 15% weight loss in three months. Neurological exams revealed normal reflexes, strength, tone, coordination, and movement. Discharge medication included triple therapy for *H. pylori*, sucralfate, clonidine patch, and ondansetron.

Six days later, she presented to the emergency room and was transferred back to the regional children's hospital for pancreatitis and hypertension with additional history of fleeting blurry vision and pruritus of the left face. Workup included a neurology consult, brain imaging, EGD with biopsy, and echocardiogram, all unremarkable. Neuropathic facial pain was added to her diagnoses. Treatment continued unchanged.

In follow-up office visit two days later, the patient's mother insisted she was having lower extremity weakness, shaking episodes that looked like seizures, and hypersensitivity of the face and head. An urgent referral to neurology resulted in hospitalization at the regional children's hospital. Neurological exam showed slightly decreased strength of the left upper extremity and bilateral lower extremities, pronator drift, and gait weakness on the left side. Video EEG, EMG, and nerve conduction studies were unrevealing. Wilson's disease was ruled out. The patient was found to have a vitamin D deficiency, normal cortisol, and negative ANA.

Nine days later in follow-up with the primary care provider, tremors were witnessed and the patient had intense pain of the bilateral upper extremities, chest, and low back. Urgent referral to pediatric neurology resulted in an order for MRI of the whole spine with and without contrast which was performed eight days later. The next day, the radiology results were described to the patient (increased signal in the medulla oblongata, between C2 and C5, and possible diagnosis of syringomyelia). Three days later she saw a pediatric neurosurgeon who suspected a multilevel spinal cord tumor and referred her to a tertiary care children's hospital department of neurosurgery. Due to difficulty scheduling an outpatient consultation, the patient presented to the emergency room nine days later and was admitted for a possible multilevel spinal cord tumor.

5. Outcome

At the tertiary care children's hospital, CSF from lumbar puncture was NMO positive with 18 WBC, 3 RBC, gram stain and culture negative, IgG index 0.6, oligoclonal bands negative, ACE 1.1, and NMDA receptor antibody negative. MRI of the cervical spine revealed confluent ill-defined, partly enhancing, abnormal intramedullary signal from the pontomedullary junction through the lower cervical cord with no optic nerve abnormality (no syringomyelia or spinal cord tumor). She was also diagnosed with extensive cervical myelopathy and dystonia. She was started on carbamazepine, two days of IV IG, and five days of IV methylprednisone and discharged on a prednisone taper.

Eight days later she followed up with pediatric neurology and started mycophenolate with the goal of a 1000 mg BID. She was noted to have Secondary Paroxysmal Kinesigenic Dyskinesia (PKD).

Six weeks later in a follow-up with her primary care physician, she had gained 34 pounds and was doing well on mycophenolate, carbamazepine, and prednisone.

6. Patient Perspective

Mother's perspective: I knew something was wrong with my daughter. It was frustrating to have to ask for testing. I am glad that we finally got a diagnosis. Now my daughter is much better.

7. Discussion

Physicians involved in the management of this patient were diligent in efforts to reveal the underlying cause of intractable nausea and vomiting. Several factors contributed to the difficulty of determining the correct underlying diagnosis. (1) Nausea and vomiting were the presenting problem for one month. (2) The patient's neurological symptoms presented late and were vague and diffuse with only subtle findings on physical exam. While her mother reported "shaking spells," the tremors observed appeared to be a stress response. (3) The normal CT and MRI of the brain were falsely reassuring that a demyelinating disorder or other neurological disease was not the underlying cause. (4) The patient developed neck pain late in the course of her illness. The combination of tremors, paresthesias, nonspecific muscle tenderness, and weakness led to whole spine MRI. The cervical spine MRI revealed the abnormal findings which allowed subsequent diagnosis.

This patient's diagnostic workup also demonstrates a critical point about interpretation of abnormal spinal cord images: a false diagnosis of spinal cord tumor can result in unnecessary biopsy of the spinal cord. Fortunately, the neurosurgeon referred the patient to a tertiary care setting where further evaluation resulted in the correct diagnosis and treatment.

Neuromyelitis optica (NMO) is an uncommon disease syndrome of the central nervous system (CNS) that affects the optic nerves and spinal cord. Individuals with NMO develop optic neuritis (pain in the eye and vision loss) and transverse myelitis (weakness, numbness, and sometimes paralysis of the arms and legs), along with sensory disturbances and loss of bladder and bowel control [1–5].

NMO is distinguished from multiple sclerosis by positive serum autoantibody NMO-IgG, which targets aquaporin 4 [6–11]. Over the last nine years, the aquaporin 4 serum test has allowed identification of a wider spectrum of clinical and radiological characteristics associated with NMO.

In 2006 [3], diagnostic criteria were developed for a related clinical syndrome, NMOSD (NMO Spectrum Disorder). This requires NMO-IgG seropositive status in association with a limited form of NMO or a "signature clinical syndrome," such as intractable nausea, vomiting, or hiccoughs [5, 12, 13].

This patient demonstrates several typical findings of NMO, presented here to encourage clinicians to identify this unusual constellation of symptoms. NMO should be considered in the differential for intractable nausea and vomiting [13]. Analysis of a multicenter study by Mealy et al. [14] provides the best current characteristics of patients with NMO and NMOSD. This study examined 187 patients who were diagnosed with NMO or NMODS at three nationally known medical centers distributed across the US.

Our patient shares several characteristics with patients in the multicenter study. As in other autoimmune disorders, females predominate (6.5 : 1) [14]. African Americans were overrepresented at 37% [14], while they represent only 13.2% of the US population [15]. Additionally, of those patients in the study with brain stem lesions (n = 30/187), 80% (n = 24/30) were of African descent [14]. The disproportionate prevalence of NMO in African Americans and their increased incidence of brain stem lesions deserve further study. However, while our patient was only 17, the median age of onset in the study group was 40 years (range: 3–81) [14].

Other common manifestations of NMO were also noted in this patient [5]. For example, most patients with transverse myelitis due to NMO have extensive longitudinal involvement ($\geq$3 vertebral segments), as did our patient. Additionally there are reported cases of generalized pruritus early in the disease [9, 16, 17]; this patient had focal pruritus of the left cheek which became hyperpigmented due to inflammation and scratching. This was the only clue to the itching she was experiencing. This patient also developed hypertension.

NMO has yet to receive funding for a national multicenter consortium; however, a five-year multicenter analysis in 2012 [14] revealed several key features of the disease that this patient demonstrates. Pediatricians and other primary care providers should be sensitized to the unusual presenting symptoms of NMO to optimize early detection and treatment. Early detection and treatment seem to improve prognosis and reduce relapse rate.

Conflict of Interests

The authors declare that there is no conflict of interests regarding the publication of this paper.

References

[1] Office of Communications and Public Liaison, National Institute of Neurological Disorders and Stroke, and National Institutes of Health, *NINDS Neuromyelitis Optica Information Page*, 2015, http://www.ninds.nih.gov/disorders/neuromyelitis_optica/neuromyelitis_optica.htm.

[2] D. M. Wingerchuk, W. F. Hogancamp, P. C. O'Brien, and B. G. Weinshenker, "The clinical course of neuromyelitis optica (devic's syndrome)," *Neurology*, vol. 53, no. 5, pp. 1107–1114, 1999.

[3] D. M. Wingerchuk, V. A. Lennon, S. J. Pittock, C. F. Lucchinetti, and B. G. Weinshenker, "Revised diagnostic criteria for neuromyelitis optica," *Neurology*, vol. 66, no. 10, pp. 1485–1489, 2006.

[4] M. A. Lana-Peixoto, "Devic's neuromyelitis optica: a critical review," *Arquivos de Neuro-Psiquiatria*, vol. 66, no. 1, pp. 120–138, 2008.

[5] M. Matiello, A. Jacob, D. M. Wingerchuk, and B. G. Weinshenker, "Neuromyelitis optica," *Current Opinion in Neurology*, vol. 20, no. 3, pp. 255–260, 2007.

[6] B. G. Weinshenker and D. M. Wingerchuk, "The two faces of neuromyelitis optica," *Neurology*, vol. 82, no. 6, pp. 466–467, 2014.

[7] S. L. Galetta and J. Bennett, "Neuromyelitis optica is a variant of multiple sclerosis," *Archives of Neurology*, vol. 64, no. 6, pp. 901–903, 2007.

[8] D. M. Wingerchuk, V. A. Lennon, C. F. Lucchinetti, S. J. Pittock, and B. G. Weinshenker, "The spectrum of neuromyelitis optica," *Lancet Neurology*, vol. 6, no. 9, pp. 805–815, 2007.

[9] M. Muto, M. Mori, Y. Sato et al., "Current symptomatology in multiple sclerosis and neuromyelitis optica," *European Journal of Neurology*, vol. 22, no. 2, pp. 299–304, 2015.

[10] P. V. A. Lennon, D. M. Wingerchuk, T. J. Kryzer et al., "A serum autoantibody marker of neuromyelitis optica: distinction from multiple sclerosis," *The Lancet*, vol. 364, no. 9451, pp. 2106–2112, 2004.

[11] P. Huppke, M. Blüthner, O. Bauer et al., "Neuromyelitis optica and NMO-IgG in European pediatric patients," *Neurology*, vol. 75, no. 19, pp. 1740–1744, 2010.

[12] C. Trebst, S. Jarius, A. Berthele et al., "Update on the diagnosis and treatment of neuromyelitis optica: recommendations of the Neuromyelitis Optica Study Group (NEMOS)," *Journal of Neurology*, vol. 261, no. 1, pp. 1–16, 2014.

[13] M. Apiwattanakul, B. F. Popescu, M. Matiello et al., "Intractable vomiting as the initial presentation of neuromyelitis optica," *Annals of Neurology*, vol. 68, no. 5, pp. 757–761, 2010.

[14] M. A. Mealy, D. M. Wingerchuk, B. M. Greenberg, and M. Levy, "Epidemiology of neuromyelitis optica in the United States: a multicenter analysis," *Archives of Neurology*, vol. 69, no. 9, pp. 1176–1180, 2012.

[15] Centers for Disease Control and Prevention, "Minority health: Black and African American populations," 2015, http://www.cdc.gov/minorityhealth/populations/REMP/black.html.

[16] R. Govindarajan and E. Salgado, "What is the true clinicopathologic spectrum of neuromyelitis optica?" *JAMA Neurology*, vol. 70, no. 2, pp. 272–273, 2013.

[17] L. Elsone, T. Townsend, K. Mutch et al., "Neuropathic pruritus (itch) in neuromyelitis optica," *Multiple Sclerosis*, vol. 19, no. 4, pp. 475–479, 2013.

37

Goldenhar Syndrome Associated with Extensive Arterial Malformations

Renee Frances Modica, L. Daphna Yasova Barbeau, Jennifer Co-Vu, Richard D. Beegle, and Charles A. Williams

University of Florida, Gainesville, FL, USA

Correspondence should be addressed to Renee Frances Modica; modicar@peds.ufl.edu

Academic Editor: Ozgur Cogulu

Goldenhar Syndrome is characterized by craniofacial, ocular and vertebral defects secondary to abnormal development of the 1st and 2nd branchial arches and vertebrae. Other findings include cardiac and vascular abnormalities. Though these associations are known, the specific anomalies are not well defined. We present a 7-month-old infant with intermittent respiratory distress that did not improve with respiratory interventions. Echocardiogram suggested a double aortic arch. Cardiac CT angiogram confirmed a right arch and aberrant, stenotic left subclavian artery, dilation of the main pulmonary artery, and agenesis of the left thyroid lobe. Repeat echocardiograms were concerning for severely dilated coronary arteries. Given dilation, a rheumatologic workup ensued, only identifying few weakly positive autoantibodies. Further imaging demonstrated narrowing of the aorta below the renal arteries and extending into the common iliac arteries and proximal femoral arteries. Given a physical exam devoid of rheumatologic findings, only weakly positive autoantibodies, normal inflammatory markers, and presence of the coronary artery dilation, the peripheral artery narrowings were not thought to be vasculitic. This case illustrates the need to identify definitive anomalies related to Goldenhar Syndrome. Although this infant's presentation is rare, recognition of specific vascular findings will help differentiate Goldenhar Syndrome from other disease processes.

1. Introduction

Goldenhar Syndrome (GS) or oculo-auricular-vertebral dysplasia (OAVD) is a rare condition characterized by typical ocular and auricular malformations. Associated findings may include cardiac and vascular anomalies. We present a 7-month-old infant with GS who had extensive vascular findings including internal carotid artery (ICA) agenesis, right aortic arch, and vascular ring, as well as coronary artery dilation and narrowing of the infrarenal aorta, common iliacs, and proximal femoral arteries. This is the first case report of an infant with GS with the novel findings of coronary artery dilation and narrowing of peripheral arteries, which may be confused with infantile vasculitis.

2. Case Report

This is a 7-month-old African American male born from a nonconsanguineous pregnancy to a 17-year-old primigravida who was group B strep and chlamydia positive and had spontaneous rupture of membranes. Pregnancy was remarkable for polyhydramnios and preterm labor resulting in premature SVD at 35 weeks' gestation. There was no medication or known teratogenic exposures or illnesses during pregnancy. At delivery, heart rate was initially 60 but improved with positive pressure ventilation. APGARs were 3, 8, and 9 at 1, 5, and 10 minutes, respectively.

The patient's family history was negative for any known birth defects. Both parents had normal craniofacial development. This is the only child from this couple but there are five normal paternal 1/2 siblings. The infant was transferred to our institution for evaluation of respiratory distress and congenital malformations. The newborn examination revealed left hemifacial microsomia, absence of left pinna, and difficulty opening the left eye raising concern for palsy. The right ear was normal as well as the cervical region without masses or sinuses. There was asymmetric crying faces; however, eyes were normal without epibulbar dermoids or coloboma

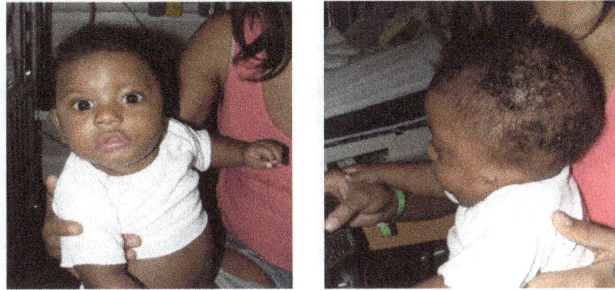

FIGURE 1: Patient with GS at 8 months of life with features of left hemifacial microsomia and left anotia.

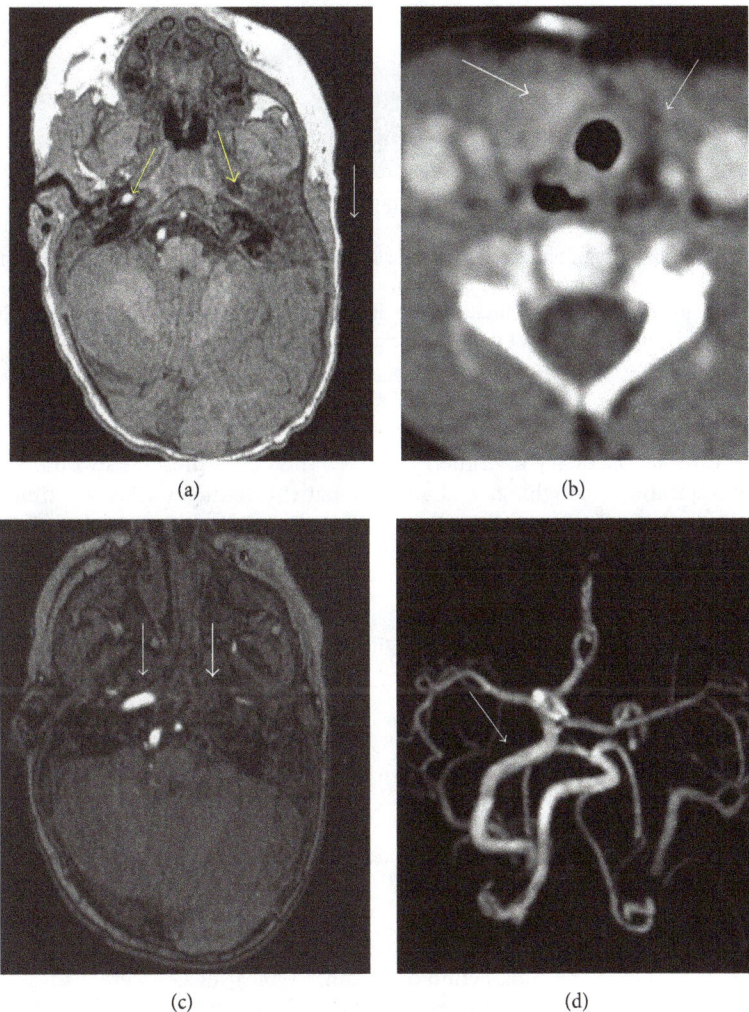

(a)

(b)

(c)

(d)

FIGURE 2: (a) Axial T1 weighted MR of the brain without contrast through the level of the external auditory canals demonstrates absence of the left external ear and external auditory canal (thin white arrow). There is also absence of the left internal carotid artery (thick yellow arrow). The right internal carotid artery is shown for comparison (thin yellow arrow). (b) Axial postcontrast CT of the neck at the level of the thyroid gland shows a normal right thyroid lobe (thick white arrow) with absence of the left thyroid lobe (thin white arrow). (c) Axial noncontrast time of flight MRA of the brain demonstrates a normal right internal carotid artery at its petrous segment (thin white arrow). There is absence of the left internal carotid artery (thick white arrow). (d) Three-dimensional reformation of the MRA of the brain demonstrates a normal right internal carotid artery (thin white arrow). The left internal carotid artery is absent.

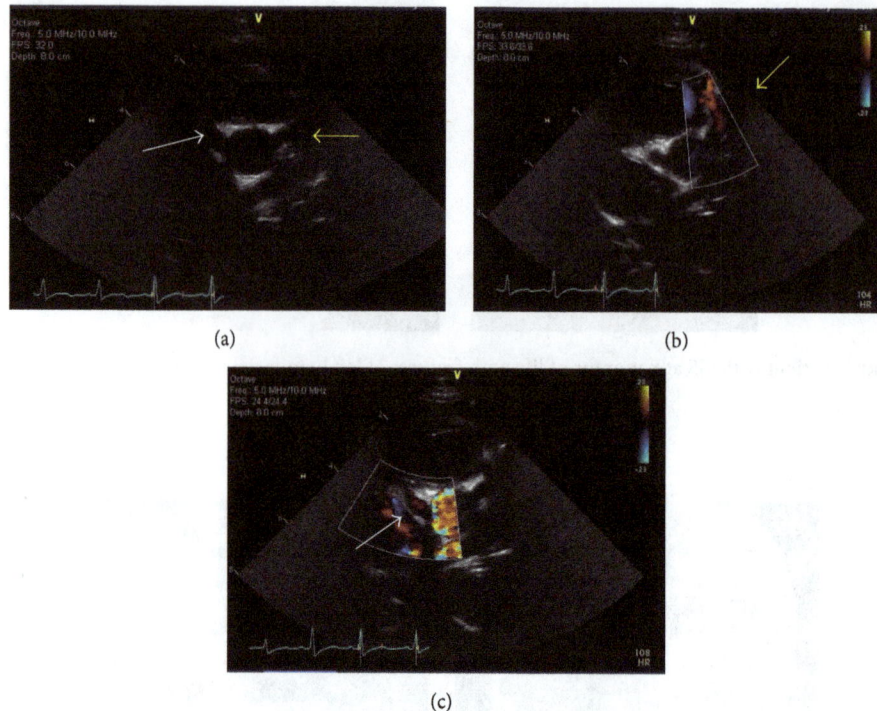

FIGURE 3: Presurgical transthoracic echocardiographic images of the right and left coronary arteries. (a) 2D transthoracic echocardiographic coronary images prior to cardiac surgery demonstrate dilated proximal right coronary artery (white arrow) and left main coronary artery (yellow arrow). (b) 2D and color Doppler transthoracic image of the dilated left main and left anterior descending coronary arteries (yellow arrow). (c) 2D and color Doppler transthoracic image of the dilated right coronary artery (white arrow).

of the eyelids. There was no obvious maxillary asymmetry. He had noisy upper airway respirations, coughing, and an abnormal cry reflecting tracheomalacia. The extremities had normal range of motion, joint, and muscle development without finger, toe, or nail abnormalities. Chest, abdomen, genitalia, and sacral areas appeared normal and the skin had no hemangiomas or birthmarks.

Bone conduction ABR was normal for each ear as well as normal air conduction testing of the right ear; however air conduction testing could not be performed in the left ear, given atresia of the external ear canal. He was also noted to have a soft 1/6 systolic murmur. An echocardiogram suggested a double aortic arch with a dominant right arch and mild branch pulmonary stenosis. A gated cardiac CT angiogram confirmed a right arch and an aberrant left subclavian artery that was markedly stenotic, dilation of the distal main pulmonary artery, and agenesis of the left thyroid lobe. Neonatal MRI of the brain demonstrated subarachnoid blood products but the brain was anatomically normal. Ophthalmological exam demonstrated findings consistent with retinopathy of prematurity.

Initial work-up by genetics showed a normal chromosome single nucleotide polymorphism (SNP) microarray, normal abdominal ultrasound, and babygram without evidence of spinal malformation or other bony abnormalities. Follow-up with genetics was recommended to monitor for growth and development; however family failed to present for outpatient appointments.

The infant presented to the emergency department and inpatient setting numerous times within the first several months of life with complaints of noisy breathing, stridor, and respiratory distress. He often required admission with viral illness that he acquired within the first year of life. During one admission, at age 7 months, he underwent bronchoscopy and was noted to have laryngotracheomalacia with dynamic collapse of the mid trachea, extrinsic compression of the mid trachea, and mild bronchomalacia of the left mainstem bronchus.

He was reevaluated by genetics at 8 months of age. He had anotia on the left with only a nubbin of tissue present, without pits or accessory tags (Figure 1). A repeat MRI of the brain (Figure 2) demonstrated complete absence of the auricle and external auditory canal, and dysmorphic incus and malleus within the internal ear. Unilateral and ipsilateral absence of the left internal carotid artery with absence of the carotid canal typical of GS were also noted. MRI of the head and neck also confirmed left thyroid agenesis and absence versus hypoplasia of the left trigeminal nerve.

From a cardiovascular standpoint, at 8 months of age, two follow-up echocardiograms showed severely dilated right and left coronary artery systems in addition to previously identified cardiac anomalies. No pericardial effusion was seen on either echo. The proximal right coronary artery measured 0.3–0.4 cm (Z-scores 4.98–9.3). The left main coronary artery diameters were 0.38 cm–0.43 cm (Z-scores of 6.14–6.97) (Figure 3). Follow-up CT angiogram of the chest

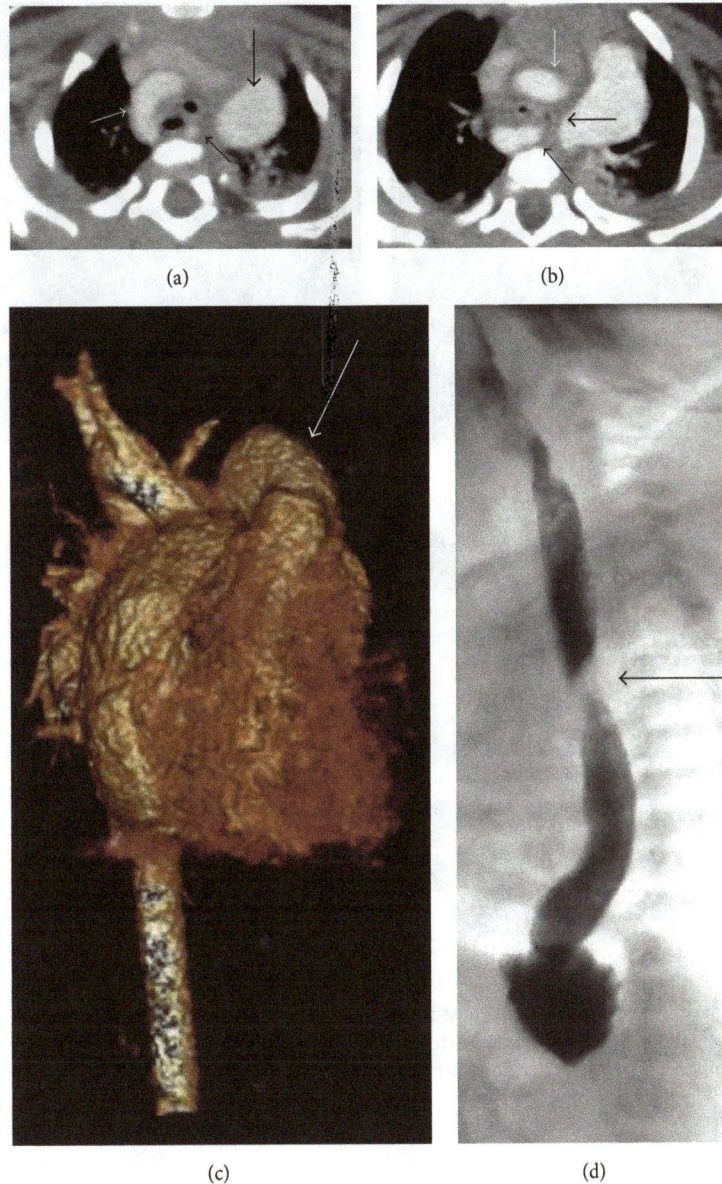

FIGURE 4: (a) Axial postcontrast CTA of the chest demonstrates a right aortic arch (white arrow). The aberrant left subclavian artery is seen extending posterior to the esophagus (thin black arrow) which helps form the complete vascular ring. The pulmonary artery was enlarged in this patient (thick black arrow). (b) Axial postcontrast CTA of the chest at a slice inferior to (a) demonstrates the ascending aorta projecting to the right (white arrow) and the aberrant left subclavian artery arising from the descending aorta and traveling posterior to the esophagus (thin black arrow). The complete vascular ring causes mass effect and narrowing of the esophagus and trachea (thick black arrow). (c) 3D surface rendered reformation of the CTA of the chest viewed in the anteroposterior dimension clearly demonstrates the right aortic arch (thick white arrow). (d) Fluoroscopic image of a barium esophagram demonstrates mass effect on the posterior esophagus (thick black arrow) created by the aberrant left subclavian artery.

(Figures 4 and 5) confirmed right aortic arch with stenotic and aberrant left subclavian artery forming a complete vascular ring compressing the lower esophagus. There were diminutive proximal right and left bronchi, "crisscrossed" branch pattern of the pulmonary arteries (the left pulmonary artery arises from the main pulmonary artery and more superiorly than the right pulmonary artery). The right and left coronary arteries are diffusely dilated with normal origins and without fistula.

Given his dilated coronary arteries, pediatric rheumatology was consulted to evaluate for vasculitic disease. No historical or physical findings for Kawasaki's disease, Lupus, or other vasculitic disorders were noted including lack of fever, lymphadenopathy, hepatosplenomegaly, edema, rash, arthritis, asymmetric pulses, mucocutaneous findings, nailbed telangiectasia, digital ulcers, Raynaud's phenomenon, bruits, or ocular injection. However, given the lack of explanation for his coronary artery dilation,

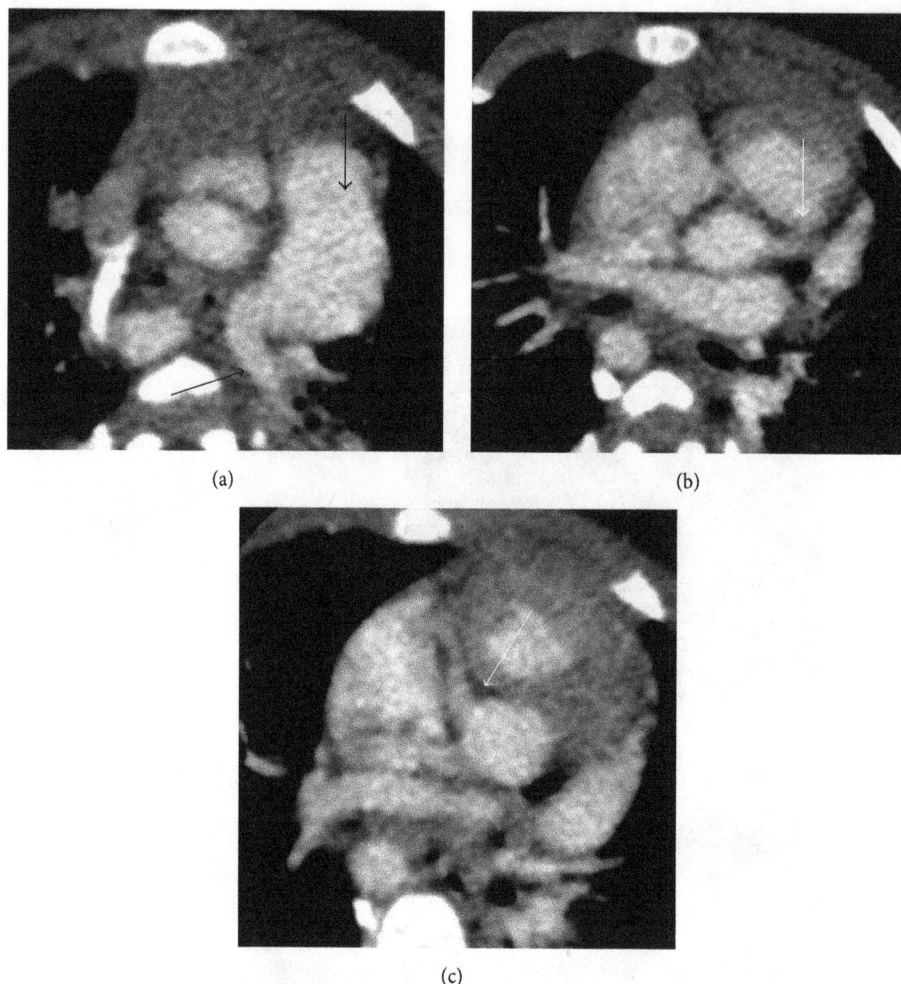

(a)

(b)

(c)

FIGURE 5: Multiple slices from a postcontrast CTA of the chest from superior to inferior demonstrate enlargement of the pulmonary artery (thick black arrow) and crisscross pattern of the pulmonary arteries (thin black arrow). There is dilatation of the origins of the left coronary artery (thick white arrow) and right coronary artery (thin white arrow).

further work-up was recommended. Notably, he was found to have weakly positive ANA (1 : 40, speckled) and weakly positive Smith antibody (26 units) on autoimmune testing. His other autoantibody screening demonstrated negative P-ANCA, C-ANCA, dsDNA, SM-RNP antibody, SS-A and SS-B, and anti-cardiolipins IgG and IgM. His von willebrand antigen, DRVVT, PT, PTT, CRP, ESR, C3, C4, and quantitative immunoglobulins were all normal. MRA of the abdomen and pelvis (Figure 6) was performed and demonstrated symmetric narrowing without beading or inflammation of the aorta below the renal arteries and extending into the common iliac arteries and proximal femoral arteries. Upper and lower extremity deep venous ultrasounds were also found to be normal. Upon retrospective review of his neonatal echocardiogram he did have dilated coronary arteries at birth. Given the lack of physical exam features for rheumatic disease, only weakly positive autoantibodies, normal inflammatory markers, and congenital presence of the coronary artery dilation, the peripheral artery narrowing were not thought to be vasculitic in nature.

The infant had repair of the vascular ring at 9 months of age without complications however; he has continued to demonstrate stridor at baseline, likely from his laryngotracheomalacia. Postsurgical echocardiograms continued to show dilation of his coronary arteries. The repeat right coronary artery diameters by echo were 0.28–0.33 cm (Z-scores of 4.47–5.94) and the left middle coronary artery diameters were 0.35 cm–0.39 cm (Z-scores 4.52–5.47), which are similar to his previous studies (Figure 7).

3. Discussion

GS is generally thought to be due to a developmental abnormality of 1st and 2nd branchial arches and vertebral bodies resulting in the triad of craniofacial microsomia and ocular and vertebral abnormalities. Given this typical triad, it has also become known as oculo-auriculo-vertebral dysplasia (OAVD) [1]. The diagnosis of this condition is mostly based on these characteristic clinical findings but supportive radiologic and laboratory results can be helpful. Ophthalmologic

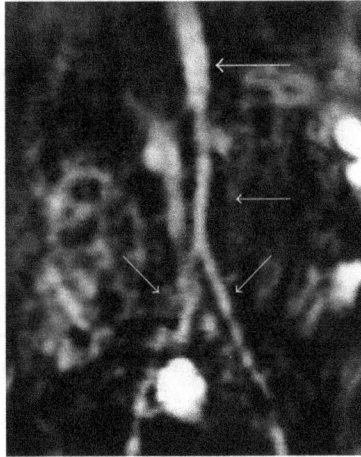

FIGURE 6: Coronal view of a postcontrast MRA of the abdomen demonstrates normal caliber of the abdominal aorta above the renal arteries (thick white arrow). There is symmetric narrowing of the abdominal aorta below the level of the renal arteries extending into the iliac arteries (thin white arrows). Of note, the beaded appearance of the iliac arteries is artifactual.

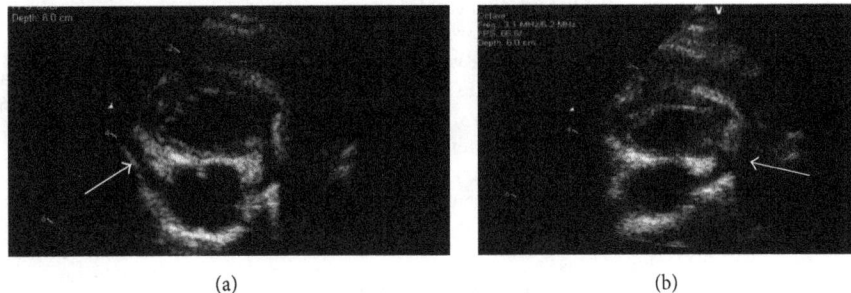

(a)   (b)

FIGURE 7: Postsurgical transthoracic echocardiographic images of the right and left coronary arteries. (a) 2D and color Doppler transthoracic image of the persistently dilated right coronary artery (white arrow). (b) 2D and color Doppler transthoracic image of the persistently dilated left main coronary artery (yellow arrow).

and otorhinolaryngologic examinations are also important [12]. GS occurs in conjunction with cardiac and vascular anomalies although no single cardiac or vascular anomaly is characteristic. Tetralogy of Fallot (TOF) and ventricular septal defects (VSD) are the most common cardiac anomalies reported and agenesis of the internal carotid artery (ICA) is one of the more common vascular anomalies [2]. ICA agenesis ipsilateral to the hemifacial microsomia is more common than contralateral [6].

Despite being classically described as a craniofacial disorder involving bilateral or hemifacial underdevelopment and ocular changes, other less proximate abnormalities have been reported since its initial description. These include other organ systems such as cardiopulmonary [2–5, 7], vascular [2–6], and renal and genitourinary abnormalities [5, 9–11] (Table 1).

A literature review of GS syndrome does report unilateral ICA findings as well as vascular ring, but, to our knowledge, there are no reports of GS with such extensive arterial abnormalities as described in this infant [5, 6]. Due to the presence of the associated other cardiac abnormalities typical of GS as well as the extensive and symmetric nature of these arteriographic findings, we think that the vascular changes

in our patient are probably part of the GS disorder. In our case there was no correlation of the laterality of the vascular findings to the facial deformities, which has been reported in other less typical findings of GS. It is likely that patients with GS may have peripheral vascular changes but MRAs have not been routinely ordered on these patients due to lack of clinical need or suspicion. Of note, Rad had reported one case of bilateral renal artery stenosis that was limited without extension distally [5].

In spite of our patient's extensive findings of abnormal vasculature, his prenatal exam only demonstrated slight murmur. Otherwise, his pulses were normal and vascular exam was without bruits. The MRA was ordered looking for vasculitis due to the presence of dilated coronary arteries without clear explanation such as a fistula. Patients' vasculitides that present in infancy with coronary artery involvement include Polyarteritis Nodosa (PAN), systemic onset juvenile arthritis (SOJIA), and Kawasaki disease (KD) [8, 13–15]. PAN is a non-ANCA associated necrotizing inflammation of the medium sized blood vessels that typically presents with skin ulcerations, arthritis, GI vasculitis, nephritis, and orchitis as well as anemia, thrombocytosis, and elevated inflammatory markers. On angiography, the vasculitis is frequently

TABLE 1

System [ref.]	Description of finding	Findings unique to this case
Auricular [1]	Anotia, microtia, conductive hearing loss, and preauricular skin tags	
Ophthalmologic [1]	Epibulbar dermoids and coloboma of the eyelids	
Facial [1]	Hemifacial microsomia and cleft lip and palate	Severe microtia in the absence of overt hemifacial microsomia
Cardiac [2–5]	(i) Tetralogy of Fallot (ii) Ventricular septal defect (iii) Abnormalities of the aortic arch (hypoplasia, right aortic arch, right circumflex aortic arch, vascular ring, coarctation of the aorta, and aberrant right subclavian artery) (iv) Complete transposition of great arteries (v) Persistent Patent Ductus Arteriosus (isolated or in combination with other anomalies) (vi) Isolation of the left innominate artery with bilateral Patent Ductus Arteriosus (vii) Dextrocardia (viii) Dysplastic valves	Coronary artery dilation
Vascular malformations [2–6]	(i) Agenesis of the internal carotid artery (ii) Hypoplastic external carotid arteries (iii) Persistent left superior vena cava (iv) Isolated left innominate artery (v) Vascular ring (vi) Bilateral renal artery stenosis (vii) Hypoplastic pulmonary artery and its branches (viii) Aberrant right subclavian artery	(i) Narrowing of infrarenal aorta, common iliacs, and proximal femoral arteries (ii) Crisscross branch pattern of the pulmonary arteries
Pulmonary [2, 7, 8]	(i) Incomplete lobulation (ii) Unlobed lungs (iii) Hypoplasia of the lung (typically on the ipsilateral side of the facial anomalies) (iv) Pulmonary hypoplasia and agenesis (v) Laryngotracheomalacia	
Renal [5, 9]	(i) Ectopic and/or fused kidneys (ii) Multicystic kidney	
Genitourinary [9–11]	(i) Ureteropelvic junction obstruction (ii) Ureteral duplication (iii) Vesicoureteral reflux	

segmental and may form microaneurysms. Patients with SOJIA may have dilated coronary arteries but typically have quotidian fevers, salmon colored evanescent migratory rash, lymphadenopathy, hepatosplenomegaly, and inflammatory CBC as well as arthritis. In Kawasaki disease patients typically present with fever, mucocutaneous changes, lymphadenopathy, ocular injection, and dilated coronary arteries with vascular brightness.

GS has associated malformations that have yet to be explained by one theory [16]. Chromosomal abnormalities, vascular pathogenesis that disturbs placental or embryonic blood supply, disturbance of neural crest cells, environmental influences, teratogens, and maternal diabetes have all been suggested as possible etiologies; however, the cause of GS remains unknown [12, 16–20]. Family reports on occasion have suggested autosomal dominant or recessive inheritance [10, 16, 19]. Chromosome disorders or single gene defects have been implicated but not proven as causative of the syndrome.

Affected children typically have normal chromosomes and normal family histories and recurrence in a family is rare. This suggests that GS may be a stochastic, spontaneous event rather than an inherited one. Sometimes teratogens such as thalidomide, primidone, tamoxifen, cocaine, and retinoic acid have been implicated and there does seem to be an increased incidence of GS among the children of Gulf War veterans [19].

With regard to theories of vascular pathogenesis, Ottaviano et al. state that there is a close link between the structures from where the carotid vessels and the ear structures originate [20]. They state that the vascular malformations might derive from a vascular deficiency of the cephalic mesodermal cells with subsequent alteration of the development of the I and II branchial arches. Experiments in lambs from Escobar and Liechty demonstrated a possible link between late gestational vascular disruptions and subsequent craniofacial anomalies [21]. They showed that interruption of the carotid blood flow in the late gestation period produces phenotypic craniofacial anomalies similar to those seen in GS [20, 21]. They suggest that the early lack of blood flow in the cephalic region at the I and II branchial arches could influence the appearance of the OAV spectrum.

It is unclear what led to the more pervasive vascular abnormalities in our patient involving narrowing of the infrarenal aorta, common iliac arteries, and proximal femoral arteries. Although the etiology is unclear, peripheral arterial narrowing and coronary artery dilation may be a new reportable finding associated with GS. These findings may warrant the need for more extensive vascular screening for patients with GS.

Conflict of Interests

The authors declare that there is no conflict of interests regarding the publication of this paper.

References

[1] C. S. Ashokan, A. Sreenivasan, and G. K. Saraswathy, "Goldenhar syndrome—review with case series," Journal of Clinical and Diagnostic Research, vol. 8, no. 4, pp. ZD17–ZD19, 2014.

[2] M. E. M. Pierpont, J. H. Moller, R. J. Gorlin, and J. E. Edwards, "Congenital cardiac, pulmonary, and vascular malformations in oculoauriculovertebral dysplasia," Pediatric Cardiology, vol. 2, no. 4, pp. 297–302, 1982.

[3] J. Morrison, H. C. Mulholland, B. G. Craig, and N. C. Nevin, "Cardiovascular abnormalities in the oculo-auriculo-vertebral spectrum (Goldenhar syndrome)," American Journal of Medical Genetics, vol. 44, no. 4, pp. 425–428, 1992.

[4] C. M. Digilio, F. Calzolari, R. Capolino et al., "Congenital heart defects in patients with oculo-auriculo-vertebral spectrum (Goldenhar syndrome)," American Journal of Medical Genetics Part A, vol. 146, no. 14, pp. 1815–1819, 2008.

[5] E. M. Rad, "Goldenhar syndrome with right circumflex aortic arch, severe coarctation and vascular ring in a twin pregnancy," Annals of Pediatric Cardiology, vol. 7, no. 3, pp. 217–220, 2014.

[6] E. Ventura, F. Ormitti, G. Crisi, and E. Sesenna, "Goldenhar syndrome associated with contralateral agenesis of the internal carotid artery," The Neuroradiology Journal, vol. 27, no. 2, pp. 150–153, 2014.

[7] W. Jacobs, A. Vonk Noordegraaf, R. P. Golding, J. G. van den Aardweg, and P. E. Postmus, "Respiratory complications and Goldenhar syndrome," Breathe, vol. 3, no. 3, pp. 305–308, 2007.

[8] S. Ozen, A. Pistorio, S. M. Iusan et al., "EULAR/PRINTO/PRES criteria for Henoch-Schönlein purpura, childhood polyarteritis nodosa, childhood Wegener granulomatosis and childhood Takayasu arteritis: Ankara 2008. Part II: final classification criteria," Annals of the Rheumatic Diseases, vol. 69, no. 5, pp. 798–806, 2010.

[9] N. D. Soni, D. B. Rathod, and A. D. Nicholson, "Goldenhar syndrome with unusual features," Bombay Hospital Journal, vol. 54, no. 2, p. 334, 2012.

[10] M. Mutanabbi, M. A. Rahman, A. A. Mamun, M. A. Helal, M. B. Billah, and K. A. Islam, "Goldenhar syndrome—a case report," Mymensingh Medical Journal, vol. 23, no. 3, pp. 586–589, 2014.

[11] M. L. Ritchey, J. Norbeck, C. Huang, M. A. Keating, and D. A. Bloom, "Urologic manifestations of Goldenhar syndrome," Urology, vol. 43, no. 1, pp. 88–91, 1994.

[12] A. L. B. Pinheiro, L. C. Araújo, S. B. Oliveira, M. C. C. Sampaio, and A. C. Freitas, "Goldenhar's syndrome—case report," Brazilian Dental Journal, vol. 14, no. 1, pp. 67–70, 2003.

[13] J. H. Stone, "Polyarteritis nodosa," in CURRENT Diagnosis & Treatment Rheumatology, J. B. Imboden, D. B. Hellman, and J. H. Stone, Eds., chapter 35, New York, NY, USA, 3rd edition, 2013.

[14] T. Kawakami, "A review of pediatric vasculitis with a focus on juvenile polyarteritis nodosa," American Journal of Clinical Dermatology, vol. 13, no. 6, pp. 389–398, 2012.

[15] T. L. Canares, D. M. Wahezi, K. M. Farooqi, R. H. Pass, and N. T. Ilowite, "Giant coronary artery aneurysms in juvenile polyarteritis nodosa: a case report," Pediatric Rheumatology, vol. 10, article 1, 2012.

[16] J. K. Hartsfield, "Review of the etiologic heterogeneity of the oculo-auriculo-vertebral spectrum (Hemifacial Microsomia)," Orthodontics & Craniofacial Research, vol. 10, no. 3, pp. 121–128, 2007.

[17] S. Preis, F. Majewski, R. Hantschmann, H. Schumacher, and H. G. Lenard, "Goldenhar, Möbius and hypoglossia-hypodactyly anomalies in a patient: syndrome or association?" European Journal of Pediatrics, vol. 155, no. 5, pp. 385–389, 1996.

[18] T. W. Sadler and S. A. Rasmussen, "Examining the evidence for vascular pathogenesis of selected birth defects," American Journal of Medical Genetics Part A, vol. 152, no. 10, pp. 2426–2436, 2010.

[19] J. K. Sharma, S. K. Pippal, S. K. Raghuvanshi, and A. Shitij, "Goldenhar-Gorlin's syndrome: a case report," Indian Journal of Otolaryngology and Head & Neck Surgery, vol. 58, no. 1, pp. 97–101, 2006.

[20] G. Ottaviano, F. Calzolari, and A. Martini, "Goldenhar syndrome in association with agenesia of the internal carotid artery," International Journal of Pediatric Otorhinolaryngology, vol. 71, no. 3, pp. 509–512, 2007.

[21] L. F. Escobar and E. A. Liechty, "Late gestational vascular disruptions inducing craniofacial anomalies: a fetal lamb model," Journal of Craniofacial Genetics and Developmental Biology, vol. 18, no. 3, pp. 159–163, 1998.

38

Troubling Toys: Rare-Earth Magnet Ingestion in Children Causing Bowel Perforations

Parkash Mandhan, Muthana Alsalihi, Saleem Mammoo, and Mansour J. Ali

Department of Pediatric Surgery, Hamad General Hospital, Hamad Medical Corporation, P.O. Box 3050, Doha, Qatar

Correspondence should be addressed to Parkash Mandhan; kidscisurg@icloud.com

Academic Editor: Vjekoslav Krzelj

Ingestion of foreign bodies in the pediatric population is common and magnet ingestion is known to cause a significant morbidity. Rare-earth magnets are small 3–6 mm diameter spherical powerful magnets that are sold as popular desk toys for adults and were previously found in construction toys in attractive colors for children to play with. We describe 2 young healthy children who ingested rare-earth magnets Buckyballs while playing with these magnetic toys and later presented in emergency with acute abdomen. Abdominal imaging revealed several (26 and 5) pieces of rare-earth magnets in the bowel loops. Emergency surgical exploration revealed multiple gastrointestinal perforations and fistula formation at sites of bowel entrapment in between strong magnets apposed to one another. We highlight the potential dangers of rare-earth magnets in children and suggest increasing public awareness about risks involved in rare-earth magnets ingestion by children to overcome this serious public health issue.

1. Introduction

Ingestion of various types of foreign bodies such as coins, toy parts, jewelry pieces, needles and pins, fish and chicken bones, and button-type batteries is common among children [1]. Reports of magnet ingestion are increasing rapidly globally and over 150 cases have been reported over 22 countries in 2012 [2–4]. Rare-earth magnets, also known as Buckyballs (Maxfield and Oberton, New York, NY), are small 3–6 mm diameter spherical powerful magnets that are sold as popular "desk toys" for adults and were previously found in construction toys in attractive colors for children to play with. Although the US Consumer Product Safety Commission, the American Academy of Pediatrics, and the North American Society for Pediatric Gastroenterology have highlighted growing concerns over these high-powered magnets [4, 5], the current popularity of these magnets as toys and also as body ornamentation for tongue and lip piercing has heightened the safety concern of these magnets in all pediatric age groups resulting in a serious public health issue.

We describe 2 young healthy children who inadvertently ingested multiple pieces of rare-earth magnets while playing with these magnets and developed serious complication requiring emergency surgical intervention. We recommend more public awareness and information to parents and physicians about the potential risks of these magnetic toys.

2. Case 1

A 2-year-old girl was admitted through accident and emergency room with a short history of abdominal pain. The initial clinical and laboratory assessment of patient was unremarkable and a plain X-ray of abdomen showed 26 pieces of rare-earth magnets joined to each other in linear fashion in the left upper quadrant (Figure 1(a)). Further exploration from parents revealed that prior to this she was playing with a box of rare-earth magnets with her 5-year-old brother. The patient was kept under close observation and a repeat abdominal X-ray after 6 hours showed that all pieces of rare-earth magnets still joined together and are present in the left upper part of abdomen. After 12 hours, the patient developed vomiting and showed tachycardia, mild dehydration, and guarding in the midabdomen. Another X-ray of abdomen showed 26 magnetic pieces forming a ring in the left upper abdomen

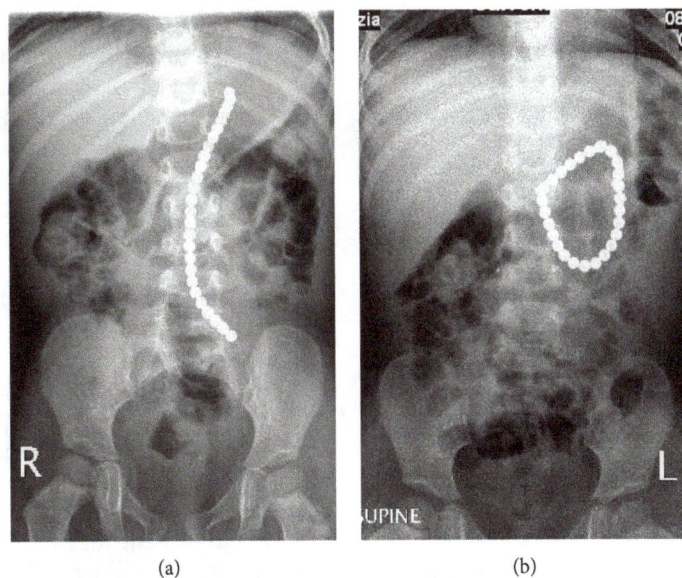

(a)   (b)

FIGURE 1: (a) Plain X-ray of abdomen of 2-year-old girl showing ingested 26 pieces of rare-earth magnets joined together in linear fashion. (b) Repeated plain abdominal X-ray of the same patient after 36 hours showing ingested rare-earth magnets forming a ring in the left upper abdomen with no free air and/or obstructive bowel pattern.

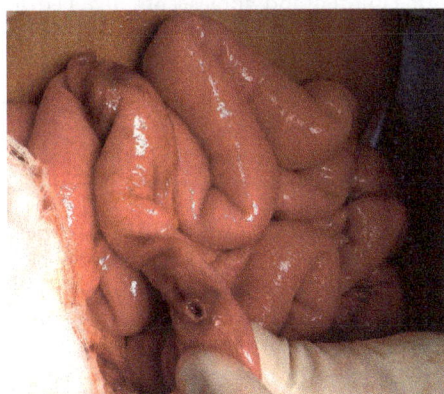

FIGURE 2: Operative findings of the same patient showing loops of jejunum, which were entrapped in between multiple rare-earth magnets resulting in pressure necrosis and bowel perforation.

with no pneumoperitoneum and/or obstructive bowel pattern (Figure 1(b)). After discussion with parents, the child was taken to operating room for laparoscopy and proceeds to remove the magnets. Laparoscopy showed multiple small bowel loops adherent to each other forming a mass in the left upper quadrant. The procedure was converted to open through umbilical port site. On careful examination, it was observed that loops of jejunum are entrapped in between multiple magnetic pieces inside the jejunum resulting in pressure necrosis and perforation of jejunum at two sites (Figure 2). Through this enterotomy site, 14 pieces of magnets were retrieved and the remaining 12 pieces were not palpable in the small and large bowel. A table X-ray showed these missing pieces of magnets in the stomach, which were palpated and retrieved through a gastrostomy. Her postoperative

course was unremarkable and she was reviewed in clinic after 2 weeks. Six months after initial surgery, the patient was brought back to accident and emergency room with symptoms of bowel obstruction, which was confirmed by the radiology images. After adequate resuscitation and a period of observation, the patient was taken to operating room for emergency reexploration of abdomen, which showed multiple adhesions resulting in bowel obstruction requiring adhesiolysis. The patient's postoperative recovery was slow and was discharged after full recovery. She has been reviewed in our follow-up clinic and has remained stable.

3. Case 2

A 4-year-old boy had mild occasional abdominal pain 3 days after ingestion of rare-earth magnets while playing. He was brought to accident and emergency room and his initial examination was unremarkable. A plain X-ray of abdomen showed 5 pieces of rare-earth magnets in the right lower quadrant joined together (Figure 3). The patient was admitted and parents were informed about the risks related to rare-earth magnet ingestion and offered early surgical intervention to retrieve the magnets but the family refused and opted to observe the spontaneous passage. After 24 hours of observation, the parents were counseled again for potential risks and after that the child was taken to operating room where initial laparoscopy revealed adhesive loops of small bowel and a perforation in the distal ileum. The procedure was converted to open through supraumbilical port site and 5 pieces of rare-earth magnets were retrieved through the perforated ileum. Patient's postoperative course was uneventful and he has been reviewed regularly in the follow-up clinic.

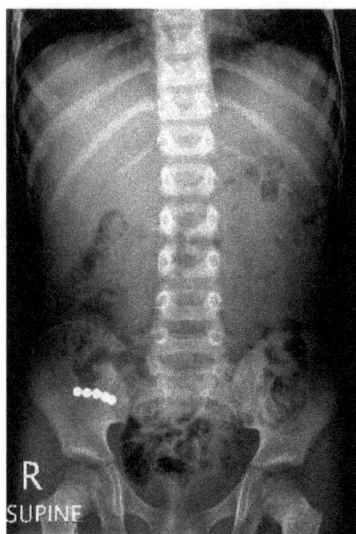

FIGURE 3: Plain X-ray of abdomen of 4-year-old boy showing ingested 5 pieces of rare-earth magnets joined together due to strong magnetic force.

4. Discussion

Multiple magnet ingestion in young children poses a serious health risk [3, 6]. When ingested inadvertently, a single piece of rare-earth magnet is expected to behave like other foreign objects and often observed to pass spontaneously, whereas ingestion of multiple magnet pieces is known to cause potential complications [4]. New generation of powerful rare-earth magnets consists of alloys of neodymium iron boron or samarium cobalt, which results in strong magnetic force. These magnets are capable of attracting each other through up to 6 layers of bowel wall and are strong enough to reposition the intestines in order to meet [7]. In one reported case, a 2-year old died of sepsis before rare-earth magnet ingestion was discovered and treated [8]. In our study, both children developed bowel perforations in a short period of time after ingestion of magnets possibly due to pressure necrosis of trapped bowel in between forceful magnetic attraction of rare-earth magnets. Both children required emergency surgery to remove multiple pieces of magnets. Even though the recovery from initial surgery was smooth in both cases, one patient represented within six months with bowel obstruction requiring second surgery. This highlights that the early intervention to remove multiple pieces of such powerful magnets may not reduce the high risk of complication related to ingestion of rare-earth magnets.

The number of magnets ingested by children has been described from 2 to 5 and only in few cases the incident of ingestion has been reported to be witnessed [6, 9–11]. In our study, one child ingested 26 and other 5 pieces of magnets and parents of both children were not aware of the ingestion. It is anticipated that, due to young age and lack of witness, the time interval between the ingestion and the date of intervention varied, which may have contributed to the perforation and fistula formation. Other contributory factors include the nature of magnets as recently engineered

magnets contain iron, boron, and neodymium powders that are five to 10 times stronger than plain iron magnets [12]. Therefore, the bowel walls that are compressed between these strong magnets nearly disappear resulting in fistula formation, leakage, and peritonitis.

In the past, children with a variety of psychological conditions such as autism, developmental delays, history of pica, schizoid characteristics, behavioral problems, mental retardation, reactive attachment, and anxiety were considered to be at high risk for accidental ingestion of such objects [9]. At present, the incidence of this problem no longer remains confined to these children as both of our patients were well developed with no psychosocial condition. The possible causes for the increase of ingestion of such magnets include easy availability, attractive colors, small size, and making of these magnets along with poor visible risk information on boxes/toys and lack of national warnings. In our patients, the younger patient ingested multiple pieces of rare-earth magnets while her elder sibling was playing with her and the second child owned these magnets and ingested them while playing. A visible and strong readable warning over the package along with release of periodic information about such cases from national and regional consumer product safety authorities in local print and electronic media about the risks for children and adolescents involved in the use of toys/material with high-powered rare-earth magnets will enhance the awareness about this serious public health issue and will significantly contribute to the prevention of such cases.

5. Conclusion

Ingestion of multiple rare-earth magnets leads to serious gastrointestinal morbidity even with early intervention. Concerns regarding magnet ingestion in young children have increased because of the current popularity of new generation high-powered rare-earth magnets, and our two cases highlight the potential hazards and associated gastrointestinal complications of ingestion of such magnets in the young children.

Conflict of Interests

The authors declare that there is no conflict of interests regarding the publication of this paper.

Acknowledgment

The authors gratefully acknowledge the Medical Research Centre, Hamad Medical Corporation, Doha, Qatar, for their support in publishing this paper.

References

[1] M. M. Tavarez, R. A. Saladino, B. A. Gaines, and M. D. Manole, "Prevalence, clinical features and management of pediatric magnetic foreign body ingestions," *The Journal of Emergency Medicine*, vol. 44, no. 1, pp. 261–268, 2013.

[2] J. C. Brown, K. F. Murray, and P. J. Javid, "Hidden attraction: a menacing meal of magnets and batteries," *The Journal of Emergency Medicine*, vol. 43, no. 2, pp. 266–269, 2012.

[3] S. Chandra, G. Hiremath, S. Kim, and B. Enav, "Magnet ingestion in children and teenagers: an emerging health concern for pediatricians and pediatric subspecialists," *Journal of Pediatric Gastroenterology & Nutrition*, vol. 54, no. 6, p. 828, 2012.

[4] A. C. de Roo, M. C. Thompson, T. Chounthirath et al., "Rare-earth magnet ingestion-related injuries among children, 2000–2012," *Clinical Pediatrics*, vol. 52, no. 11, pp. 1006–1013, 2013.

[5] US Consumer Product Safety Commission, "CPSC Warns High-Powered Magnets and Children Make a Deadly Mix," 2011, http://www.cpsc.gov/en/Newsroom/News-Releases/2012/CPSC-Warns-High-Powered-Magnets-and-Children-Make-a-Deadly-Mix/.

[6] D. Gregori, B. Morra, and A. Gulati, "Magnetic FB injuries: an old yet unresolved hazard," *International Journal of Pediatric Otorhinolaryngology*, vol. 76, supplement 1, pp. S42–S48, 2012.

[7] B. E. Wildhaber, C. le Coultre, and B. Genin, "Ingestion of magnets: innocent in solitude, harmful in groups," *Journal of Pediatric Surgery*, vol. 40, no. 10, pp. E33–E35, 2005.

[8] Family Voices: Kenny. Kids in Danger, 2005, http://www.kidsindanger.org/family-voices/kenny/.

[9] A. E. Oestreich, "Worldwide survey of damage from swallowing multiple magnets," *Pediatric Radiology*, vol. 39, no. 2, pp. 142–147, 2009.

[10] B. K. Lee, H. H. Ryu, J. M. Moon, and K. W. Jeung, "Bowel perforations induced by multiple magnet ingestion," *Emergency Medicine Australasia*, vol. 22, no. 2, pp. 189–191, 2010.

[11] H. Naji, D. Isacson, J. F. Svensson, and T. Wester, "Bowel injuries caused by ingestion of multiple magnets in children: a growing hazard," *Pediatric Surgery International*, vol. 28, no. 4, pp. 367–374, 2012.

[12] S. McCormick, P. Brennan, J. Yassa, and R. Shawis, "Children and mini-magnets: an almost fatal attraction," *Emergency Medicine Journal*, vol. 19, no. 1, pp. 71–73, 2002.

39

Acute Peripheral Facial Palsy after Chickenpox: A Rare Association

Helena Ferreira, Ângela Dias, and Andreia Lopes

Departamento de Pediatria, Centro Hospitalar do Alto Ave, Rua dos Cutileiros, Creixomil, 4835-044 Guimarães, Portugal

Correspondence should be addressed to Helena Ferreira; helena-of@hotmail.com

Academic Editor: Piero Pavone

Chickenpox, resulting from primary infection by the varicella-zoster virus, is an exanthematous disease very common during childhood and with good prognosis. However, serious complications, namely, neurological syndromes, may develop during its course, especially in risk groups, including adolescents. Peripheral facial palsy is a rare neurologic complication that has been previously described. *Conclusion.* We report the case of a teenager with peripheral facial palsy as a complication of chickenpox, aiming to increase the awareness of this rare association.

1. Introduction

Varicella-zoster virus (VZV) is a human herpesvirus which leads to the onset of two distinct diseases: varicella (or chickenpox) and herpes zoster (or shingles). Primary VZV infection results in chickenpox, which normally manifests itself as a generalized exanthematous rash. The virus then becomes latent in dorsal root ganglia and can manifest itself later in life as shingles, which is characterized by a painful rash with blisters limited to one or more adjacent sensory dermatomes [1–4]. Generally, chickenpox is a benign and self-limited infection with good prognosis; however, severe complications may arise [3, 5]. The most common complication is bacterial superinfection of the skin, lungs, or bones [3, 6]. Neurological complications develop in up to 0.03% of the cases [4, 7, 8]. The main neurological syndromes are encephalitis, acute cerebellar ataxia, myelitis, and meningitis [2]. Peripheral facial palsy (PFP) is a rare neurologic complication of chickenpox, which may develop five days before to sixteen days after appearance of exanthema [7, 9].

Information about PFP as a complication of chickenpox is scarce and there are no guidelines about its optimal clinical management.

Here, we report a case of PFP following chickenpox and discuss the association between these clinical entities.

2. Case Report

A 15-year-old girl was admitted into the pediatric emergency department with drooping of the left corner of the mouth and inability to close the right eyelid for 3 days.

Her personal and family history were unremarkable.

Two weeks before she had developed a dental pain and underwent antibiotic treatment for 3 days, suspended by self-initiative due to the appearance of fever and an exanthematous rash compatible with chickenpox, she did not undergo acyclovir treatment.

Furthermore, there was no clinical history of associated headache, nausea, vomiting, visual disturbances, neurological focal deficits, muscular strength, sensibility asymmetries, or other symptoms suggestive of an additional central nervous system involvement. Retroauricular pain, hyperacusis, decreased production of tears, or altered taste was also denied. There was no history of previous cold exposure.

The patient was afebrile and her vital signs were within the normal range, namely, her blood pressure which was 110/75 mmHg (below the 90th percentile for gender, age, and height). There were multiple crusted lesions scattered all over the body. She had no vesicular eruption over the external pinna, ear canal, or pharynx. Otoscopy revealed a gray and translucent tympanic membrane in the neutral position. There were no signs of otitis or mastoiditis or evidence of ear trauma. No evidence of dental abscess was found. The ophthalmological examination revealed symmetrical pupillary reflexes, normal eye movements, and preserved convergence. The neurological examination showed asymmetries in the ability to perform eyelid closure and asymmetries in labial movements, which were not evident at rest due to a normal facial symmetry. The observed decreased ability to close the right eyelid and concomitant drooping of the left corner of the mouth were compatible with a right PFP as a neurological complication of chickenpox.

As chickenpox and PFP are two clinical diagnoses and this adolescent had pathognomonic signs and symptoms of chickenpox complicated by PFP, no other serologic or imaging studies were performed.

She was treated with acyclovir (20 mg/kg/dose, 4 times/ day, during 5 days), artificial tears, and physical rehabilitation. During follow-up, a complete recovery of the initial deficits and a restoration of normal functions were registered.

3. Discussion

Chickenpox is a highly infectious acute, febrile, and exanthematous disease, affecting a great percentage of people during their lifetime, with greater incidence during childhood [3]. Because of its characteristic rash and distribution, along with epidemiologic information, the diagnosis is mainly clinical. Laboratory diagnosis is facilitated by the accessibility of the virus in superficial skin lesions but it is only justifiable if clinical doubt exists [3].

Chickenpox has generally a benign course although it can be associated with several complications, depending on immune status, presence of chronic diseases, and age [5]. Neurological complications associated with chickenpox are rather uncommon, being estimated in 1–3 per 10.000 cases [4]. The expected proportion of neurological complications among hospitalized children varies between 13.9% and 20.4% [5]. Encephalitis, acute cerebellar ataxia, myelitis, and meningitis are the most common neurological complications reported [2]. More uncommon are Guillain-Barré syndrome, meningoencephalitis, ventriculitis, optic neuritis, delayed contralateral hemiparesis, peripheral motor neuropathy, cerebral angiitis, Reye's syndrome, and facial palsy [4, 8].

The prevalence of neurological complications of chickenpox is highly variable, and few studies have been published in the pediatric population. A study with sixty cases of children and adults with neurological complications due to chickenpox reported encephalitis in 23.3% of those patients, cerebellar ataxia in 21.7%, meningitis in 8.3%, stroke in 13.3%, and PFP in 8.3% [10]. In a more recent study with pediatric patients only, the main neurological complication was cerebritis in 44.7%, followed by seizures in 22.3% and by meningoencephalitis, meningitis, and encephalitis in 10.5%. PFP was diagnosed in just 5.2% of children [5].

PFP may occur before, during, or after exanthema appearance. This peripheral neuropathy can be isolated or bilateral and can have different degrees of functional impairment [7–9, 11].

The relationship between PFP and chickenpox is neither common nor completely understood. Two possible mechanisms exist: direct nerve lesion due to direct viral toxicity or nerve damage associated with immunologically mediated inflammatory response [11].

Established guidelines for the treatment of varicella-zoster related neurological complications do not exist and therefore the treatment must be individualized for each patient. In the majority of the published reports, the pediatric patients were treated with acyclovir and/or steroids [7–9, 11].

In the present case, given the minimal neurological compromise, the treatment was carried out using oral acyclovir without steroids and artificial tears along with physical rehabilitation. After 5 days of treatment the adolescent had significantly recovered from her previous deficits, which supports the efficacy of the applied therapeutic measures.

Although scarce, the available reports on the prognosis of PFP associated with chickenpox show a good prognosis and 80% of the afflicted patients recover completely even without treatment. Yet, acyclovir and/or steroids might accelerate the expected recovery [8, 9].

Some investigations have been developed to determine the epidemiologic effect of varicella vaccine introduction in vaccination programs. These studies confirm that after the inclusion of this vaccine in the childhood vaccination schedule, the incidence of this disease has diminished drastically, not only in vaccinated individuals but also in the unvaccinated ones, due to herd immunity. The authors have also shown that the rates of hospitalization markedly declined as well as the complicated forms of chickenpox [12, 13]. A countrywide sentinel surveillance system was initiated in Germany after implementation of routine varicella vaccination. In that survey the number of reported varicella cases as well as chickenpox complications decreased by 63% and 81%, respectively, and neurologic complications accounted for only 0.03% of all cases [14].

In Portugal, this vaccine is not included in the national vaccination program. Consequently, the vaccination rate is very low, not being enough to generate herd immunity. Thus, prevalence remains high, and complications continue to emerge. In an attempt to reduce varicella complications, it is essential to vaccinate high-risk groups and to initiate antiviral drugs to those who develop the disease.

In conclusion, VZV can be a causative agent of PFP in the pediatric population. Despite being rare, this neurological complication of chickenpox should be kept in mind. The antiviral treatment should be highlighted as a fundamental therapeutic measure which can reduce the duration of symptoms and avoid possible complications following infection by the VZV.

Abbreviations

Kg: Kilogram
mmHg: Millimeters of mercury
mg: Milligram
PFP: Peripheral facial palsy
VZV: Varicella-zoster virus.

Disclosure

The paper does not contain clinical studies or patient data.

Conflict of Interests

The authors declare that they have no conflict of interests regarding the publication of this paper.

References

[1] M. A. Albrecht, "Clinical features of varicella -zoster virus infection: chickenpox," 2013, http://www.uptodate.com/online.

[2] C. Amlie-Lefond and B. Jubelt, "Neurologic manifestations of varicella zoster virus infections," *Current Neurology and Neuroscience Reports*, vol. 9, no. 6, pp. 430–434, 2009.

[3] A. A. Gershon, "Varicella-zoster virus infections," *Pediatrics in Review*, vol. 29, no. 1, pp. 5–11, 2008.

[4] J. W. Gnann Jr., "Varicella-zoster virus: a typical presentations and unusual complications," *Journal of Infectious Diseases*, vol. 186, no. 1, pp. S91–S98, 2002.

[5] E. Bozzola, A. E. Tozzi, M. Bozzola et al., "Neurological complications of varicella in childhood: case series and a systematic review of the literature," *Vaccine*, vol. 30, no. 39, pp. 5785–5790, 2012.

[6] M. Riaza Gómez, M. de la Torre Espi, S. Mencia Bartolome, J. C. Molina Cabanero, and A. Tamariz-Martel Moreno, "Complications of varicella in children," *Anales Españoles de Pediatría*, vol. 50, pp. 259–262, 1999.

[7] C. Yilmaz and H. Çaksen, "Severe neurological complications of chickenpox: report of four cases," *European Journal of General Medicine*, vol. 2, no. 4, pp. 177–179, 2005.

[8] G. Rama Rao, A. Amareswar, Y. Kishan Kumar, and R. Rani, "Isolated facial palsy in varicella," *Indian Journal of Dermatology, Venereology and Leprology*, vol. 74, no. 3, pp. 261–262, 2008.

[9] E. Ödemis, S. Türkay, A. Tunca, and A. Karadag, "Acute peripheral facial palsy during chickenpox in a child," *Journal of Pediatric Neurology*, vol. 2, no. 4, pp. 245–246, 2004.

[10] H. Shiihara, "Neurological complications of varicella-zoster virus (VZV) infection," *No To Hattatsu*, vol. 25, no. 2, pp. 128–134, 1993.

[11] M. Muñoz-Sellart, C. García-Vidal, S. Martnez-Yelamos, J. Niub, and P. Fernndez-Viladrich, "Peripheral facial palsy after varicella. Report of two cases and review of the literature," *Enfermedades Infecciosas y Microbiologia Clinica*, vol. 28, no. 8, pp. 504–508, 2010.

[12] M. García Cenoz, J. Castilla, J. Chamorro et al., "Impact of universal two-dose vaccination on varicella epidemiology in Navarre, Spain, 2006 to 2012," *Eurosurveillance*, vol. 18, no. 32, 2013.

[13] A. Siedler and U. Arndt, "Impact of the routine varicella vaccination programme on varicella epidemiology in Germany," *Euro Surveillance*, vol. 15, no. 13, 2010.

[14] M. Spackova, M. Muehlen, and A. Siedler, "Complications of varicella after implementation of routine childhood varicella vaccination in Germany," *Pediatric Infectious Disease Journal*, vol. 29, no. 9, pp. 884–886, 2010.

40

Inflammatory Bowel Disease in a Child with Sickle Cell Anemia

Khaled Alqoaer, Mohammed M. Ahmed, and Efteraj S. Alhowaiti

Pediatric Department, Prince Salman North West Armed Forces Hospital, P.O. Box 100, Tabuk 71411, Saudi Arabia

Correspondence should be addressed to Khaled Alqoaer; dralquaer@hotmail.com

Academic Editor: Paul A. Rufo

Sickle cell anemia (SCA) is a chronic haemoglobinopathy that can affect many organs in the body including gastrointestinal tract. However, colonic involvement is very rare and usually in the form of ischemic colitis. We are reporting an 11-year-old Saudi girl with SCA who presented with persistent diarrhea and was found to have inflammaftory bowel disease.

1. Introduction

Homozygous sickle cell anemia (SCA) is an autosomal recessive chronic haemoglobinopathy characterized by abnormal globin chain of hemoglobin (Hb) content of the red blood cells that result in "sickle" shapes, attraction of RBCs to each other, and polymerization when in a low oxygen environment. The RBC polymerization leads to manifestations such as chronic occlusion of blood vessels (vasoocclusion), reduced blood flow to vital organs (ischemia), and alterations of the immune system. The gastrointestinal manifestation of SCA varies [1, 2]. We are reporting a child with SCA who presented with chronic colitis resembling inflammatory bowel disease.

2. The Case

An 11-year-old Black Saudi female with homozygous sickle cell (SS) disease (SCD) presented with chronic diarrhea for more than one-year duration. Her bowel motions were mostly watery but occasionally were mixed with little blood. It was occurring up to six to eight times per day, in moderate volume, and occasionally disturbed her sleep at night. This diarrhea was associated with poor appetite and poor weight gain. She also had a history of urgency and tenesmus most of the time. The patient had history of mild intermittent periumbilical colicky abdominal pain for same duration. She and her parents denied any history of vomiting, abdominal distension, recurrent or persistent fever, joint pain or swelling, skin rash, or mouth ulcers.

The patient has a history of frequent admissions in the past due to vasooclusive and hemolytic crisis and received blood transfusion many times for this reason. Laparoscopic cholecystectomy was done at the age of eight years. She is the second child for young healthy consanguineous parents. One older brother died with sickle cell disease complicated by stroke. She has another two brothers and one sister all alive and well. On physical examination, she looked pale but not jaundiced. She has mild finger clubbing, normal skin examination, and no lymphadenopathy. Her weight was 18 kg and height was 127 cm, both far below the third percentile for her age. Her vital signs were all within normal limits. The perianal examination revealed no abnormalities. The rest of physical examination was unremarkable. Her initial laboratory workup showed white blood count of 19000 cells/cm^2 (85% neutrophils and eosinophils 0%), hemoglobin 7.8 g/dL, and platelets 631000/mm^3 with reticulocyte 10.7%. Her erythrocyte sedimentation rate (ESR) was 60 mm and C-reactive protein was 10 mg/dL. The serum albumin was low (26 g/L) and total protein was 63 g/L. All serum electrolytes, urea, and creatinine were within normal limits. Serum immunoglobulins (IgG, IgA, and IgM) were normal. Screening for celiac disease using serum antiendomysial antibodies test was negative. Liver enzymes and bilirubin were within normal limits. Several stool analyses and cultures were negative for virus, ova, or parasite and were negative for *Clostridium difficile* cytotoxin as well. The serology tests for human immunodeficiency virus were negative. Barium meal and follow through study revealed a mild irregularity with nodular hypertrophy of the terminal ileum while gastrografin

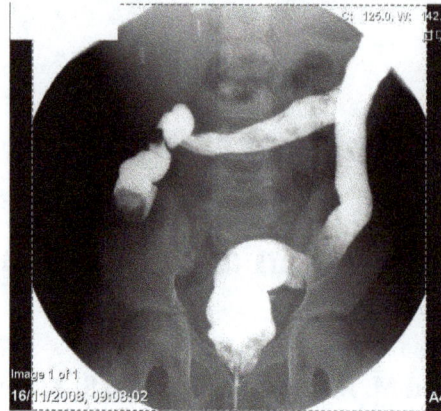

FIGURE 1: Gastrografin enema examination demonstrates loss of haustral folds in the colon with small ulcerations.

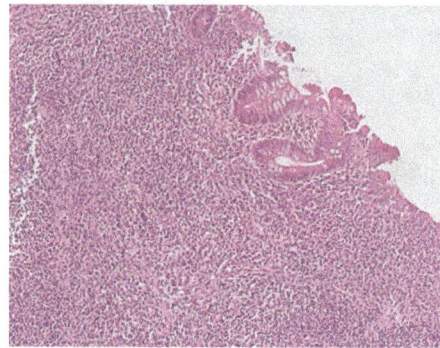

FIGURE 2: Ileal biopsy showed villus flattening with heavy infiltration of admixture of inflammatory cells rich in plasma cells.

enema (Figure 1) showed mucosal thickening of the entire colon with loss of haustral folds. The patient underwent upper endoscopic and colonoscopic examinations. Upper gastrointestinal endoscopy and histology were normal. Colonoscopy revealed nodular terminal ileum with otherwise normal mucosa. The entire colon was abnormal and had a picture of pancolitis in form of friable and edematous mucosa with diffuse erythema and decreased vascular markings. Few scattered pseudopolyps could be seen in the colon as well. The biopsies from terminal ileum (Figure 2) showed scattered hyperplastic lymphoid follicles with germinal centers. One fragment shows complete villus flattening with heavy infiltration of admixture of inflammatory cells rich in plasma cells. Colonic biopsies (Figure 3) showed focally ulcerated colonic mucosa replaced by fibroblastic and inflammatory granulation tissue. The lamina propria contained focally branched and distorted glands and heavy infiltration by lymphocytes, plasma cells, and eosinophils with the presence of scattered lymphoid follicles. The muscularis mucosa was thickened and inflamed. No granuloma could be seen at any level.

The patient was managed as an inflammatory bowel disease case (indeterminate type). She was started initially on oral sulfasalazine (1.5 g daily) but oral corticosteroid (prednisolone 40 mg daily) had to be added later on because of poor response. The patient started to improve and show signs of remission. She did well after that with no more diarrhea or abdominal pain and started to have better appetite. Her ESR went down to 5 mm and her serum albumin started to rise up. Prednisolone dose was tapered till discontinued. She was kept on the same dose of sulfasalazine as maintenance therapy. She was seen regularly in the clinic for more than six months with no significant relapse so far.

3. Discussion

SCA is a systemic disease that can affect many organs in the body including gastrointestinal tract. However, colonic involvement is very rare. Our patient represents a rare combination of SCA and chronic colitis. Review of the literature revealed only a single report of such association. Terry et al. [3] described four patients with SCA (one child) who presented with persistent diarrhea and chronic colitis. Those patients were diagnosed later on with ulcerative colitis based on clinical, radiological, and histopathological findings. The differential diagnosis of colitis in SCA patients should include ischemic and infectious colitis. In our patient, no organism could be isolated despite multiple cultures and examination of stool, blood, and urine. Furthermore, the histopathological and radiological findings were not supporting this possibility. Ischemic colitis had been reported in the literature emphasizing the liability of SCA patient to occlusion of blood vessels (vasoocclusion) and ischemia. However, ischemic colitis is not that common among sicklers and only eight cases were

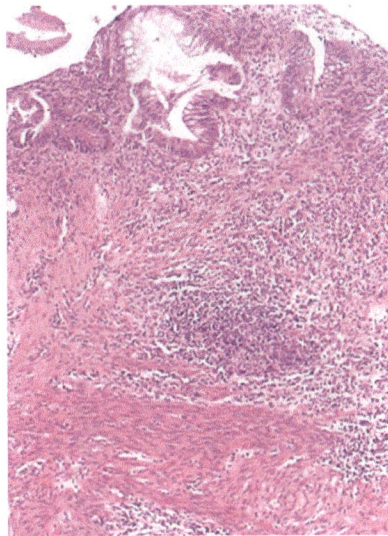

FIGURE 3: Colonic biopsy showed focally branched and distorted glands and heavy infiltration by lymphocytes, plasma cells, and eosinophils. The muscularis mucosa is thickened and inflamed.

reported so far [2, 4–10]. This is likely because the colon has an abundant collateral blood supply and low oxygen extraction. The bowel can tolerate up to a 75% reduction of mesenteric blood flow for up to 12 hours with no ischemic changes [11].

The typical features of ischemic colitis include acute abdominal pain that persist despite conservative management associated with colonic changes in the form of segmental distribution of disease, abrupt transition between injured and uninjured mucosa, and rectal sparing. Colonic biopsies in several cases clearly demonstrated sickling within the vasculature of the diseased colonic segment [8].

Our patient presented with long standing chronic diarrhea which is unusual for ischemic colitis. In addition, the involvement of the entire colon that was seen on radiological, endoscopic, and histopathological evaluation makes ischemic colitis less likely. We do believe that the whole picture would be explained by inflammatory bowel disease especially after marked improvement with immunomodulation therapy. However, because inflammatory bowel disease is less common in children—particularly among Africans and Arabs—[12–14] and in addition to the complexity of SCA, further studies are needed to evaluate and explain more the relationship between these two disorders.

Conflict of Interests

The authors declare that there is no conflict of interests regarding the publication of this paper.

References

[1] E. C. Ebert, M. Nagar, and K. D. Hagspiel, "Gastrointestinal and Hepatic Complications of Sickle Cell Disease," *Clinical Gastroenterology and Hepatology*, vol. 8, no. 6, pp. 483–489, 2010.

[2] C. L. Stewart and G. E. Ménard, "Sickle cell-induced ischemic colitis," *Journal of the National Medical Association*, vol. 101, no. 7, pp. 726–728, 2009.

[3] S. I. Terry, A. Rajendran, B. Hanchard, and G. R. Serjeant, "Ulcerative colitis in sickle cell disease," *Journal of Clinical Gastroenterology*, vol. 9, no. 1, pp. 55–57, 1987.

[4] T. P. Gage and J. M. Gagnier, "Ischemic colitis complicating sickle cell crisis," *Gastroenterology*, vol. 84, no. 1, pp. 171–174, 1983.

[5] F. W. van der Neut, A. van Enk, and M. M. van de Sandt, "Maternal death due to acute necrotizing colitis in homozygous sickle cell disease," *The Netherlands Journal of Medicine*, vol. 42, no. 4, pp. 132–133, 1993.

[6] A. A. Moukarzel, M. Rajaram, A. Sundeep, L. Guarini, and F. Feldman, "Sickle cell anemia: severe ischemic colitis responding to conservative management," *Clinical Pediatrics*, vol. 39, no. 4, pp. 241–243, 2000.

[7] A. Karim, S. Ahmed, L. J. Rossoff, R. Siddiqui, A. Fuchs, and A. S. Multz, "Fulminant ischaemic colitis with atypical clinical features complicating sickle cell disease," *Postgraduate Medical Journal*, vol. 78, no. 920, pp. 370–372, 2002.

[8] B. T. Green and M. S. Branch, "Ischemic colitis in a young adult during sickle cell crisis: case report and review," *Gastrointestinal Endoscopy*, vol. 57, no. 4, pp. 605–607, 2003.

[9] S. Sada, L. Benini, C. Pavan et al., "Ischemic colitis sustained by sickle cell trait in young adult patient," *The American Journal of Gastroenterology*, vol. 100, no. 12, pp. 2818–2821, 2005.

[10] A. Qureshi, N. Lang, and D. H. Bevan, "Sickle cell "girdle syndrome" progressing to ischaemic colitis and colonic perforation," *Clinical and Laboratory Haematology*, vol. 28, no. 1, pp. 60–62, 2006.

[11] S. J. Boley, W. Freiber, P. R. Winslow, M. L. Gliedman, and F. J. Veith, "Circulatory response to acute reduction of superior mesenteric arterial flow," *Physiologist*, vol. 12, article 180, 1969.

[12] E. V. Loftus Jr., "Clinical epidemiology of inflammatory bowel disease: incidence, prevalence, and environmental influences," *Gastroenterology*, vol. 126, no. 6, pp. 1504–1517, 2004.

[13] M. I. El Mouzan, A. M. Abdullah, and M. T. Al Habbal, "Epidemiology of juvenile-onset inflammatory bowel disease in Central Saudi Arabia," *Journal of Tropical Pediatrics*, vol. 52, no. 1, pp. 69–71, 2006.

[14] J. M. White, S. O'Connor, H. S. Winter et al., "Inflammatory bowel disease in African American children compared with other racial/ethnic groups in a multicenter registry," *Clinical Gastroenterology and Hepatology*, vol. 6, no. 12, pp. 1361–1369, 2008.

41

Management of Large Erupting Complex Odontoma in Maxilla

Colm Murphy,[1] John Edward O'Connell,[1] Edward Cotter,[2] and Gerard Kearns[1]

[1]*Department of Oral and Maxillofacial Surgery, Our Lady's Children's Hospital, Crumlin, Dublin 12, Ireland*
[2]*Hermitage Medical Clinic, Suite 10, Old Lucan Road, Dublin 20, Ireland*

Correspondence should be addressed to Colm Murphy; colmmmurphy@rcsi.ie

Academic Editor: Amalia Schiavetti

We present the unusual case of a large complex odontoma erupting in the maxilla. Odontomas are benign developmental tumours of odontogenic origin. They are characterized by slow growth and nonaggressive behaviour. Complex odontomas, which erupt, are rare. They are usually asymptomatic and are identified on routine radiograph but may present with erosion into the oral cavity with subsequent cellulitis and facial asymmetry. This present paper describes the presentation and management of an erupting complex odontoma, occupying the maxillary sinus with extension to the infraorbital rim. We also discuss various surgical approaches used to access this anatomic area.

1. Introduction

Odontomas are benign tumours of odontogenic origin [1–3]. They are described as mixed tumours containing both epithelial and mesenchymal elements [3]. These calcified lesions are classified into compound and complex types. Compound odontomas may appear as tooth like structures containing enamel, dentine, cementum, and pulp and may be single or multiple [4]. Complex odontomas appear as a disorganized amorphous mass of calcified hard tissues [4, 5]. Both lesions usually present in the first two decades of life [4]. Clinical presentation may be as an impacted tooth, alveolar swelling, or incidental radiographic finding. Complex odontomas tend to occur in the posterior mandible or maxilla and only rarely reach a considerable size [6]. Radiographically, the complex odontoma appears as a dense amorphous irregular mass with well-demarcated borders [6].

The differential diagnosis for mixed odontogenic tumours includes compound and complex odontoma, ameloblastic fibroma, and ameloblastic fibroodontoma [6, 7]. Compound odontomas are recognizable as orderly tooth like structures. A complex odontoma may bear resemblance to osteoblastoma, ossifying fibroma, and osteomata [6]. Ameloblastic fibroodontoma presents as a mixed radiolucent-radiopaque lesion and may resemble a developing odontoma. Ameloblastic fibroma is a separate entity and presents as a radiolucent lesion [6, 7].

Complex odontomas present less frequently than compound odontomas. In addition, eruption through the mucosa is rare [7]. To our knowledge, there have only been 20 reported cases of erupting odontoma in the literature, of which 11 were complex odontomas [8].

2. Case Report

A 13-year-old boy was referred to the department of oral and maxillofacial surgery in a tertiary referral centre and presented with a right facial cellulitis, and a hard mass was palpable in his right maxilla The patient reported that the symptoms had begun 1 week previously but that he had noticed a mass in the right maxillary molar area 6 months previously. The infection was treated with empirical intravenous antibiotic therapy. Extraoral examination revealed a hard swelling over the right maxilla, with an associated intraoral calcified mass and missing molar teeth. There was no associated sensory nerve deficit. Plain radiographs and computed tomography demonstrated an extensive calcified lesion in the right maxilla, extending to the infraorbital rim (Figures 1 and 2). An incisional biopsy was taken and histopathological examination suggested the presence of odontoma or fibrous dysplasia.

Surgical removal of the lesion was planned using a transoral approach under general anaesthesia. A mucoperiosteal

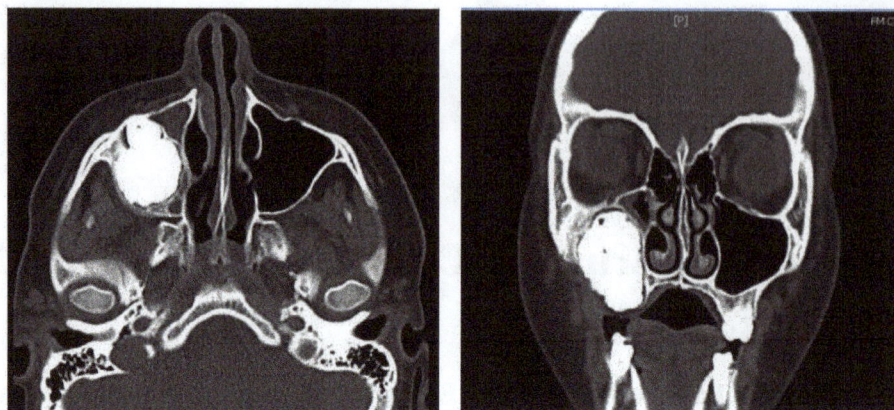

FIGURE 1: Axial and coronal CT images demonstrating the extent of the lesion in the right maxillary antrum.

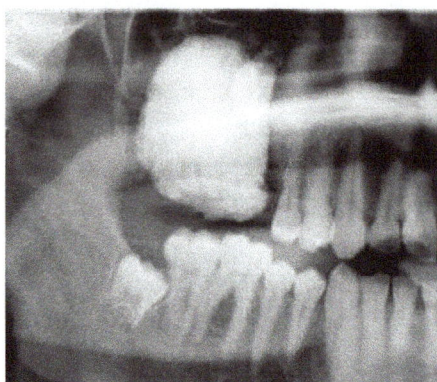

FIGURE 2: Orthopantomogram.

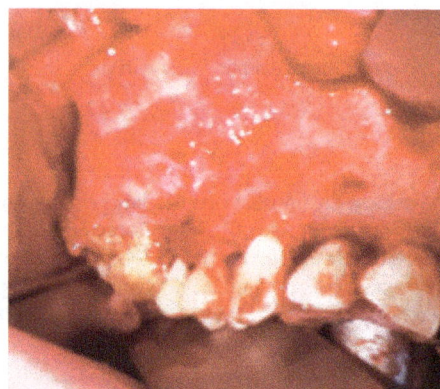

FIGURE 3: Intraoperative photo of lesion.

flap was raised and the tumour was identified (Figure 3). The lesion was found to be eroding into the infraorbital rim. An upper lip split incision was made to facilitate complete removal of the tumour and maintain the integrity of the orbital floor and allow safe dissection and release of the infraorbital nerve. The tumour was enucleated intact using an osteotome and a periosteal elevator, while maintaining continuity of the infraorbital rim and orbital floor. The ipsilateral buccal fat pad was mobilised and advanced to repair the maxillary defect, following tumour removal.

Histopathological examination confirmed the diagnosis of complex odontoma. The patient made an uneventful recovery and had no sensory nerve deficit. The extraoral incision has healed well with minimal scarring; the patient is pleased with the appearance and healing of his extraoral incision (Figure 4). Prosthetic impressions were taken to facilitate construction of a maxillary obturator. To date, the patient has been followed up for a period of 36 months. There has been no clinical or radiographic evidence of recurrence. He will be considered for autogenous bone grafting and placement of osseointegrated dental implants and an overlying fixed prosthesis in the future.

3. Discussion

Odontomas are the most common odontogenic tumour [1–3]. They are characterized by slow growth and nonaggressive behaviour. They usually present in children and young adults in the 2nd decade of life [9, 10]. Complex odontomas are commonly found in the maxillary sinus and posterior mandible and can grow to a large size but rarely cause jaw deformity [1]. The treatment for odontomas is enucleation. Recurrences are rare.

The mechanism of eruption of odontoma is different to tooth eruption as Osteomata lack root formation and a periodontal ligament [4]. The increasing size may lead to resorption of the edentulous part of the alveolar process with subsequent exposure in the oral cavity [7]. This is the most likely explanation in our case due to the extensive nature of the lesion. Therefore, it could be suggested that, rather than erupting, the tumour simply erodes the adjacent bone leading to exposure in the oral cavity.

The surgical removal of benign tumours from the maxillary sinus has traditionally been carried out via a transoral approach with Caldwell-Luc antrostomy through the lateral sinus wall. However, large tumours, which occupy the entire

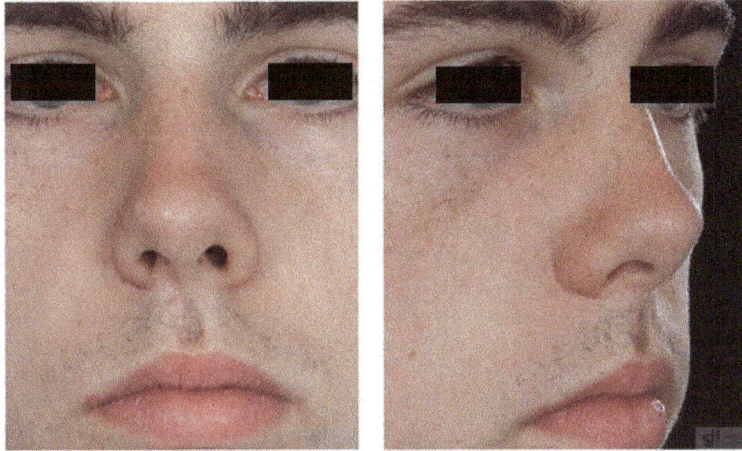

FIGURE 4: Postoperative photo demonstrating satisfactory appearance of extraoral incision.

antrum or cause significant deformity, may require a more extensive approach to facilitate surgical access. Korpi et al. [2] have advocated the use of the Le Fort 1 downfracture to gain access to the posterior maxilla for removal of complex odontoma. They suggest that this approach decreases the risk of bony defects, thus preventing oroantral fistula formation, and reduces facial deformity [2]. The maxilla can be repositioned in its original position with titanium miniplates and screws. However, we feel that downfracture of the maxilla is less predictable when there has been significant bone resorption and expansion due to a large tumour as it was in this present case.

The most common approach for management of maxillary odontogenic neoplasms is a transoral approach [7]. Labial and palatal mucoperiosteal flaps may be raised to allow adequate exposure. A transcutaneous approach may be required to facilitate the safe and adequate removal of more extensive maxillary odontogenic tumours. Extensions to the orbital floor and beyond the posterior wall of the maxillary sinus are examples [6].

In this present case, an upper lip split was performed to both adequately expose the tumour and maintain the integrity of the orbital floor, as well as allowing safe dissection and release of the infraorbital nerve. The patient suffered no sensory nerve deficit and the extraoral skin incision healed satisfactorily.

4. Conclusion

This case highlights the extensive nature and rare presentation of erupting complex odontomas. They may increase in size after calcification and lead to complications following eruption [4]. They may present with facial cellulitis or, more rarely, facial deformity. Surgical removal is the treatment of choice with preservation of adjacent structures. In cases with larger tumours, an extraoral skin incision may be successfully used to allow access to and removal of the lesion.

Conflict of Interests

The authors declare that they have no conflict of interests.

References

[1] B. R. Chrcanovic, F. Jaeger, and B. Freire-Maia, "Two-stage surgical removal of large complex odontoma," *Oral and Maxillofacial Surgery*, vol. 14, no. 4, pp. 247–252, 2010.

[2] J. T. Korpi, V. T. Kainulainen, G. K. B. Sándor, and K. S. Oikarinen, "Removal of large complex odontoma using Le fort 1 Osteotomy," *Journal of Oral and Maxillofacial Surgery*, vol. 67, no. 9, pp. 2018–2021, 2009.

[3] C. J. Perumal, A. Mohamed, A. Singh, and C. E. E. Noffke, "Sequestrating giant complex odontoma: a case report and review of the literature," *Journal of Oral and Maxillofacial Surgery*, vol. 12, no. 4, pp. 480–484, 2013.

[4] M. Soluk Tekkesin, S. Pehlivan, V. Olgac, N. Aksakall, and C. Alatl, "Clinical and histopathological investigation of odontomas: review of the literature and presentation of 160 cases," *Journal of Oral and Maxillofacial Surgery*, vol. 70, no. 6, pp. 1358–1361, 2012.

[5] G. I. Prodromidis, K. I. Tosios, and I. G. Koutlas, "Cemento-osseous dysplasia-like lesion and complex odontoma associated with an impacted third molar," *Head and Neck Pathology*, vol. 5, no. 4, pp. 401–404, 2011.

[6] R. E. Marx and D. Stern, *Oral and Maxillofacial Pathology, A Rational for Diagnosis and Treatment*, Quinntessence Books, 2003.

[7] C. C. Ragalli, J. L. Ferreria, and F. Blasco, "Large erupting complex odontoma," *International Journal of Oral and Maxillofacial Surgery*, vol. 29, no. 5, pp. 373–374, 2000.

[8] G. Serra-Serra, L. Berini-Aytés, and C. Gay-Escoda, "Erupted odontomas: a report of three cases and review of the literature," *Medicina Oral, Patologia Oral y Cirugia Bucal*, vol. 14, no. 6, pp. E299–E303, 2009.

[9] J. A. Regezi, *Oral Pathology Clinical Pathologic Correlations*, Saunders, 4th edition, 2002.

[10] B. M. Owens, N. J. Schuman, and H. H. Mincer, "Dental odontomas: a retrospective study of 104 cases," *Journal of Clinical Pediatric Dentistry*, vol. 21, no. 3, pp. 261–264, 1997.

42

Huge Intrathoracic Malignant Peripheral Nerve Sheath Tumor in an Adolescent with Neurofibromatosis Type 1

Jong Hyung Yoon,[1] Hyun-Sung Lee,[1,2] Jong In Chun,[1] Seog-Yun Park,[1,3] Hyeon Jin Park,[1] and Byung-Kiu Park[1]

[1] Center for Pediatric Oncology, National Cancer Center, 323 Ilsan-ro, Ilsandong-gu, Goyang-si, Gyeonggi-do 410-769, Republic of Korea
[2] Center for Lung Cancer, National Cancer Center, 323 Ilsan-ro, Ilsandong-gu, Goyang-si, Gyeonggi-do 410-769, Republic of Korea
[3] Department of Pathology, National Cancer Center, 323 Ilsan-ro, Ilsandong-gu, Goyang-si, Gyeonggi-do 410-769, Republic of Korea

Correspondence should be addressed to Byung-Kiu Park; bkpark@ncc.re.kr

Academic Editor: Maria Moschovi

Malignant peripheral nerve sheath tumor (MPNST) is a rare soft tissue malignancy usually found in patients with neurofibromatosis type 1 (NF1) with a poor outcome. Although MPNST can be found in any part of the body including head and neck or extremities, intrathoracic MPNST with or without NF1 is uncommon, especially in children or adolescents. Reported herein is a case of huge intrathoracic MPNST in a 16-year-old girl with NF1, and a brief review of the literature.

1. Introduction

Malignant peripheral nerve sheath tumor (MPNST) is a rare soft tissue malignancy generally encountered during adulthood and only 10–20% is found in children and adolescents [1–4]. Many cases of this tumor arise in the patients with neurofibromatosis type 1 (NF1) with a poor outcome [1, 3, 4]. Although MPNST can be found in any part of the body including extremities, head and neck, trunk, or retroperitoneum [1, 2], intrathoracic MPNST with or without NF1 is uncommon, only with several reported adult cases [5–15]. In children or adolescents, only a few cases have been reported up to date [16–20].

Here, we report our experience in a rare case of huge intrathoracic MPNST in a 16-year-old adolescent with NF1. A review of the pertinent literature is included.

2. Case Presentation

A 16-year-old girl visited our hospital because of progressive chest discomfort and respiratory difficulties that started a month prior to the visit. Physical examination performed during her visit revealed multiple café-au-lait spots and cutaneous neurofibromas indicating NF1 in the patient as well as in the patient's mother. Her height and weight were 153 cm (5–10 percentile) and 48.4 kg (10–25 percentile), respectively. Her Tanner stage was 4. Her blood pressure, pulse rate, respiratory rate, and body temperature were 136/66 mmHg, 114/min, 24/min, and 36.5°C, respectively. Her chest radiography and chest computed tomography (CT) images revealed a large mass occupying the right thoracic cavity with multiple pleural nodules suggesting metastasis (Figures 1(a) and 1(b)). Scoliosis was associated with the tumor and multiple neurofibromas on magnetic resonance imaging of the whole spine (Figure 1(c)). The findings were suggestive of highly malignant tumor on positron emission tomography (PET)/CT imaging (Figure 1(d)) with a maximum standardized uptake value (SUV_{max}) of 6.9. Her *NF1* gene mutation analysis revealed no known overt mutation except silent mutation in C369G without change of amino acids.

She underwent immediate surgery (grossly total resection of the tumor and chest wall reconstruction with patch graft) without diagnostic biopsy because total resection of the tumor seemed feasible. Intraoperatively, the tumor was encapsulated and showed adhesion to pleura with somewhat

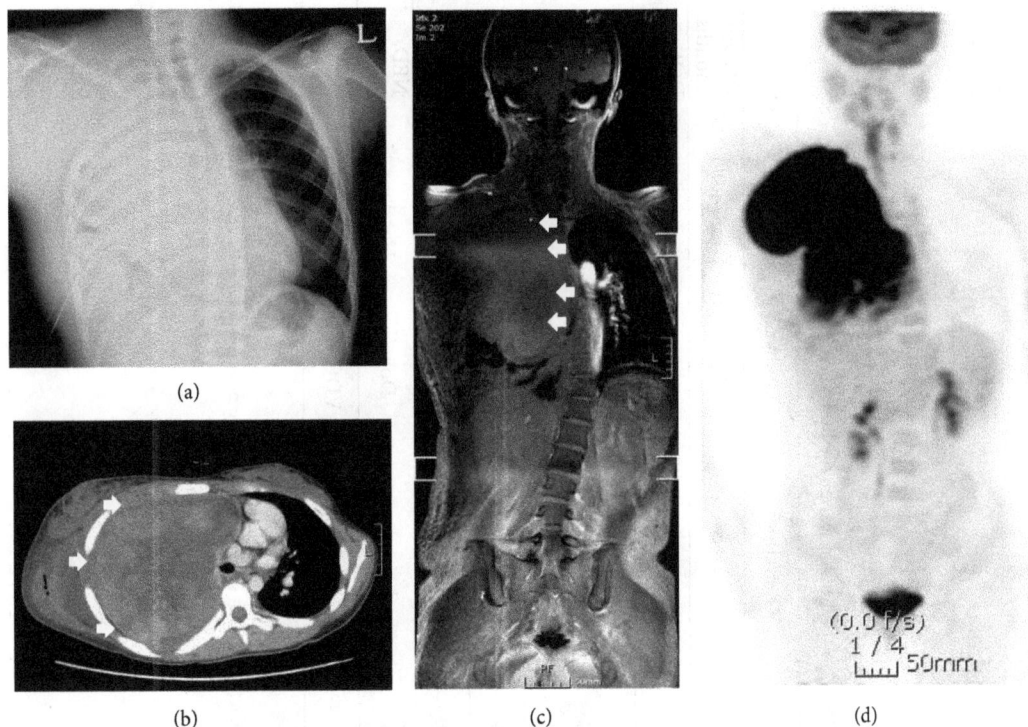

FIGURE 1: The patient's chest radiography shows a large thoracic mass with total collapse of right lung (a). Her chest CT scan (b) and spine MR imaging (c) also show a large intrathoracic hyperdense mass (white arrows) in the right chest, resulting in prominent scoliosis and cardiac deviation. Her ^{18}F-FDG PET/CT scan showed highly increased FDG uptake (SUV$_{max}$ = 6.9) in this mass, suggesting highly malignant tumor (d).

of effusion and incomplete fissure. Brachial plexus, vagus nerve, and phrenic nerve were functionally saved without tumor involvement. Macroscopically, the resected tumor was $22 \times 17 \times 9$ cm in size (Figure 2(a)). Pulmonary metastasis was not detected in intraoperative findings. Microscopic features of the tumor showed many spindle-shaped cells with pale, eosinophilic cytoplasm (Figure 2(b)). Immunohistochemically, tumor cells expressed neuron-specific enolase (Figure 2(c)) and CD68 (focal) but not desmin, CD34, and smooth muscle actin, which were consistent with a diagnosis of MPNST.

After the surgery, she received 6,600 cGy of tomotherapy to the right whole lung field and pleura. Subsequently, she received 6 courses of chemotherapy consisting of vincristine, doxorubicin, and cyclophosphamide, alternating with ifosfamide and etoposide (VDC/IE) [21]. However, her residual pleural metastasis showed no definite response to adjuvant therapies and showed rapid progression with newly appearing pulmonary nodules. She developed a large amount of malignant pericardial effusion associated with enlarged pulmonary metastases after the sixth course of chemotherapy. Despite supportive measures including pericardiocentesis, she died of progressive disease at 9 months after the surgery.

3. Discussion

NF1, formerly called von Recklinghausen disease, is an autosomal dominant neurocutaneous disorder, with an estimated incidence of 1 in 3000 births [4, 16]. NF1 is commonly associated with higher incidence in many kinds of benign or malignant tumors, such as optic pathway glioma, chronic myeloid leukemia, or pheochromocytoma, neurofibroma, and MPNST [22], and is related to mutations in *NF1* gene located in chromosome 17q11.2. Because *NF1* gene product named neurofibromin acts as a negative regulator in Ras signal transduction pathway, mutation in *NF1* gene is related to tumor development and results in malignancies [22, 23].

MPNST is a rare soft tissue malignancy comprising about 5–10% of all soft tissue sarcomas [1–4]. Its incidence in healthy people is approximately 0.001%, but its incidence is much higher in NF1 patients (2~5%) [3, 4]. Inversely, MPNST is one of the most common malignancies in NF1 patients and 50% of MPNST arises in NF1 patients [1–3]. MPNST can be found in any part of the body, including extremities (40%), trunk (22%), head and neck (20%), and retroperitoneal visceral area (15%) [1, 2]. However, intrathoracic or mediastinal MPNST is very rare. Although 14 cases of intrathoracic MPNST with (8) or without (6) NF1 were reported previously in English-language literature, most of them were in adult patients with a median age of 40 (54.5 without and 39.5 with NF1) years [5–15] and only four cases with NF1 (including one with angiosarcoma component) and two without NF1 of children or adolescents have been reported (Table 1) [16–20]. We were unable to find differences between the patients with and without NF1 because of limited number of the patients. Despite its rarity, intrathoracic MPNSTs in patients

TABLE 1: Reported cases of children and adolescents with intrathoracic MPNST in the English-language literature.

Reference	Age (years)	Sex	Symptoms	Location	Metastasis	NF1	Operation	Chemotherapy	Radiotherapy (cGy)	Outcome
Elli et al., 2007 [16]	13[1]	Male	LUQ pain, weight loss	Lt paravertebral	—	Yes	Total resection	VICE, Ep, and A	Local, 4680	DOD, 14 months
Komori et al., 2003 [17]	12	Female	Chest pain, dyspnea	Rt paravertebral	N/A	No	Partial resection	N/A	N/A	DOD, 15 months
Muwakkit et al., 2006 [18]	2.5	Male	Malaise, fatigue, anorexia, and palpitations upon exertion	Rt pulmonary	N/A	No	Total resection and lobectomy	VDC	Not done	N/A
Imazu et al., 2006 [19]	12	Female	Neck swelling[2]	Rt paraclavicular	—	Yes	Total resection	Not done	Not done	NED, 12 months
Moharir et al., 2010 [20]	8	Male	Weight loss, respiratory symptoms	Lt hemithorax	—	No	Subtotal resection	Done	Not done	DOD, 2.5 months
Moharir et al., 2010 [20]	12	Female	None (incidental)	Rt paraspinal	—	Yes	Total resection	Done	Not done	NED, 2 years
Present case	16	Female	Chest pain, respiratory problem	Rt anterior	Lung	No	Total resection	VDC/IE	Rt lung and pleura, 6600	DOD, 9 months

[1] His tumor was diagnosed with MPNST associated with some angiosarcoma components.
[2] Her tumor was located at cervicothoracic lesion.

A: actinomycin-D; C: cyclophosphamide; D: doxorubicin; DOD: died of disease; E: etoposide; Ep: epirubicin; I: ifosfamide; Lt: left; LUQ: left upper quadrant; N/A: not assessed; NED: no evidence of disease; NFI: diagnosis of neurofibromatosis type 1; Rt: right; V: vincristine.

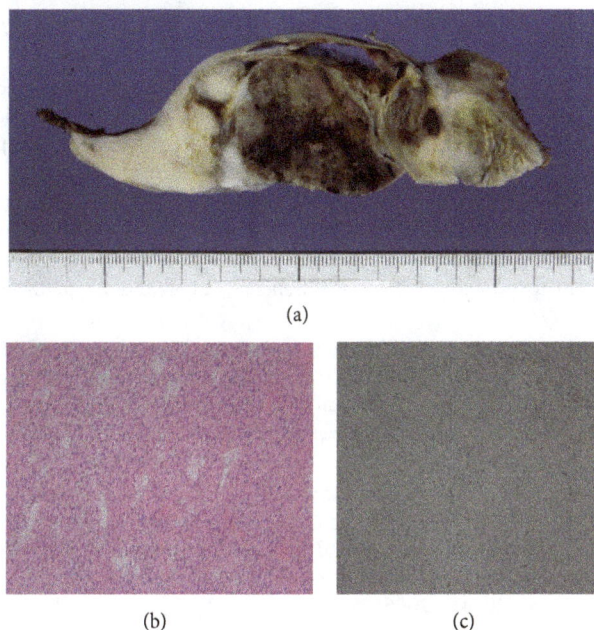

FIGURE 2: Macroscopic appearance of the cut surface of the resected tumor shows some hemorrhage and necrosis in the center. It was 22 × 17 × 9 cm in size (a). Microscopically, the tumor is composed of homogenous spindle cells (hematoxylin and eosin, ×100) (b). Immunohistochemical stains showing positivity to neuron-specific enolase (c), consistent with MPNST.

with NF1 are thought to be originated from the plexiform neurofibromas (PNs) of thoracic nerves or vagus nerve [13]. Four (including one with angiosarcoma component) of them with NF1 had no metastasis at diagnosis, and only two survived longer than 12 months. Our patient had a tumor huge in size compared to those of previous reports with multiple pleural nodules suggesting metastasis at diagnosis, which indicates delayed diagnosis despite her NF1 stigmata. It is well known that MPNST associated with NF1 shows a poor response to chemotherapy or radiotherapy and the prognosis with residual tumor or metastasis is dismal [1, 2, 18]. Although doxorubicin/ifosfamide- (AI-) based chemotherapy is known to be somewhat effective for adult MPNST and some pediatric cases [4, 23, 24], there is no known standard chemotherapy regimen for treatment of MPNST. Since MPNST with NF1 usually shows poor response to conventional chemotherapy we used 5-drug chemotherapy to treat our patient because VDC/IE regimen for the Ewing sarcoma or rhabdomyosarcoma may show a better response to MPNST than AI-based regimen [4, 21, 23, 24]. However, our patient also showed no response of tumor to adjuvant therapies and died of disease progression.

Wide excision of the tumor is one of the most important prognostic factors in MPNST [2]. Because some of the large intrathoracic malignant tumors cannot be removed completely due to adjacent critical vital organs, early detection of intrathoracic MPNST is very important for long-term survival of the patients with NF1 [20]. Although some assessment guidelines for children with NF1 including annual

clinical evaluation of spine were suggested [25], no specific evaluation strategy for surveillance of MPNST in the patients with NF1 is known [20, 22]. Because MPNST in NF1 patient is usually transformed from PNs and they have similar initial symptoms and signs, it is very important to distinguish small MPNST from PN for early detection of MPNST [20]. Recently, some reports suggest that ^{18}FDG-PET/CT (with various cutoff SUV_{max} of 2.5~3.5) can be a useful diagnostic tool for early detection and good prognosis of MPNST in NF1 patients [20, 26, 27]. However, considering no solid cutoff value of SUV_{max} and risk of radiation exposure after ^{18}FDG-PET/CT, further investigation for adequate schedule or strategy using PET/CT for early detection and rapid intervention of MPNST in NF1 should be warranted.

The authors report a rare case of huge intrathoracic MPNST in a 16-year-old girl with NF1. Considering its location and poor prognosis without complete resection, a screening strategy for early detection and intervention of MPNST in NF1 should be investigated.

Conflict of Interests

The authors declare that there is no conflict of interests regarding the publication of this paper.

References

[1] S. R. Grobmyer, J. D. Reith, A. Shahlaee, C. H. Bush, and S. N. Hochwald, "Malignant peripheral nerve sheath tumor: molecular pathogenesis and current management considerations," *Journal of Surgical Oncology*, vol. 97, no. 4, pp. 340–349, 2008.

[2] M. Carli, A. Ferrari, A. Mattke et al., "Pediatric malignant peripheral nerve sheath tumor: the Italian and German Soft Tissue Sarcoma Cooperative Group," *Journal of Clinical Oncology*, vol. 23, no. 33, pp. 8422–8430, 2005.

[3] H. A. Demir, A. Varan, B. Yalçin, C. Akyüz, T. Kutluk, and M. Büyükpamukçu, "Malignant peripheral nerve sheath tumors in childhood: 13 cases from a single center," *Journal of Pediatric Hematology/Oncology*, vol. 34, no. 3, pp. 204–207, 2012.

[4] A. Ferrari, G. Bisogno, and M. Carli, "Management of childhood malignant peripheral nerve sheath tumor," *Pediatric Drugs*, vol. 9, no. 4, pp. 239–248, 2007.

[5] R.-S. Lai, S.-L. Lin, S.-S. Hsu, and M.-T. Wu, "Intrathoracic paraspinal malignant peripheral nerve sheath tumor," *Journal of the Chinese Medical Association*, vol. 69, no. 1, pp. 37–41, 2006.

[6] B. H. Chao, K. A. Stogner-Underwood, J. Kiev, and T. J. Smith, "Intrathoracic malignant peripheral nerve sheath tumor in neurofibromatosis 1," *Journal of Clinical Oncology*, vol. 26, no. 13, pp. 2216–2218, 2008.

[7] R. Kawachi, H. Takei, G. Furuyashiki, Y. Koshi-Ishi, and T. Goya, "A malignant peripheral nerve sheath tumor of the mediastinum in a patient with neurofibromatosis type 1: report of a case," *Surgery Today*, vol. 38, no. 10, pp. 945–947, 2008.

[8] J. Shimizu, Y. Arano, T. Murata et al., "A case of intrathoracic giant malignant peripheral nerve sheath tumor in neurofibromatosis type i (von recklinghausen's disease)," *Annals of Thoracic and Cardiovascular Surgery*, vol. 14, no. 1, pp. 42–47, 2008.

[9] V. Kolarov, J. Stanić, Z. Eri, B. Zvezdin, M. Kojičić, and S. Hromis, "Intrathoracic malignant peripheral nerve sheath

tumor with poor outcome: a case report," *Bosnian Journal of Basic Medical Sciences*, vol. 10, no. 4, pp. 328–330, 2010.

[10] J. H. Park, K. H. Choi, H. B. Lee, Y. K. Rhee, Y. C. Lee, and M. J. Chung, "Intrathoracic malignant peripheral nerve sheath tumor in von Recklinghausen's disease," *Korean Journal of Internal Medicine*, vol. 16, no. 3, pp. 201–204, 2001.

[11] T. Shimoyama, K. Yoshiya, Y. Yamato, T. Koike, and K. Honma, "Long-term survival after removal of a malignant peripheral nerve sheath tumor originating in the anterior mediastinum," *General Thoracic and Cardiovascular Surgery*, vol. 57, no. 6, pp. 310–314, 2009.

[12] K. Asai, K. Suzuki, H. Shimota, T. Takahashi, K. Yamashita, and T. Kazui, "Malignant peripheral nerve sheath tumor of the mediastinum: a temporary aortic transection approach," *Journal of Thoracic and Cardiovascular Surgery*, vol. 128, no. 4, pp. 615–617, 2004.

[13] A. Abbas, H. Jones, G. T. Kingston, and A. Zurek, "Malignant peripheral nerve sheath tumour presenting as a pneumothorax," *British Journal of Radiology*, vol. 84, no. 1006, pp. e197–e199, 2011.

[14] M. Inoue, T. Mitsudomi, T. Osaki, T. Oyama, J. Haratake, and K. Yasumoto, "Malignant transformation of an intrathoracic neurofibroma in von Recklinghausen's disease," *Scandinavian Cardiovascular Journal*, vol. 32, no. 3, pp. 173–175, 1998.

[15] H. Ogino, M. Hara, M. Satake et al., "Malignant peripheral nerve sheath tumors of intrathoracic vagus nerve," *Journal of Thoracic Imaging*, vol. 16, no. 3, pp. 181–184, 2001.

[16] M. Elli, B. Can, M. Ceyhan et al., "Intrathoracic malignant peripheral nerve sheath tumor with angiosarcoma in a child with NF1," *Tumori*, vol. 93, no. 6, pp. 641–644, 2007.

[17] M. Komori, H. Yabuuchi, T. Kuroiwa, Y. Nagatoshi, Y. Ichinose, and Y. Hachitanda, "Thoracic malignant peripheral nerve sheath tumour mimicking a pleural tumour: a rare pedunculated appearance," *Pediatric Radiology*, vol. 33, no. 8, pp. 578–581, 2003.

[18] S. A. Muwakkit, C. Rodriguez-Galindo, A. I. El Samra et al., "Primary malignant peripheral nerve sheath tumor of the lung in a young child without neurofibromatosis type 1," *Pediatric Blood and Cancer*, vol. 47, no. 5, pp. 636–638, 2006.

[19] M. Imazu, Y. Nakamura, H. Nakatani et al., "Cervicothoracic malignant peripheral nerve sheath tumor in a 12-year-old girl with neurofibromatosis type 1," *European Journal of Pediatric Surgery*, vol. 16, no. 4, pp. 285–287, 2006.

[20] M. Moharir, K. London, R. Howman-Giles, and K. North, "Utility of positron emission tomography for tumour surveillance in children with neurofibromatosis type 1," *European Journal of Nuclear Medicine and Molecular Imaging*, vol. 37, no. 7, pp. 1309–1317, 2010.

[21] C. A. S. Arndt, D. S. Hawkins, W. H. Meyer, S. F. Sencer, J. P. Neglia, and J. R. Anderson, "Comparison of results of a pilot study of alternating vincristine/doxorubicin/cyclophosphamide and etoposide/ifosfamide with IRS-IV in intermediate risk rhabdomyosarcoma: a report from the children's oncology group," *Pediatric Blood and Cancer*, vol. 50, no. 1, pp. 33–36, 2008.

[22] B. R. Korf, "Malignancy in neurofibromatosis type 1," *Oncologist*, vol. 5, no. 6, pp. 477–485, 2000.

[23] J. R. Kroep, M. Ouali, H. Gelderblom et al., "First-line chemotherapy for malignant peripheral nerve sheath tumor (MPNST) versus other histological soft tissue sarcoma subtypes and as a prognostic factor for MPNST: an EORTC Soft Tissue

and Bone Sarcoma Group study," *Annals of Oncology*, vol. 22, no. 1, pp. 207–214, 2011.

[24] L. Granowetter, R. Womer, M. Devidas et al., "Dose-intensified compared with standard chemotherapy for nonmetastatic ewing sarcoma family of tumors: a children's oncology group study," *Journal of Clinical Oncology*, vol. 27, no. 15, pp. 2536–2541, 2009.

[25] R. E. Ferner, S. M. Huson, N. Thomas et al., "Guidelines for the diagnosis and management of individuals with neurofibromatosis," *Journal of Medical Genetics*, vol. 44, no. 2, pp. 81–88, 2007.

[26] V. S. Warbey, R. E. Ferner, J. T. Dunn, E. Calonje, and M. J. O'Doherty, "FDG PET/CT in the diagnosis of malignant peripheral nerve sheath tumours in neurofibromatosis type-1," *European Journal of Nuclear Medicine and Molecular Imaging*, vol. 36, no. 5, pp. 754–757, 2009.

[27] W. Brenner, R. E. Friedrich, K. A. Gawad et al., "Prognostic relevance of FDG PET in patients with neurofibromatosis type-1 and malignant peripheral nerve sheath tumours," *European Journal of Nuclear Medicine and Molecular Imaging*, vol. 33, no. 4, pp. 428–432, 2006.

43

Cases of Atypical Lymphangiomas in Children

Prashant K. Minocha, Lakhan Roop, and Rambachan Persad

Department of Paediatric Surgery, San Fernando General Hospital, Trinidad, Trinidad and Tobago

Correspondence should be addressed to Prashant K. Minocha; prashant.minocha@gmail.com

Academic Editor: Piero Pavone

Background. Lymphatic malformations or lymphangiomas are rare benign hamartomas that result from maldevelopment of primitive lymphatic sacs. They are most frequently found in the neck and axilla, while intra-abdominal and mediastinal lymphangiomas are uncommon. These are primarily tumours of infancy and childhood and are successfully treated with surgical excision. *Summary of Cases.* Five cases of lymphangioma comprising three intra-abdominal lymphangiomas and two unilateral axillary lymphangiomas presenting at one institution in Trinidad W.I. between 2005 and 2012 were examined. The presentations, location, workup, treatment, and outcome of these patients were studied. *Conclusion.* This paper discusses a range of extracervical lymphangioma cases seen at San Fernando General Hospital, Trinidad W.I. We report three intra-abdominal cases and the most common clinical presentations were abdominal pain and distension. Also two axillary cases were reported, which presented as painless axillary masses. The major concerns for excision of axillary lymphangioma by parents and surgeons were cosmesis and feasibility of complete resection without disruption of developing breast tissue and axillary vessels. We believe that ultrasound scan is very good at detection of the lesion, while CT is better at determining tumour content and planning for the operation. It is our opinion that complete surgical excision can be achieved.

1. Introduction

Lymphangiomas are benign lesions characterized by proliferation of lymphatic vessels. Approximately 50% are present at birth and 90% are diagnosed before the age of 2 [1]. They are most frequently found in the neck (75%) and axilla (15%) [2], while only 10% are found in the mediastinum and abdominal cavity [3, 4] including mesentery, retroperitoneal areas, and bones [5]. Retroperitoneal lymphangiomas are extremely rare comprising 1% of all lymphangiomas [6]. Lymphangiomas are successfully treated with surgical excision; however, there have been cases of recurrence with patients who have undergone incomplete excision (Table 1).

2. Case Descriptions

2.1. Case 1. The first patient was a 6-year-old female who at 6 weeks of life had a surgically resected cystic lymphangioma of the sigmoid colon (with primary colorectal anastomosis and appendectomy). She was previously well; however, she began experiencing symptoms of intermittent periumbilical abdominal pain, accompanied by vomiting, constipation, and abdominal distension, which necessitated two separate admissions. On the first admission, she was treated for acute intestinal obstruction, which spontaneously resolved after several days at the hospital. Three months later, she presented with periumbilical pain for two days followed by vomiting, abdominal distension, and headaches. On examination, her abdomen was noted to be mildly distended, but no discrete masses were palpated. She had no family history of malignancy or congenital malformations. On this admission, her haemoglobin (Hb) was found to be 5 gm/dL and she required transfusion of 250 mLs of packed red cells. Her posttransfusion Hb increased to 9.5 gm/dL. Abdominal X-ray did not show any bowel dilation or air fluid levels. Given the patient's past surgical history, there was a high index of suspicion for recurrence of the intra-abdominal lymphangioma. Other differentials included intestinal obstruction and mesenteric adenitis. A computed tomography (CT) scan of the abdomen with IV (intravenous) contrast was performed which showed a cystic mass on the colon and she had surgical intervention. Findings of the surgery included a retroperitoneal cystic

TABLE 1: Comparison of cases.

Case	Age	Gender	Site of lymphangioma	Signs/symptoms on presentation	Treatment	Response to treatment
Case 1	6 yrs	F	Retroperitoneal	Periumbilical pain, vomiting, abdominal distension, and constipation	Surgical excision	Recurrence following resection at 6 weeks of life resulting in second surgery at 6 years. Yearly follow-up with USS for the past 9 years; no recurrence
Case 2	4 yrs	M	Retroperitoneal	Periumbilical pain, constipation, abdominal distension, and left flank firmness	Complete surgical excision	Yearly follow-up with USS for the past 8 years; no recurrence
Case 3	4 yrs	F	Mesenteric	Progressive abdominal distension	Complete surgical excision	Yearly follow-up with USS for the past 3 years; no recurrence
Case 4	8 yrs	F	Left axillary	Axillary swelling	Complete surgical excision with conservation of developing breast tissue	Yearly follow-up with USS for the past 3 years. No recurrence and normal symmetrical breast development
Case 5	14 months	M	Right axillary	Swelling on the anterior chest wall since birth with increasing size	Observation for the first year followed by complete surgical excision due to progressive increase in size	Yearly follow-up with USS for the past 2 years; no recurrence

M: male and F: female.

lymphangioma enclosing a 50 mL organized clot in the left iliac fossa, multiple peritoneal adhesions, mesenteric windows, adhesions enclosing small bowel into artificial sac, and a ventral incisional hernia. Histology confirmed cystic lymphangioma. The patient has been followed up with regular ultrasound scans (USS) for the past 9 years and there has been no evidence of recurrence or intestinal obstruction thus far.

2.2. Case 2. A 4-year-old male presented with 2-day history of periumbilical pain and a past history of occasional constipation without any significant past medical history and no family history of malignancy or congenital abnormalities. On examination he was found to have a mildly distended, nontender abdomen with diffuse left flank firmness, but no discrete mass was appreciated. The patient continued to have colicky abdominal pain but no constipation or vomiting. CT scan abdomen with IV contrast was performed which showed a 30 cm by 10 cm left sided isodense retroperitoneal mass attached to the lower pole of left kidney (Figure 1). Based on imaging, the possible differential diagnoses included neuroblastoma and cystic lymphangioma. The patient underwent an exploratory laparotomy which revealed a 20 cm by 30 cm multiloculated cystic mass arising retroperitoneally from the coeliac plexus of lymph. The hilum of the cyst was anterior to splenic artery displacing pancreas laterally to the right. The histology of the specimen confirmed intra-abdominal cystic lymphangioma. Yearly follow-up with USS for the past 8 years has shown no recurrence thus far.

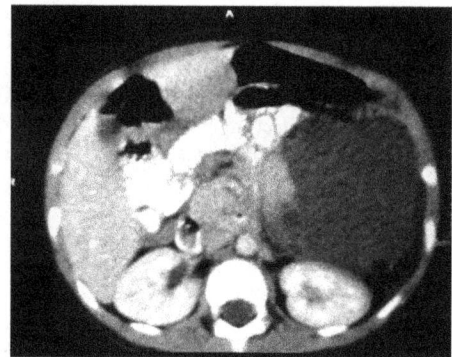

FIGURE 1: CT of the abdomen showing a 30 cm × 10 cm left sided isodense retroperitoneal mass.

2.3. Case 3. The patient was a 4-year-old female who was referred from a rural health center with 2-week history of progressive abdominal distension. She was otherwise asymptomatic with a positive history of passing stool and flatus. There was no significant past medical history or history of prior abdominal surgery or trauma. She had no family history of malignancy or congenital abnormalities. On abdominal examination, a mass arising from the pelvis was palpable. An abdominal USS revealed a 14 cm by 7 cm by 12 cm fluid filled structure in the left half of the abdomen extending into the pelvic cavity (Figure 2). Abdominal CT with IV contrast showed a 13 cm by 8 cm by 12 cm cystic abdominal mass

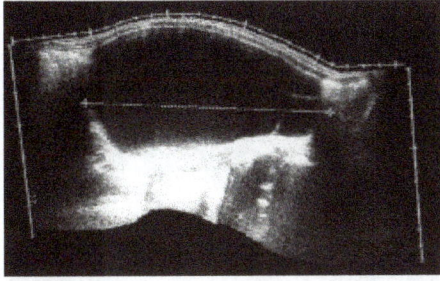

FIGURE 2: Abdominal ultrasound showing a 14 cm by 7 cm by 12 cm fluid filled structure in the left half of the abdomen.

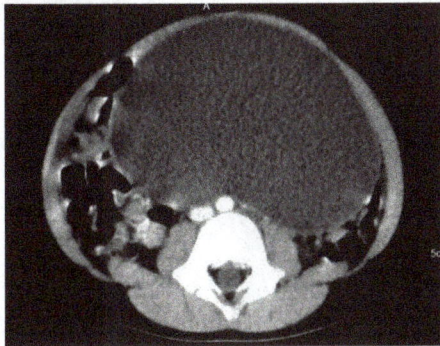

FIGURE 3: Abdominal CT showing a 13 cm × 8 cm × 12 cm cystic abdominal mass.

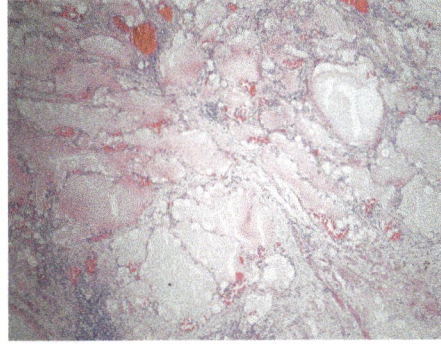

FIGURE 4: Histology showing a mixture of lymph vessels and smooth muscle, with lymphatic channels containing blood and lymphoid cells (magnification ×100).

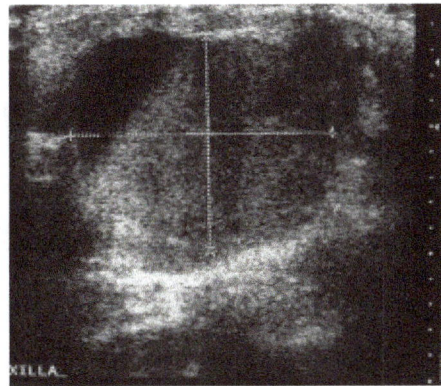

FIGURE 5: Ultrasound of the chest showing a heterogeneous solid cystic mass in the left axilla.

that appeared to arise from the pelvis extending into the abdomen and displacing the bowel bilaterally (Figure 3). Two days subsequent to admission, the patient had exploratory laparotomy and cystectomy. A 15 cm by 12 cm mesenteric cyst containing chocolate coloured fluid was found at the splenic hilum surrounded by a jejunal loop and bordered by the tail of the pancreas. She had uneventful recovery with no evidence of recurrence to date. Histology showed a mixture of lymph vessels and smooth muscle, features suggestive of lymphangioma (Figure 4).

2.4. Case 4. The patient was an 8-year-old female who presented with a 4-day history of a swelling to the left side of her chest that was increasing in size and she was otherwise asymptomatic. She had no medical problems and no significant family history. Interestingly, she was known to have a lymph node in the same area 7 years prior and was scheduled for surgical excision, but it resolved and hence no surgery was done at that time. On examination, she was found to have a 3 cm by 3 cm firm, smooth mass in her left axilla with no surrounding lymphadenopathy. USS of the chest showed a heterogeneous solid and cystic mass in the left axilla (Figure 5). The patient had needle aspiration which revealed a bloody aspirate and this was followed by a course of oral antibiotics; however, the swelling failed to resolve. CT scan of the chest with contrast done subsequently demonstrated a left axillary cystic mass with no intrathoracic extension (Figure 6). She had complete surgical excision of the cystic mass. However, the proximity of the lesion to developing

breast tissue posed a challenge to surgical resection. Follow-up in clinic for the past 3 years has shown symmetrical development of breasts with no deformity to the left breast. Histology confirmed the diagnosis of lymphangioma.

2.5. Case 5. This male patient was referred to us at birth with a right chest swelling (Figure 7). USS of the chest revealed a predominantly cystic mass with septations in the right lateral chest wall near the right axilla, 5 cm by 4 cm (Figure 8). Differential diagnoses included axillary lymphangioma and unilateral gynaecomastia and he was scheduled for regular follow-up at our outpatient clinic. The patient had no medical problems and no significant family history. Monthly follow-up revealed that the mass was progressively decreasing in size. However at one-year follow-up, mother noticed an increase in size with the mass measuring 6 cm by 5 cm on physical examination. The patient was scheduled for elective surgical excision pending CT scan. Chest CT with contrast revealed 8 cm by 7 cm by 3 cm enhancing mixed density mass in the right chest wall abutting the pectoralis major muscle (Figure 9). Surgical excision performed at 14 months showed 7 cm by 7 cm cystic mass in the right axilla. The surgical site healed well and follow-up with USS for the past 2 years has been uneventful thus far. Histology confirmed the diagnosis of lymphangioma.

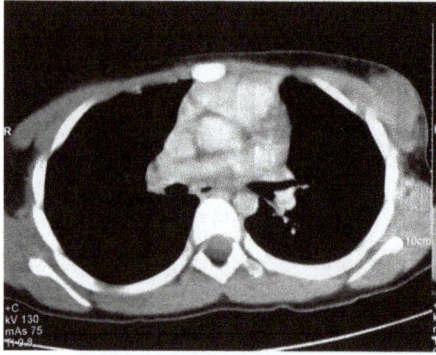

FIGURE 6: CT of the chest showing several soft tissue lesions noted laterally and anterior to the left pectoralis major measuring 4 cm × 3 cm × 1 cm.

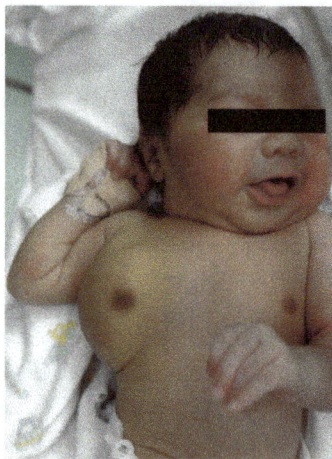

FIGURE 7: Picture showing right chest swelling shortly after birth.

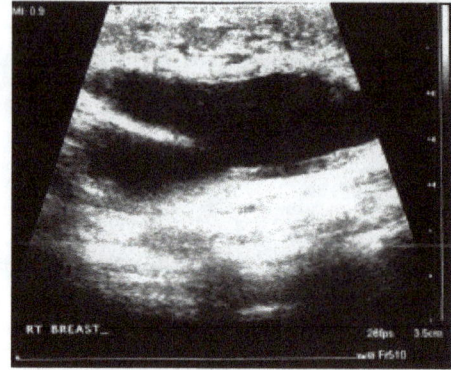

FIGURE 8: Ultrasound of the chest/axilla showing a cystic mass with septations in the right lateral chest wall near the right axilla, 5 cm × 4 cm.

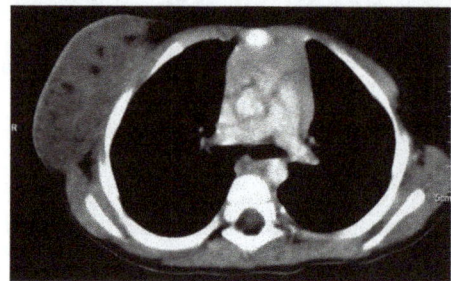

FIGURE 9: CT of the chest showing an 8 cm × 7 cm × 3 cm enhancing mixed density mass in the right chest wall.

3. Discussion

Lymphatic malformations or lymphangiomas are congenital anomalies composed of dilated lymphatic channels. They are filled with a proteinaceous fluid and generally do not have connections to the normal lymphatic system [7]. Lesions can be macrocystic (>1 cm), microcystic (<1 cm), or mixed [8, 9]. Lymphangiomas can be divided into lymphangioma circumscriptum, which are superficial, cutaneous lesions, and cavernous lymphangioma, which are more deep-seated.

Cavernous lymphangiomas occur in areas of loose connective tissue, areola, and are found primarily during infancy, and most are diagnosed by the age of 2 [1]. They are commonly located in the head, neck, and axilla and are rarely intra-abdominal. It is believed that lymphangiomas arise due to failure of connection between primitive lymphatic sacs and the surrounding lymphatic channels due to abnormalities in embryonic development [10]. This results in dilated lymphatic sacs and subsequent lymphangioma formation. Other possible hypotheses propose acquired factors such as trauma, fibrosis, and inflammatory etiologies [10].

Abdominal cystic lymphangioma (ACL) may occur anywhere along the course of the gastrointestinal tract and visceral organs. ACL has been found to occur in the small bowel mesentery in 80% of cases, while retroperitoneal location appears to be less common [11]. Abdominal distension, abdominal pain, and other symptoms of intestinal obstruction may accompany ACL, but the incidence of proven intestinal obstruction is actually quite low. Abdominal pain (72.3%) and distension (34%) are the most commonly experienced symptoms with ACL [12, 13]. Abdominal pain was noted in two of the cases, while abdominal distension was observed in all three cases of intra-abdominal lymphangioma. ACL may be asymptomatic and may be found incidentally during imaging for another pathology [8].

Axillary lymphangiomas typically present as painless swellings, which are soft, compressible, nontender, and transilluminant and are without a bruit on physical examination [14]. Axillary swellings may pose a diagnostic challenge initially with some patients being misdiagnosed as lipoma, neurofibroma, haematoma, gynaecomastia, and dermoid cyst [15]. The patient in case 4 was initially thought to have unilateral gynaecomastia at birth, but USS soon after made the diagnosis evident. Although children may present with axillary swellings at different ages, it is believed that the lymphatic malformation is present from birth. It is especially difficult to get complete excision of axillary lymphangiomas without disrupting developing breast tissue in females. In such cases, parents should be extensively counseled on cosmetic outcome.

Axillary lymphangiomas can be complicated by infection usually secondary to a respiratory tract infection. Infected lesions become red and tender and the patient may become pyretic. In some cases, they may turn into abscesses and require incision and drainage [14]. Another common complication of axillary lymphangioma is spontaneous bleeding into the cyst [14] as seen in case 4. ACL may also be complicated by infection or haemorrhage within the cyst [13] also seen in case 1. We believe that haemorrhage within cysts may have been responsible for patient's anaemia in case 1.

Radiological investigations greatly aid in the preoperative diagnosis of lymphangioma with ultrasound scan (USS) being used as the initial mode of investigation, detecting the lesion in 100% of cases in one study [16]. In cases of axillary lymphangioma, USS helps in differentiating glandular from cystic tissue [15]. Macrocystic lymphangiomas typically appear as anechoic cavities with septae and debris on gray scale USS [7]. Ultrasound scan is primarily used to monitor size and determine extent preceding excision [7]. However, computed tomography (CT) scan is significantly better at determining tumour content [13]. CT is especially helpful in determining the relations to major vessels and other surrounding structures and hence is essential in planning the surgery [13]. Lymphangiomas appear as low attenuation and fluid-filled masses on CT. Fluid-fluid levels can occasionally be seen representing acute or subacute bleeding into the cyst [7]. Magnetic resonance imaging (MRI) is an excellent modality to assess lesion extent in terms of tissue planes, airway compression, mediastinal extension, and potential solid organ and bone involvement [7]. Abdominal X-ray is noncontributory in diagnosing ACL but can detect intestinal obstruction associated with ACL [11]. The combination of both USS and CT seems to provide as much information as that obtained from MRI in ACL.

Surgical excision is known to be the gold standard for treatment of all types of lymphangioma and hence was the mode of treatment in all of the above cases. However, incomplete surgical resection is linked with recurrence as seen in case 1. Recurrence rate accounts for 10% of cases due to difficulty in resecting the entire cyst wall and is especially so for retroperitoneal cysts due to close relationship to vital retroperitoneal structures which make resection very hazardous or even impossible [11]. Postoperative complications in cases of ACL include peritonitis, haemorrhage, abscess, and torsion, which is a rare postoperative complication [10]. Wound infection, haemorrhage, hypertrophied scar, and lymphatic discharge from the wound are postoperative complications of axillary lymphangioma excision [14].

Use of sclerosing agent such as bleomycin at the time of operations remains controversial but may have some benefit in management of extra-abdominal lymphangioma [11]. Ozeki et al. recently reported some success in the use of propranolol in the treatment lymphatic malformation. Cases of diffuse intractable lymphangiomatosis showed very promising results with the use of propranolol, which is thought to cause downregulation of the Raf mitogen activated protein kinase signaling pathway, with reduced expression of vascular endothelial growth factor (VEGF) [17]. This led to a decrease in size of up to 30.6% in patients treated with propranolol [18].

Laparoscopic resection of ACL is not well documented in children but Son and Liem strongly advocate that laparoscopic surgery is both safe and feasible in resection of ACL in children. In their study of 47 children with ACL, there were no reports of mortality or intestinal obstruction postoperatively and there was a conversion rate of only 6.8%. They suggest that many cases can in fact be performed by a single port technique [13].

The diagnosis of lymphangioma is confirmed by histology, which shows benign cystic proliferation of lymphatic tissue. However typically they do not communicate with the lymphatic system (Figure 4). Immunohistochemistry may be used to differentiate intra-abdominal hemangioma from lymphangioma in cases of diagnostic uncertainty. Lymphatic malformations are thin walled vessels lined by lymphatic endothelial cells that are immunohistochemically positive for endothelial markers D2-40 and lymphatic vessel endothelial receptor 1 [9].

There is very limited regional data regarding lymphangioma. Only two regional publications exist, *Intrathoracic cystic hygroma in an infant with respiratory failure*, Balkaran et al. (Trinidad) [19], and *Orbital lymphangioma in a child: a diagnostic dilemma*, Mowatt and Crossman (Jamaica) [20]. No published regional data regarding axillary and intra-abdominal cystic lymphangioma could be found in our literature search. We do hope that this paper may serve to increase understanding of presentation and treatment of lymphangioma in the Caribbean region.

4. Conclusion

This paper discusses a range of extracervical lymphangioma cases seen at San Fernando General Hospital, Trinidad. We report three intra-abdominal cases, and the most common clinical presentations were abdominal pain and distension. Also two axillary cases were reported, which presented as painless axillary masses. The major concerns for excision of axillary lymphangioma by parents and surgeons were cosmesis and feasibility of complete resection without disruption of developing breast tissue and axillary vessels. We believe that ultrasound scan is very good at detection of the lesion, while CT is better at determining tumour content and planning for the operation. It is our opinion that complete surgical excision can be achieved.

Conflict of Interests

The authors declare that they have no conflict of interests.

Acknowledgment

The authors thank Dr. Wesley Greaves, Head of Department of Pathology, San Fernando General Hospital.

References

[1] T. Bhavsar, D. Saeed-Vafa, S. Harbison et al., "Retroperitoneal cystic lymphangioma in an adult: a case report and review of

the literature," *World Journal of Gastrointestinal Pathophysiology*, vol. 15, pp. 171–176, 2010.

[2] M. A. Kosir, R. E. Sonnino, and M. W. L. Gauderer, "Pediatric abdominal lymphangiomas: a plea for early recognition," *Journal of Pediatric Surgery*, vol. 26, no. 11, pp. 1309–1313, 1991.

[3] A. Alqahtani, L. T. Nguyen, H. Flageole, K. Shaw, and J.-M. Laberge, "25 years' experience with lymphangiomas in children," *Journal of Pediatric Surgery*, vol. 34, no. 7, pp. 1164–1168, 1999.

[4] B. J. Hancock, D. St-Vil, F. I. Luks, M. Di Lorenzo, and H. Blanchard, "Complications of lymphangiomas in children," *Journal of Pediatric Surgery*, vol. 27, no. 2, pp. 220–224, 1992.

[5] C. H. Lugo-Olivieri and G. A. Taylor, "CT differentiation of large abdominal lymphangioma from ascites," *Pediatric Radiology*, vol. 23, no. 2, pp. 129–130, 1993.

[6] K. A. Gonen, R. Abali, M. Oznur, and C. Erdogan, "Lymphangioma: surrounding the ovarian vein and ovary," *BMJ Case Reports*, Article ID 200020, 2013.

[7] A. M. Cahill and E. L. F. Nijs, "Pediatric vascular malformations: pathophysiology, diagnosis, and the role of interventional radiology," *CardioVascular and Interventional Radiology*, vol. 34, no. 4, pp. 691–704, 2011.

[8] J. B. Mulliken, J. Glowacki, and H. G. Thomson, "Hemangiomas and vascular malformations in infants and children: a classification based on endothelial characteristics," *Plastic and Reconstructive Surgery*, vol. 69, no. 3, pp. 412–422, 1982.

[9] A. M. Vogel and B. W. Warner, "Toward an understanding of lymphatic malformations," *Gastroenterology & Hepatology*, vol. 9, no. 3, pp. 195–196, 2013.

[10] P. J. Karkera, G. R. Sandlas, R. R. Ranjan, K. Kesan, A. R. Gupta, and R. K. Gupta, "Intra-abdominal cystic lymphangiomas in children: a case series," *Archives of International Surgery*, vol. 2, no. 2, 2013.

[11] R. Méndez-Gallart, A. Bautista, E. Estévez, and P. Rodríguez-Barca, "Abdominal Cystic lymphangiomas in pediatrics: surgical approach and outcomes," *Acta Chirurgica Belgica*, vol. 111, no. 6, pp. 374–377, 2011.

[12] T. S. Chang, R. Ricketts, C. R. Abramowksy et al., "Mesenteric cystic masses: a series of 21 pediatric cases and review of the literature," *Fetal and Pediatric Pathology*, vol. 30, no. 1, pp. 40–44, 2011.

[13] T. N. Son and N. T. Liem, "Laparoscopic management of abdominal lymphatic cyst in children," *Journal of Laparoendoscopic & Advanced Surgical Techniques*, vol. 22, no. 5, pp. 505–507, 2012.

[14] B. Mirza, L. Ijaz, M. Saleem, M. Sharif, and A. Sheikh, "Cystic hygroma: an overview," *Journal of Cutaneous and Aesthetic Surgery*, vol. 3, pp. 139–144, 2010.

[15] F. Ekmez, O. Pirgon, H. Bilgin, and G. Aydemir, "Cystic hygroma of the breast in a 5 year old boy presenting as a gynecomastia," *European review for medical and pharmacological sciences*, vol. 16, no. 4 supplement, pp. 55–57, 2012.

[16] A. Makni, F. Chebbi, F. Fetirich et al., "Surgical management of intra-abdominal cystic lymphangioma. Report of 20 cases," *World Journal of Surgery*, vol. 36, no. 5, pp. 1037–1043, 2012.

[17] C. H. Storch and P. H. Hoeger, "Propranolol for infantile haemangiomas: insights into the molecular mechanisms of action," *British Journal of Dermatology*, vol. 163, no. 2, pp. 269–274, 2010.

[18] M. Ozeki, K. Kanda, N. Kawamoto et al., "Propranolol as an alternative treatment option for pediatric lymphatic malformation," *Tohoku Journal of Experimental Medicine*, vol. 229, no. 1, pp. 61–66, 2012.

[19] B. N. Balkaran, P. Maharaj, and P. Pitt-Miller, "Intrathoracic cystic hygroma in an infant with respiratory failure," *West Indian Medical Journal*, vol. 46, no. 4, pp. 128–129, 1997.

[20] L. Mowatt and G. Crossman, "Orbital lymphangioma in a child: a diagnostic dilemma," *West Indian Medical Journal*, vol. 61, no. 7, pp. 764–766, 2012.

44

Colonic Necrosis in a 4-Year-Old with Hyperlipidemic Acute Pancreatitis

Tiffany J. Patton,[1] Timothy A. Sentongo,[1] Grace Z. Mak,[2] and Stacy A. Kahn[1]

[1]Department of Pediatrics, Section of Pediatric Gastroenterology, University of Chicago, Wyler Pavilion C-474, 5839 S. Maryland Avenue, MC 4065, Chicago, IL 60637, USA
[2]Department of Pediatrics, Section of Pediatric Surgery, The University of Chicago Hospitals, 5841 S. Maryland Avenue, MC 4062, Chicago, IL 60637, USA

Correspondence should be addressed to Tiffany J. Patton; tiffany.patton@uchospitals.edu

Academic Editor: Daniel K. L. Cheuk

Here we report the case of a 4-year-old male with severe acute pancreatitis due to hyperlipidemia, who presented with abdominal pain, metabolic abnormalities, and colonic necrosis. This colonic complication was secondary to the extension of a large peripancreatic fluid collection causing direct serosal autodigestion by pancreatic enzymes. Two weeks following the initial presentation, the peripancreatic fluid collection developed into a mature pancreatic pseudocyst, which was percutaneously drained. To our knowledge, this is the youngest documented pediatric case of colonic necrosis due to severe pancreatitis and the first descriptive pediatric case of a colonic complication due to hyperlipidemia-induced acute pancreatitis.

1. Introduction

Colonic complications of pancreatitis, that is, necrosis, fistulae, and strictures, are uncommon in adults but are rarely reported in children [1]. Mechanistic theories of colonic involvement in acute pancreatitis include mesenteric ischemia, thrombosis/compression of mesenteric arteries, local enzymatic digestion, and disseminated intravascular coagulation [2]. An extensive PubMed search identified two reports of colonic necrosis associated with acute pancreatitis in children, one ascribed to hypotension and the other to direct extension of necrotizing pancreatitis in an immunocompromised patient [3, 4]. Here we present a child with previously undiagnosed hyperlipidemia who presented with colonic necrosis from an adjacent peripancreatic fluid collection associated with severe acute pancreatitis.

2. Case Presentation

A 4-year-old male with no known medical problems presented to a local emergency room with a 3-day history of decreased oral intake, nausea, nonbloody, nonbilious emesis, and abdominal pain. Laboratory assessment revealed lipemic serum with triglycerides of 7449 mg/dL (normal 30–149 mg/dL), anemia (hematocrit 19%), hyponatremia (sodium 129 mEq/L), metabolic acidosis (carbon dioxide 12 mEq/L), azotemia (blood urea nitrogen 73 mg/dL, creatinine 1.8 mg/dL), amylase 248 IU/L (normal 28–100 IU/L), and lipase 360 U/L (normal 13–60 U/L). A contrast abdominal CT scan demonstrated a large retroperitoneal mass appearing to arise from the left adrenal gland with normal pancreatic appearance. The patient was transferred to the University of Chicago Pediatric Intensive Care Unit for further management and diagnostic workup.

On admission the patient was febrile (39.4°C) and tachycardic (132 beats/min) with weight, height, and BMI at the 83rd, 33rd, and 97th percentiles, respectively. On physical exam his abdomen was distended with hypoactive bowel sounds and a palpable mass in the left upper quadrant; no xanthomata or lipemia retinalis was noted. The laboratory findings were comparable to the previous with the addition of amylase 79 U/L (normal 28–100 U/L), lipase 99 U/L (normal 11–65 U/L), and fasting triglycerides 6060 mg/dL.

Due to concern for malignancy, the patient underwent an extensive workup to rule out solid tumors. On repeat chest/abdominal CT scan, a diffusely enlarged pancreas

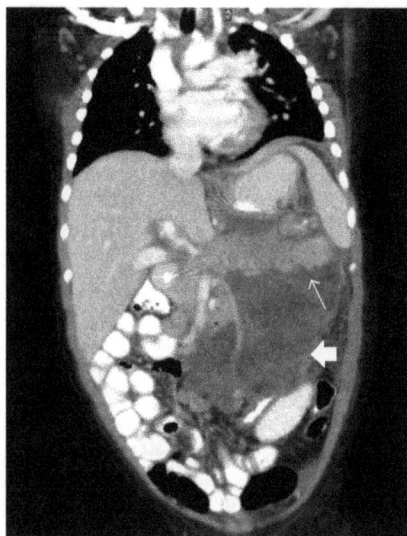

FIGURE 1: Abdominal CT (coronal view): 10 cm × 8.4 cm left-sided peritoneal mass (broad arrow) with significant inflammation of the pancreas (thin arrow).

without areas of necrosis or calcifications was noted. Additionally, the mass was described as a large infiltrative low density lesion extending from the left retroperitoneum around the pancreas, bilateral renal spaces, down to the perirectal area without obvious metastatic lesions within the lungs or abdomen (Figure 1). The patient underwent an exploratory laparotomy with tissue histology to better characterize the origin of the mass. Intraoperatively, a significant amount of ascites and the retroperitoneal mass were identified in the left paracolic gutter with necrotic extension to the omentum and onto the left colon at the splenic flexure. The mass was also noted within the lesser sac, anterior to the pancreas, and extending into the pelvis. A large portion of the retroperitoneal mass and adherent omentum was resected, in addition to the necrotic portion of the splenic flexure, and a diverting transverse colostomy was performed. The mass pathology revealed extensive fat necrosis and reactive inflammation of the omentum without any identifiable tumor cells. The resected bowel segment had extensive serosal fat necrosis and reactive inflammatory changes, but viable mucosa and muscular wall with no perforation on pathologic examination. Additionally, bone marrow biopsies and infectious studies were negative. Two weeks later, a repeat abdominal CT scan revealed a large mature pseudocyst in the site of the former fluid collection, which was then percutaneously drained by interventional radiology (amylase level of 173 U/L).

We concluded that the patient had undiagnosed type I familial hypertriglyceridemia, presenting initially as chylomicronemia syndrome, resulting in acute pancreatitis with a large peripancreatic fluid accumulation causing colonic necrosis due to direct pancreatic enzyme serosal digestion. The patient was initially managed with total parenteral nutrition and kept NPO (nil per os) with subsequent advancement to a low-fat diet and colonic reanastomosis following a 3-month period. To date his hypertriglyceridemia has been

controlled with a low-fat diet supplemented with omega-3 fatty acid ethyl esters.

3. Discussion

Colonic complications, such as necrosis, fistulae, and strictures, have been reported in 15% of adults with severe pancreatitis [1]. To date only two reports with differing etiologies have been published describing colonic necrosis associated with acute pancreatitis in children [3, 4]. Current literature describes three separate mechanisms for the etiology of pancreatitis associated colonic injury. First, the direct spread of pancreatic enzymes and peripancreatic inflammatory tissue can involve the colonic serosa, causing local inflammation and fat necrosis. Second, thrombosis/compression of the mesenteric and submucosal vessels can lead to infarction of the mucosa and deeper layers of the colon [4, 5]. Third, hypotensive episodes in severe acute pancreatitis can lead to a "low flow state" causing ischemia of the colon particularly at the splenic flexure at the junction of the middle and left colic arteries [2]. Given the related findings within the present case, we suspect that the direct extension of peripancreatic fluid and its pancreatic enzyme content were responsible for the adjacent colonic necrosis in our patient.

In adults, pancreatitis associated colonic necrosis may be diagnosed at a median of 25 (range 1–55) days following symptomatic onset and has a mortality rate of 54% [1]. While the pediatric mortality rate for pancreatitis associated colonic necrosis is unknown, it is generally accepted that the mortality rate in pediatric acute pancreatitis (~2–11.1%) is often due to concurrent systemic illness [6]. In the present case, colonic necrosis was discovered intraoperatively 8 days following initial symptomatic onset. In all cases, colonic resection with a diverting stoma is the standard therapeutic management of colonic necrosis, as was described in our case [1].

The association of hyperlipidemia and acute pancreatitis has been well described and accounts for ~6% of acute pancreatitis episodes [5, 7]. Acute pancreatitis is associated with increased serum lipids in 50% of patients, while a triglyceride level > 1,000 mg/dL can precipitate an episode of acute pancreatitis [8]. The pathophysiology of hypertriglyceridemia-induced pancreatitis is not well established. However, it is thought to occur when pancreatic lipase digests triglycerides within pancreatic capillaries causing chylomicrons to occlude these vessels leading to pancreatic ischemia and activation of trypsinogen by free fatty acids [8]. Theoretically, the resultant hyperviscosity from chylomicrons may impair circulatory flow within smaller splanchnic vessels, predisposing to colonic complications (i.e., colonic necrosis, ischemia, and perforation). However, we do not believe that this was the etiology in our patient due to a lack of necrosis within the mucosal and intramural layers of the colonic wall.

Chylomicronemia syndrome, as identified in our patient, is defined as a plasma triglyceride level > 1000 mg/dL accompanied by one or more of the following: eruptive xanthoma, lipemia retinalis, abdominal pain, acute pancreatitis, and/or hepatosplenomegaly [9]. Familial hypertriglyceridemia is the most common primary cause of chylomicronemia in adults. Treatment of chylomicronemia involves lifestyle modification with increased physical activity, weight loss, and a low-fat diet (i.e., reduction of saturated fat to <7% of total calories). Medical therapy includes fibrates and/or n-3 polyunsaturated fatty acids, both of which are capable of reducing triglycerides by 50% [9]. For severe cases of chylomicronemia (triglycerides > 500 mg/dL and abdominal pain or pancreatitis), inpatient therapy is preferred with NPO, intravenous hydration, low dose insulin and/or heparin infusions, and gradual advancement to a low-fat diet. Accordingly, our patient remained NPO for two weeks prior to advancing to a low-fat diet with a corresponding decrease in serum triglycerides. Insulin and heparin infusions were not instituted in our patient due to a relatively rapid reduction in triglyceride levels while being NPO.

Although colonic complications are far more prevalent in the adult population, pediatricians need to be aware that they can occur in children with pancreatitis. Additionally, since the association between hyperlipidemia and pancreatitis is well established, it is important for clinicians to consider hyperlipidemic pancreatitis and its complications when faced with lactescent serum samples (and/or fasting serum triglyceride levels > 1000–2000 mg/dL) and abdominal pain even in the presence of normal or mildly elevated serum amylase and lipase. It is known that lipemia commonly interferes with the processing methods of various laboratory tests, potentially rendering test results inaccurate and difficult to interpret [10].

To our knowledge, this is the first and youngest pediatric report of colonic necrosis due to direct enzymatic contact with a peripancreatic fluid collection in acute pancreatitis secondary to hyperlipidemia. Several key features of this case should be noted. First, the patient presented with extremely high triglyceride levels although there was no significant history of hyperlipidemic symptoms. Second, absence of significantly elevated serum amylase and lipase in the setting of hyperlipemic serum may obscure the diagnosis of pancreatitis [11, 12]. Therefore in this setting, subtle but ongoing gastrointestinal symptoms including vomiting and abdominal pain warrant further evaluation including a workup for pancreatitis. Finally, although this presentation was initially concerning for malignancy (i.e., neuroblastoma, Wilms' tumor, hepatoblastoma, and lymphoma), in addition to an intraperitoneal abscess, the differential diagnosis of a retroperitoneal mass should always include complications of pancreatitis and pancreatic pseudocyst.

Disclosure

All stated authors have no financial relationships relevant to this paper to disclose.

Conflict of Interests

All stated authors have no conflict of interests to disclose.

References

[1] S. R. Mohamed and A. K. Siriwardena, "Understanding the colonic complications of pancreatitis," *Pancreatology*, vol. 8, no. 2, pp. 153–158, 2008.

[2] L. P. Van Minnen, M. G. H. Besselink, K. Bosscha, M. S. Van Leeuwen, M. E. I. Schipper, and H. G. Gooszen, "Colonic involvement in acute pancreatitis: a retrospective study of 16 patients," *Digestive Surgery*, vol. 21, no. 1, pp. 33–38, 2004.

[3] I. Yamagiwa, K. Obata, Y. Hatanaka, H. Saito, and M. Washio, "Ischemic colitis complicating severe acute pancreatitis in a child," *Journal of Pediatric Gastroenterology and Nutrition*, vol. 16, no. 2, pp. 208–211, 1993.

[4] T. Acer, B. Malbora, İ. Ötgün et al., "Fat necrosis of transverse colon and necrotizing pancreatitis in a patient with Acute Lymphoblastic Leukemia (ALL): cause of massive ascites and high fever," *Turkish Journal of Pediatrics*, vol. 55, no. 4, pp. 458–461, 2013.

[5] M. C. Aldridge, N. D. Francis, and H. A. F. Dudley, "Colonic complications of severe acute pancreatitis," *British Journal of Surgery*, vol. 76, no. 4, pp. 362–367, 1989.

[6] M. E. Lowe and J. B. Greer, "Pancreatitis in children and adolescents," *Current Gastroenterology Reports*, vol. 10, no. 2, pp. 128–135, 2008.

[7] S. Z. Husain, V. Morinville, J. Pohl et al., "Toxic-metabolic risk factors in pediatric pancreatitis: recommendations for diagnosis, management and future research," *Journal of Pediatric Gastroenterology & Nutrition*, 2015.

[8] D. Yadav and C. S. Pitchumoni, "Issues in hyperlipidemic pancreatitis," *Journal of Clinical Gastroenterology*, vol. 36, pp. 54–62, 2003.

[9] D. A. Leaf, "Chylomicronemia and the chylomicronemia syndrome: a practical approach to management," *The American Journal of Medicine*, vol. 121, no. 1, pp. 10–12, 2008.

[10] M. H. Kroll, "Evaluating interference caused by lipemia," *Clinical Chemistry*, vol. 50, no. 11, pp. 1968–1969, 2004.

[11] P. B. Lesser and A. L. Warshaw, "Diagnosis of pancreatitis masked by hyperlipemia," *Annals of Internal Medicine*, vol. 82, no. 6, pp. 795–798, 1975.

[12] W. R. Matull, S. P. Pereira, and J. W. O'Donohue, "Biochemical markers of acute pancreatitis," *Journal of Clinical Pathology*, vol. 59, no. 4, pp. 340–344, 2006.

Permissions

All chapters in this book were first published in CRIPE, by Hindawi Publishing Corporation; hereby published with permission under the Creative Commons Attribution License or equivalent. Every chapter published in this book has been scrutinized by our experts. Their significance has been extensively debated. The topics covered herein carry significant findings which will fuel the growth of the discipline. They may even be implemented as practical applications or may be referred to as a beginning point for another development.

The contributors of this book come from diverse backgrounds, making this book a truly international effort. This book will bring forth new frontiers with its revolutionizing research information and detailed analysis of the nascent developments around the world.

We would like to thank all the contributing authors for lending their expertise to make the book truly unique. They have played a crucial role in the development of this book. Without their invaluable contributions this book wouldn't have been possible. They have made vital efforts to compile up to date information on the varied aspects of this subject to make this book a valuable addition to the collection of many professionals and students.

This book was conceptualized with the vision of imparting up-to-date information and advanced data in this field. To ensure the same, a matchless editorial board was set up. Every individual on the board went through rigorous rounds of assessment to prove their worth. After which they invested a large part of their time researching and compiling the most relevant data for our readers.

The editorial board has been involved in producing this book since its inception. They have spent rigorous hours researching and exploring the diverse topics which have resulted in the successful publishing of this book. They have passed on their knowledge of decades through this book. To expedite this challenging task, the publisher supported the team at every step. A small team of assistant editors was also appointed to further simplify the editing procedure and attain best results for the readers.

Apart from the editorial board, the designing team has also invested a significant amount of their time in understanding the subject and creating the most relevant covers. They scrutinized every image to scout for the most suitable representation of the subject and create an appropriate cover for the book.

The publishing team has been an ardent support to the editorial, designing and production team. Their endless efforts to recruit the best for this project, has resulted in the accomplishment of this book. They are a veteran in the field of academics and their pool of knowledge is as vast as their experience in printing. Their expertise and guidance has proved useful at every step. Their uncompromising quality standards have made this book an exceptional effort. Their encouragement from time to time has been an inspiration for everyone.

The publisher and the editorial board hope that this book will prove to be a valuable piece of knowledge for researchers, students, practitioners and scholars across the globe.

List of Contributors

Irappa Madabhavi, Apurva Patel, Mukesh Choudhary, Suhas Aagre, Gaurang Modi, Asha Anand, Harsha Panchal, Sonia Parikh and Shreeniwas Raut
Department of Medical and Paediatric Oncology, GCRI, Ahmedabad, Gujarat 380016, India

Swaroop Revannasiddaiah
Department of Radiotherapy, Government Medical College, Haldwani, India

Roxanne Lim, Hassan Choudry, Kim Conner and Wikrom Karnsakul
Division of Pediatric Gastroenterology and Nutrition, Johns Hopkins University School of Medicine, Baltimore, MD 21287, USA

Serkan AtJcJ, Eda Kepenekli KadayJfcJ, Ayşe Karaaslan and Mustafa BakJr
Department of Pediatrics and Division of Pediatric Infectious Diseases, Marmara University Medical Faculty, Pendik Training and Research Hospital, Fevzi Cakmak Mah. Mimar Sinan Cad., Ust Kaynarca, Pendik, 34899 Istanbul, Turkey

Muhammed Hasan Toper and Cigdem Ataizi Celikel
Department of Pathology, Marmara University Medical Faculty, Pendik Training and Research Hospital, Fevzi Cakmak Mah. Mimar Sinan Cad., Ust Kaynarca, Pendik, 34899 Istanbul, Turkey

Ahmet Soysal
Department of Pediatrics and Division of Pediatric Infectious Diseases, Marmara University Medical Faculty, Pendik Training and Research Hospital, Fevzi Cakmak Mah. Mimar Sinan Cad., Ust Kaynarca, Pendik, 34899 Istanbul, Turkey
Marmara University Medical Faculty, Pendik Training and Research Hospital, Fevzi Cakmak Mah. Mimar Sinan Cad., Ust Kaynarca, Pendik, 34899 Istanbul, Turkey

Osamah Abdullah AlAyed
King Faisal Specialist Hospital Research Centre, P.O. Box 280581, Riyadh 11392, Saudi Arabia

Oluwafemi Olasupo Awe
Plastic Surgery Unit, Department of Surgery, Irrua Specialist Teaching Hospital, Irrua, Edo State, Nigeria
Plastic Surgery Unit, Department of Surgery, Ambrose Alli University, PMB 08, Ekpoma, Edo State, Nigeria

Emeka B. Kesieme
Cardiothoracic Surgery Unit, Department of Surgery, Irrua Specialist Teaching Hospital, Irrua, Edo State, Nigeria

Babatunde Kayode-Adedeji
Special Care Baby Unit, Department of Paediatrics, Irrua Specialist Teaching Hospital, Irrua, Edo State, Nigeria

Quinzy O. Aigbonoga
Plastic Surgery Unit, Department of Surgery, Irrua Specialist Teaching Hospital, Irrua, Edo State, Nigeria

S. Stabouli, N. Printza, J. Dotis, A. Matis, N. Gombakis and F. Papachristou
1st Department of Pediatrics, Aristotle University of Thessaloniki, Hippokration Hospital of Thessaloniki, 49 Kostantinoupoleos Street, 54642 Thessaloniki, Greece

D. Koliouskas
Pediatric Oncology Clinic, Hippokration Hospital of Thessaloniki, 49 Kostantinoupoleos Street, 54642 Thessaloniki, Greece

Boris Limme and Ramona Nicolescu
Department of Pediatrics, General Hospital Citadelle, Boulevard du 12 ème de Ligne 1, 4000 Liège, Belgium

Jean-Paul Misson
Department of Pediatrics, General Hospital Citadelle, Boulevard du 12 ème de Ligne 1, 4000 Liège, Belgium
Universitè de Liège, Place du 20 Août 7, 4000 Liège, Belgium

Serap Alsancak and Senem Guner
Department of Orthopedic Prosthetics and Orthotics, Vocational School of Health Services, Ankara University, Fatih Street 197/A Gazino, Kecioren, 06280 Ankara, Turkey

Panagiotis Kratimenos
Neonatal-Perinatal Medicine, St. Christopher's Hospital for Children, Drexel University College of Medicine, Philadelphia, PA, USA
Department of Pediatrics, The Unterberg Children's Hospital at Monmouth Medical Center, Drexel University College of Medicine, Long Branch, NJ, USA

Ioannis Koutroulis
Department of Emergency Medicine, St. Christopher's Hospital for Children, Drexel University College of Medicine, Philadelphia, PA, USA

Dante Marconi, Jennifer Ding, Christos Plakas and Margaret Fisher
Department of Pediatrics, The Unterberg Children's Hospital at Monmouth Medical Center, Drexel University College of Medicine, Long Branch, NJ, USA

A. Nael and P. Siaghani
Department of Pathology and Laboratory Medicine, University of California Irvine Medical Center, 101 The City Drive, Orange, CA 92868, USA

W. W. Wu
Department of Pathology and Laboratory Medicine, Memorial Sloan Kettering Cancer Center, 1275 York Avenue, New York, NY 10065, USA

K. Nael
Department of Medical Imaging, University of Arizona Medical Center, 1501 N. Campbell Avenue, P.O. Box 245067, Tucson, AZ 85724-5067, USA

Lisa Shane and S. G. Romansky
University of California Irvine, Long Beach Memorial Care Health System, 2801 Atlantic Avenue, Long Beach, CA 908068, USA

Simon Berzel, Katja Schneider and Nico Hepping
Department of Neonatology, GFO-Hospitals Bonn, St Mary's Hospital, Robert-Koch Street 1, 53115 Bonn, Germany

Emilia Stegemann
Department of Vascular Surgery, GFO-Hospitals Bonn, St Mary's Hospital, Bonn, Germany
Department of Cardiology, Pulmonology and Angiology, University Medical Centre, Dusseldorf, Germany

Hans-Joerg Hertfelder
Department of Experimental Hematology and Transfusion Medicine, University Medical Centre, Bonn, Germany

Claudia Barone, Nicolina Stefania Carucci and Claudio Romano
Pediatric Department, University of Messina, Italy

Antonella Gagliano and Eva Germanò
Division of Child Neurology and Psychiatry, Department of Pediatrics, University of Messina, Via Consolare Valeria, 98125 Messina, Italy

Loredana Benedetto
Division of Psychology, Department of Humanities and Social Sciences, University of Messina, Via Concezione, No. 6/8, 98100Messina, Italy

Gabriele Masi
IRCCS Stella Maris, Scientific Institute Child Neurology and Psychiatry, Viale del Tirreno, No. 331, 56018 Calambrone, Pisa, Italy

Elena Castilla Cabanes
Echocardiography Section, Department of Cardiology, Hospital Clínico Universitario de Zaragoza, Avenida San Juan Bosco 15, 50009 Zaragoza, Spain
Department of Cardiology, Hospital General Universitario de Elche, Camí de L'Almassera 11, Alicante, 03023 Elche, Spain

Isaac Lacambra Blasco
Echocardiography Section, Department of Cardiology, Hospital Clínico Universitario de Zaragoza, Avenida San Juan Bosco 15, 50009 Zaragoza, Spain

Yuri A. Zarate
Section of Genetics and Metabolism, University of Arkansas for Medical Sciences College of Medicine, Little Rock, AR 72205, USA
Arkansas Children's Hospital, 1 Children's Way, Slot 512-22, Little Rock, AR 72202, USA

Katherine A. Bosanko and Jaime Vengoechea
Section of Genetics and Metabolism, University of Arkansas for Medical Sciences College of Medicine, Little Rock, AR 72205, USA

Chaowapong Jarasvaraparn and Elizabeth M. McDonough
Division of Pediatric Gastroenterology, Hepatology and Nutrition, University of Arkansas for Medical Sciences College of Medicine, Little Rock, AR 72205, USA

Timothy Brooks and Laura Nolting
Department of Emergency Medicine, Palmetto Health Richland, Suite 350, 14 Medical Park, Columbia, SC 29203, USA

Eric Tibesar, Christine Karwowski, Ann Scheimann and Wikrom Karnsakul
Division of Pediatric Gastroenterology, Johns Hopkins University School of Medicine, 600 N.Wolfe Street, Baltimore, MD 21287, USA

Paula Hertel
Division of Pediatric Gastroenterology, Texas Children's Hospital, 6621 Fannin Street, Houston, TX 77030, USA

Kimberly M. Thornton, Howard Kilbride and Kristin Voos
Division of Neonatology, Children's Mercy Hospital, 2401 Gillham Road, Kansas City, MO 64108, USA
University of Missouri-Kansas City School of Medicine, 2411 Holmes Road, Kansas City, MO 64108, USA

Timothy Bennett
University of Missouri-Kansas City School of Medicine, 2411 Holmes Road, Kansas City, MO 64108, USA
Department of Obstetrics and Gynecology, Elizabeth J. Ferrell Fetal Health Center, Children's Mercy Hospital, 2401 Gillham Road, Kansas City, MO 64108, USA

Vivekanand Singh
University of Missouri-Kansas City School of Medicine, 2411 Holmes Road, Kansas City, MO 64108, USA
Department of Pathology, Children's Mercy Hospital, 2401 Gillham Road, Kansas City, MO 64108, USA

Neil Mardis
University of Missouri-Kansas City School of Medicine, 2411 Holmes Road, Kansas City, MO 64108, USA
Department of Radiology, Children's Mercy Hospital, 2401 Gillham Road, Kansas City, MO 64108, USA

Jennifer Linebarger
University of Missouri-Kansas City School of Medicine, 2411 Holmes Road, Kansas City, MO 64108, USA
Department of Pediatrics, Palliative Care Center, Children's Mercy Hospital, 2401 Gillham Road, Kansas City, MO 64108, USA

L. M. Pérez-López, M. Cabrera-González, D. Gutiérrez-de la Iglesia and G. Knörr-Giménez
Pediatric Orthopaedic Surgery Department, Sant Joan de Déu Children's Hospital, University of Barcelona, Barcelona, Spain

S. Ricart
Pediatric Rheumatology Department, Sant Joan de Déu Children's Hospital, University of Barcelona, Barcelona, Spain

Mustafa Çakan and Ahmet Koç
Department of Pediatric Hematology and Oncology, Faculty of Medicine, Marmara University, Mimar Sinan Caddesi No. 41, Pendik, 34899 Istanbul, Turkey

KJvJlcJmCerit
Department of Pediatric Surgery, Faculty of Medicine, Marmara University, Mimar Sinan Caddesi No. 41, Pendik, 34899 Istanbul, Turkey

Süheyla Bozkurt
Department of Pathology, Faculty of Medicine, Marmara University, Mimar Sinan Caddesi No. 41, Pendik, 34899 Istanbul, Turkey

Rabia Ergelen
Department of Radiology, Faculty of Medicine, Marmara University, Mimar Sinan Caddesi No. 41, Pendik, 34899 Istanbul, Turkey

Irmak Vural
Department of Pediatrics, Faculty of Medicine, Marmara University, Mimar Sinan Caddesi No. 41, Pendik, 34899 Istanbul, Turkey

Ricardo A.Mosquera, Mark McDonald and Cheryl Samuels
High Risk Children Comprehensive Care Clinic, University of Texas Health Science of Houston, 6410 Fannin Street, Suite 500, Houston, TX 77030, USA

Tamer Celik and Mustafa Komur
Pediatric Neurology, Adana Numune Research and Training Hospital, Adana, Turkey

Umit Celik, Cigdem Donmezer and Orkun Tolunay
Pediatrics, Adana Numune Research and Training Hospital, Adana, Turkey

Pelin Demirtürk
Pathology Department, Adana Numune Research and Training Hospital, Adana, Turkey

Mehmet Demirdöven
Department Of Pediatrics, School Of Medicine, Fatih University, Turkey
Fatih Üniversitesi Tıp Fakültesi, Sahil Yolu Sokak No. 16 Dragos Maltepe, 34844 Istanbul, Turkey

Hamza Yazgan, Arzu GebeGçe and Alparslan Tonbul
Department Of Pediatrics, School Of Medicine, Fatih University, Turkey

Mevlit Korkmaz
Department Of Pediatrics Surgery, School Of Medicine, Fatih University, Turkey

Nicola Bizzotto, Andrea Sandri, Dario Regis, Guillherme Carpeggiani, Franco Lavini and Bruno Magnan
Department of Orthopaedic and Trauma Surgery, Integrated University Hospital, Piazzale A. Stefani 2, 37126 Verona, Italy

David Kurahara, Marina Morie, Maya Yamane, Sarah Lam, Wallace Matthews, Keolamau Yee and Kara Yamamoto
Department of Pediatrics, John A. Burns School of Medicine, University of Hawaii, Honolulu, HI, USA

Sarra Benmiloud
Unit of Pediatric Hematology-Oncology, Department of Pediatrics, University Hospital Hassan II, Faculty of Medicine and Pharmacy, University of Sidi Mohamed Ben Abdellah, 30000 Fez, Morocco
Unit of Pediatric Hematology-Oncology, Department of Pediatrics, Mother-Child Hospital, University Hospital Hassan II, Faculty of Medicine and Pharmacy, University of Sidi Mohamed Ben Abdellah, BP 1893, Km 2.200, Sidi Hrazem Road, 30000 Fez, Morocco

Mohamed Hbibi, Sana Chaouki, Sana Abourazzak and Moustapha Hida
Unit of Pediatric Hematology-Oncology, Department of Pediatrics, University Hospital Hassan II, Faculty of Medicine and Pharmacy, University of Sidi Mohamed Ben Abdellah, 30000 Fez, Morocco

Mohamed A. Hendaus
Department of Pediatrics, Section of General Pediatrics, Hamad Medical Corporation, Doha, Qatar

Ahmad Alhammadi
Department of Pediatrics, Section of General Pediatrics, Hamad Medical Corporation, Doha, Qatar
Weill Cornell Medical College, Doha, Qatar

Mehdi M. Adeli
Weill Cornell Medical College, Doha, Qatar
Department of Pediatrics, Allergy and Immunology Section, Hamad Medical Corporation, Doha, Qatar

Fawzia Al-Yafei
Department of Pediatrics, Section of General Pediatrics, Hamad Medical Corporation, Doha, Qatar
Department of Pediatrics, Endocrinology Section, Hamad Medical Corporation, Doha, Qatar

KaeWatanabe
Department of Pediatrics, University of Florida, 1600 SW Archer Road, Gainesville, FL 32608, USA

Dhanashree A. Rajderkar
Department of Radiology, University of Florida, Gainesville, FL 32608, USA

Renee F. Modica
Department of Pediatric Immunology, Rheumatology and Infectious Disease, University of Florida, Gainesville, FL 32608, USA

G. Nayantara Rao and S. Narasimha Rao
Department of Pediatrics, Apollo Institute of Medical Sciences and Research, Hyderabad 500096, India

Jayasri Helen Gali
Department of Pulmonology, Apollo Institute of Medical Sciences and Research, Hyderabad 500096, India

Sabrina Congedi, Silvia Spadini, Chiara Di Pede, Martina Ometto, Tatiana Franceschi, Valentina De Tommasi, Caterina Agosto, Pierina Lazzarin and Franca Benini
Department of Women's and Children's Health, University of Padua, 3 Giustiniani Street, 35128 Padua, Italy
Pediatric Pain and Palliative Care Service, University of Padua, 59 Ospedale Civile Street, 35121 Padua, Italy

Sona Zaleta, Sarah Miller and Prashant Kumar
Department of Paediatrics, Timaru Public Hospital, Timaru 7910, New Zealand

Rebekah Beyers, Sevilay Dalabih and Abdallah Dalabih
Department of Child Health, University of Missouri, 400 Keene Street, Columbia, MO 65201, USA

Michael Baldwin
Department of Molecular Microbiology and Immunology, University of Missouri, Columbia, MO 65201, USA

Lidia Puchalska-Niedbał and Urszula Kulik
Department of Ophthalmology, Pomeranian Medical University, Aleja Powstaców Wielkopolskich 72, 70-111 Szczecin, Poland

Stanisław Zajączek
Cytogenetic Unit, Department of Pathology, Pomeranian Medical University, Aleja Powstaców Wielkopolskich 72, 70-111 Szczecin, Poland

Elżbieta Petriczko
Department of Paediatrics, Endocrinology, Diabetology, Metabolic Disorders and Cardiology, Pomeranian Medical University, Aleja Powstaców Wielkopolskich 72, 70-111 Szczecin, Poland

Toru Watanabe
Department of Pediatrics, Niigata City General Hospital, 463-7 Shumoku, Chuo-ku, Niigata 950-1197, Japan

Valentina Pastore and Fabio Bartoli
Pediatric Surgery Unit, Medical and Surgical Sciences Department, University of Foggia, Viale Pinto 1, 71122 Foggia, Italy

Rachel Bramson
College of Medicine, Texas A&M Health Science Center College of Medicine, Bryan, TX 77807, USA
Family Medicine, Scott and White University Clinic, College Station, TX 77845, USA

Angela Hairrell
College of Medicine, Texas A&M Health Science Center College of Medicine, Bryan, TX 77807, USA

Renee Frances Modica, L. Daphna Yasova Barbeau, Jennifer Co-Vu, Richard D. Beegle and Charles A. Williams
University of Florida, Gainesville, FL, USA

Parkash Mandhan, Muthana Alsalihi, Saleem Mammoo and Mansour J. Ali
Department of Pediatric Surgery, Hamad General Hospital, Hamad Medical Corporation, P.O. Box 3050, Doha, Qatar

Helena Ferreira, Ângela Dias and Andreia Lopes
Departamento de Pediatria, Centro Hospitalar do Alto Ave, Rua dos Cutileiros, Creixomil, 4835-044 Guimarães, Portugal

Khaled Alqoaer, Mohammed M. Ahmed and Efteraj S. Alhowaiti
Pediatric Department, Prince Salman North West Armed Forces Hospital, P.O. Box 100, Tabuk 71411, Saudi Arabia

Colm Murphy, John Edward O'Connell and Gerard Kearns
Department of Oral and Maxillofacial Surgery, Our Lady's Children's Hospital, Crumlin, Dublin 12, Ireland

Edward Cotter
Hermitage Medical Clinic, Suite 10, Old Lucan Road, Dublin 20, Ireland

Jong Hyung Yoon, Jong In Chun, Hyeon Jin Park and Byung-Kiu Park
Center for Pediatric Oncology, National Cancer Center, 323 Ilsan-ro, Ilsandong-gu, Goyang-si, Gyeonggi-do 410-769, Republic of Korea

Hyun-Sung Lee
Center for Pediatric Oncology, National Cancer Center, 323 Ilsan-ro, Ilsandong-gu, Goyang-si, Gyeonggi-do 410-769, Republic of Korea
Center for Lung Cancer, National Cancer Center, 323 Ilsan-ro, Ilsandong-gu, Goyang-si, Gyeonggi-do 410-769, Republic of Korea

Seog-Yun Park
Center for Pediatric Oncology, National Cancer Center, 323 Ilsan-ro, Ilsandong-gu, Goyang-si, Gyeonggi-do 410-769, Republic of Korea
Department of Pathology, National Cancer Center, 323 Ilsan-ro, Ilsandong-gu, Goyang-si, Gyeonggi-do 410-769, Republic of Korea

Prashant K. Minocha, Lakhan Roop and Rambachan Persad
Department of Paediatric Surgery, San Fernando General Hospital, Trinidad, Trinidad and Tobago

Tiffany J. Patton, Timothy A. Sentongo and Stacy A. Kahn
Department of Pediatrics, Section of Pediatric Gastroenterology, University of Chicago, Wyler Pavilion C-474, 5839 S. Maryland Avenue, MC 4065, Chicago, IL 60637, USA

Grace Z. Mak
Department of Pediatrics, Section of Pediatric Surgery, The University of Chicago Hospitals, 5841 S. Maryland Avenue, MC 4062, Chicago, IL 60637, USA